Examples of how to describe the clinical features of lesions or rashes

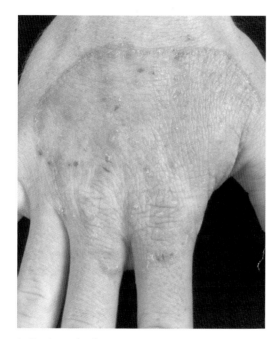

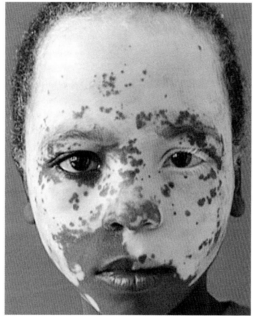

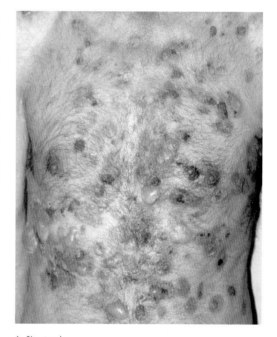

1. Site: dorsum hand
2. Erythematous
3. Chronic
4. Surface: scale
5. Raised lesion: plaques

GO TO algorithm on p. 407

1. Site: face
2. Non-erythematous
3. Chronic
4. Surface: normal
5. Flat lesion: patch
6. Colour: white

GO TO algorithm on p. 281

1. Site: trunk
2. Erythematous
3. Chronic
4. Surface: crust
5. Lesions: bullae and erosions

GO TO algorithm on p. 255

For all the patients from whom we have learnt so much over the years and to all those who we hope will benefit from this book in the future

Differential Diagnosis in Dermatology

Fourth Edition

Richard Ashton

Consultant Dermatologist Portsmouth NHS Trust,
Nobles Hospital, Isle of Man

Barbara Leppard

Retired Consultant Dermatologist, Southampton University NHS Trust

Hywel Cooper

Consultant Dermatologist, Portsmouth NHS Trust

RADCLIFFE PUBLISHING
London • New York

Radcliffe Publishing Ltd
St Mark's House
Shepherdess Walk
London N1 7BQ
United Kingdom

www.radcliffehealth.com

British Library Cataloguing in Publication Data

A catalogue record for this book is available from the British Library.

ISBN-13: 978 190936 872 9

The paper used for the text pages of this book is FSC® certified. FSC (The Forest Stewardship Council®) is an international network to promote responsible management of the world's forests.

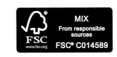

Typeset by Darkriver Design, Auckland, New Zealand
Printed and bound by Lion FPG, West Bromwich, West Midlands, UK

Contents

Preface to the fourth edition

In a review of the first edition of *Differential Diagnosis in Dermatology* in *Postgraduate Education for General Practice*, the reviewer wrote:

> Brilliant! Take for granted the superb colour photographs, the comprehensive and readable text, the clinical accuracy and acumen of the authors. What's special is the diagnostically and educationally helpful structure. This book understands that most of us haven't got photographic memories, and panic when we don't immediately recognise a skin lesion. Provided we can establish a few simple features of the rash – where it is, what colour, how long it has been there, surface characteristics – we turn to the appropriate algorithm, look at the picture for confirmation and come up with the right answer. It is such a relief I could burst into tears of gratitude.

We hope we haven't changed any of that, and that this new edition is equally user-friendly. It is designed for the primary care physician to use with the patient sitting in front of him or her.

The third edition incorporated treatment into the text and this new edition has brought that up to date, particularly with the new biologic treatments. We have invited our colleague Hywel Cooper to keep the text and treatments up to date, and we have included many new photographs, especially of rashes in black and Asian skin.

We would like to thank several colleagues for their help in keeping us up to date, especially Dr Steven Hayes (dermoscopy for general practitioners), Dr Adam Haworth (patch testing and lasers), Dr Suzanna Hoey (vascular birthmarks), Dr Jennifer Jones (scalp), Liz Jones (emollients), Mr Tim Mellor (lasers), Dr Raj Patel (genitalia) and Denise Woodd (wound dressings and leg ulcers) and all the patients who have allowed us to use their photographs in this book.

Richard Ashton
Barbara Leppard
September 2014

Introduction to dermatological diagnosis

1

BASIC BIOLOGY OF THE SKIN

THE EPIDERMIS

As the outside layer of the skin, the function of the epidermis is to produce keratin and melanin. Pathology in the epidermis produces a rash or a lesion with abnormal scale, change in pigmentation, or loss of surface integrity (exudate or erosion).

Keratin

Keratin is the end product of maturation of the epidermal cells; its function is to make the skin waterproof.

Melanin

Melanin is produced by melanocytes in the basal layer. Packets of melanin (melanosomes) are transferred from the melanocytes through their dendritic processes into the surrounding epidermal cells (*see* Fig. 1.02). Melanosomes protect the nucleus from the harmful effects of ultraviolet radiation; without this protection skin cancer may develop.

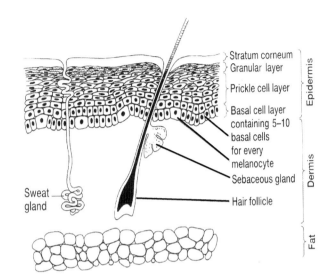

Fig. 1.01 The structure of the skin

THE DERMIS

The bulk of the dermis is made up of connective tissue: collagen, which gives the skin its strength, and elastic fibres, which allow it to stretch. Here are also the blood vessels, lymphatics, cutaneous nerves and the skin appendages (hair follicles, sebaceous glands and sweat glands). Diseases of the dermis usually result in change in elevation of the skin (i.e. papules, nodules, atrophy), and if the pathology is restricted to the dermis, then there will be no surface changes such as scale, crust or exudate. Loss or necrosis of the dermis results in an ulcer (as opposed to an erosion, which is due to loss of epidermis alone).

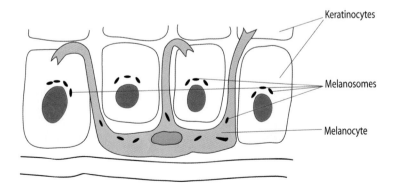

Fig. 1.02 Melanocyte in basal layer inserting melanosomes into keratinocytes

DIAGNOSIS OF SKIN DISEASE

The diagnosis of skin disease is made by following the same general principles as in any other branch of medicine. Begin by taking a history. This is followed by careful physical examination. If at this stage the diagnosis has not been made, further investigations can be carried out. Very often the non-dermatologist tends to look at a rash or skin lesion and 'guess' the diagnosis. This is quite unnecessary. In this section we have outlined a scheme to enable you to make the correct diagnosis.

HISTORY OF PRESENTING COMPLAINT

Duration of individual lesions

How long has/have the lesion/s been present? This is the most important question in the history. Acute lesions present for less than 2 weeks need to be distinguished from chronic ones.

Do the lesions come and go? Do they occur at the same site or at different sites? This question is particularly important if the diagnosis of urticaria or herpes simplex is being considered. Urticaria (*see* p. 171) can be diagnosed by a history of lesions coming and going within a 24-hour period. To establish the transitory nature of urticarial weals, draw a line around a weal and ask the patient to return the next day. You will see that the site and shape will have changed. Herpes simplex (*see* p. 108–9) and fixed drug eruptions (*see* p. 181) last around 7–14 days and usually reoccur at the same site.

Relationship to physical agents

A past history of living or working in a hot climate may be the clue you need for the diagnosis of skin cancer. Determine the patient's skin response to sun exposure. Six skin types are recognised, depending how well a patient develops a skin tan

Table 1.01 Skin types

Type 1: Always burns, never tans
Type 2: Always burns, tans minimally
Type 3: Sometimes burns, tans gradually
Type 4: Rarely burns, tans well
Type 5: Asian skin
Type 6: Black skin
Those with fair skin (types 1 and 2) are more liable to develop skin cancers.

(*see* Table 1.01). In rashes on the face and backs of the hands, ask about relationship to sun exposure. The important questions to ask are regarding the time interval after sun exposure before the rash occurs and whether the patient gets the rash through window glass on a sunny day. In solar urticaria, the rash occurs within 5 minutes of sun exposure and is gone in an hour. In polymorphic light eruption (*see* p. 100), the rash occurs several hours after sun exposure and lasts several days. In porphyria (which is very rare, *see* p. 408) the rash occurs within a few minutes and lasts several days. Rashes that occur through window glass are due to ultraviolet A rays and will need a sunblock containing titanium dioxide or zinc oxide (*see* p. 39).

Ask about irritants on the skin in hand dermatitis (*see* p. 414), e.g. detergents and oils, and about working practices and hobbies. Are the hands protected by rubber gloves or in direct contact with irritants?

Itching

Itching is a nuisance to the patient but may not help you in making a diagnosis. Severe itching, especially at night bad enough to prevent sleep, should make you think of scabies (*see* p. 248) or rarely dermatitis herpetiformis (*see* p. 246).

PAST, FAMILY AND SOCIAL HISTORY

Past history

Has the patient had a rash before and, if so, was it the same as now? If eczema is present, a history of infantile eczema, asthma or hay fever may suggest a diagnosis of atopic eczema.

Family history

Does anyone else in the family have a skin problem and is it the same as the patient's? This will indicate either that the skin disease is genetically determined, e.g. atopic eczema, ichthyosis or psoriasis, or that it is contagious, e.g. scabies, impetigo.

Social history

This should include family relationships and work practices that may give you a clue as to the cause of the problem. For instance, in cases of hand dermatitis, does the condition improve at weekends or when away on holiday?

PREVIOUS TREATMENT

What topical agents have been used and did they help? Establish whether these are ointments or creams, because the base may be as important as the active agent. Remember that topical local anaesthetics, antibiotics and antihistamines may induce a contact allergic dermatitis. A drug history is important if a drug-induced rash is considered, e.g. if there is a sudden onset of a widespread rash. If the patient has been on the drug for more than 2 months, the likelihood of it being the cause of the rash is low.

DESCRIBING SKIN LESIONS

Look first and identify:
1. sites involved
2. number of lesions
3. distribution
4. arrangement.

Feel the lesions by:
5. surface palpation – with fingertips
6. deep palpation – by squeezing between finger and thumb.

Describe a typical lesion under the following headings:
7. type of lesion
8. surface features and texture
9. colour of lesion – including erythematous or non-erythematous
10. border of lesion or rash
11. shape of lesion.

Check other sites, e.g. scalp, nails, mouth and genitalia.

1. SITES INVOLVED

Describe body areas involved.

2. NUMBER OF LESIONS

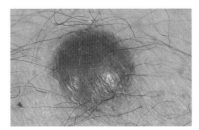 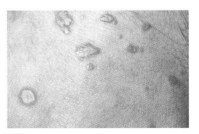

Single Fig. 1.03 Lymphoma   **Multiple** Fig. 1.04 Lichen planus

3. DISTRIBUTION

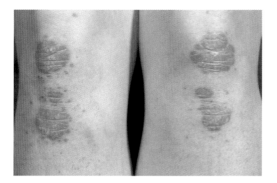

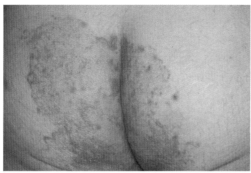

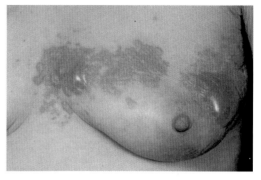

Symmetrical   Fig. 1.05 Psoriasis
Involving both sides of body to a similar extent; usually due to endogenous causes, e.g. acne, eczema, psoriasis.

Asymmetrical   Fig. 1.06 Tinea corporis on buttocks
Involving predominantly one side of the body, usually due to exogenous cause, e.g. infections or contact dermatitis.

Unilateral   Fig. 1.07 Herpes zoster
Restricted to one side of body only.

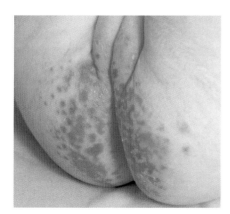

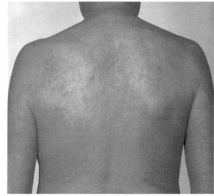

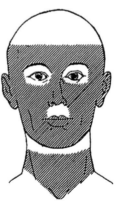
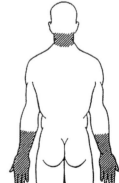

Localised   Fig. 1.08 Nappy/diaper rash
Restricted to one area of skin.

Generalised   Fig. 1.09 Erythrodermic psoriasis
Covering most of the body's surface.

Sun exposed   Fig. 1.10   Fig. 1.11
Involving the face, 'V' and back of the neck, dorsum of hands and forearms. Note: behind ears and under chin and/or eyebrows will be spared (*see* p. 85).

4. ARRANGEMENT

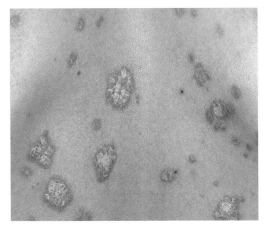

Discrete Fig. 1.12 Psoriasis
Individual lesions separated from one another by normal skin.

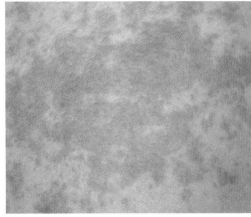

Coalescing Fig. 1.13 Eczema
Similar lesions merging together.

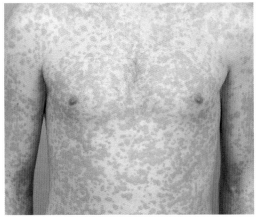

Disseminated Fig. 1.14 Psoriasis
Widespread discrete lesions.

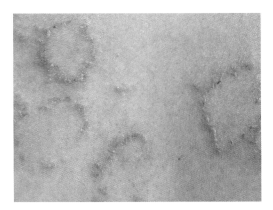

Annular Fig. 1.15 Eczema
Arranged in ring (*see* p. 209).

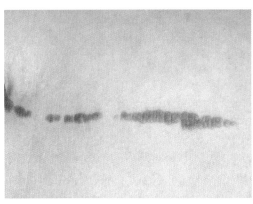

Linear Fig. 1.16 Epidermal naevus
Arranged in line (*see* p. 212).

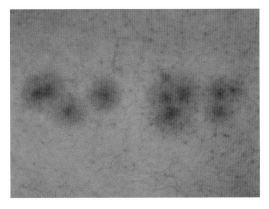

Grouped Fig. 1.17 Insect bites
Multiple similar lesions grouped together in one area.

FEEL THE LESIONS

5. SURFACE PALPATION

Feel the surface with your fingertips.

Smooth: feels like normal skin.

Uneven: found with fine scaling or some warty lesions.

Rough: feels like sandpaper, and is characteristic of solar keratosis, cutaneous horn or crust.

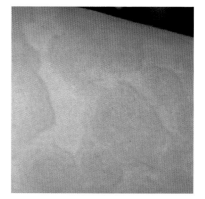

Smooth Fig. 1.18 Urticaria

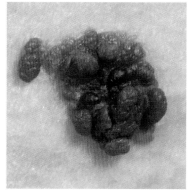

Uneven Fig. 1.19 Compound naevus

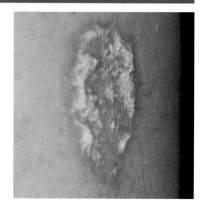

Rough Fig. 1.20 Solar keratosis

6. DEEP PALPATION

Compress the lesion between thumb and index finger.

Normal: feels the same as the normal surrounding skin.

Soft: easily compressible – feels like the lips.

Firm: only slightly compressible – feels like the tip of the nose.

Hard: not compressible – feels like bone.

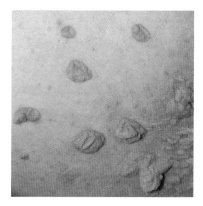

Soft Fig. 1.21 Skin tags

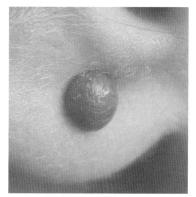

Firm Fig. 1.22 Keloid scar

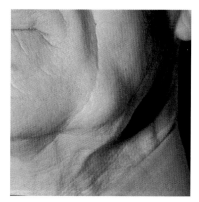

Hard Fig. 1.23 Osteoma on jaw

7. TYPE OF LESION

Assess whether the lesions are flat or raised, solid or fluid filled, or have a broken surface.

a. Flat lesions

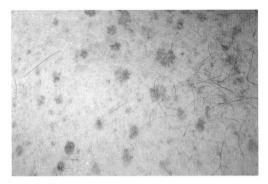

Macule ≤ 1 cm diameter   Fig. 1.24 Lentigines

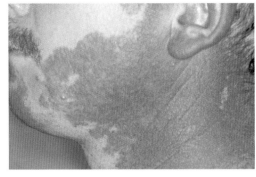

Patch > 1 cm diameter   Fig. 1.25 Port wine stain

b. Raised solid lesions

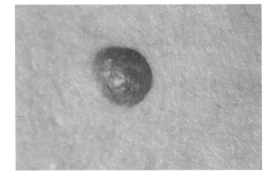

Papule ≤ 1 cm diameter
Fig. 1.26 Compound naevus

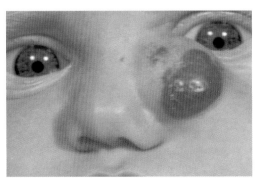

Nodule > 1 cm diameter (= thickness)
Fig. 1.27 Strawberry naevus

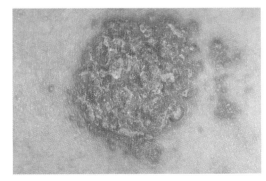

Plaque > 1 cm diameter (>> thickness)
Fig. 1.28 Discoid eczema

Flat lesions Any area of colour or surface change which cannot be felt on palpation.

Raised solid lesions

Papule Any solid lesion (≤ 1 cm size) that is raised above the surface or can be felt on palpation.

Nodule Any elevated lesions (> 1 cm diameter) which is palpable between finger and thumb, i.e. there is substance to the lesion. Often due to dermal pathology but there may or may not be surface change.

Plaque Any lesion (size > 1 cm) where the **diameter** is >> than the thickness, i.e. the lesion can be felt only with finger tips. Usually due to epidermal pathology with surface scale, crust or keratin.

c. Fluid-filled lesions

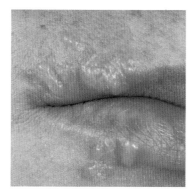

Vesicle ≤1 cm diameter   Fig. 1.29
Herpes simplex

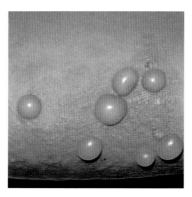

Bulla > 1 cm diameter   Fig. 1.30
Bullous pemphigoid

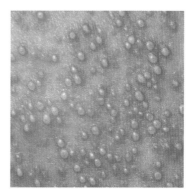

Pustule ≤1 cm diameter   Fig. 1.31

d. Lesions due to a broken surface

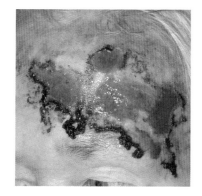

Erosion   Fig. 1.32
Loss of epidermis only

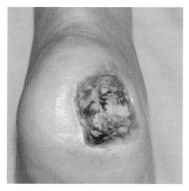

Ulcer   Fig. 1.33 Neuropathic ulcer
Loss of epidermis and dermis

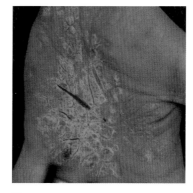

Fissure   Fig. 1.34 Psoriasis on palm
Linear split in skin

Blisters (vesicles and bullae) contain clear fluid (serum) and last for a few days only. The presence of fluid can be confirmed by pricking with a needle. The site of the blister can be within the epidermis or at the dermo-epidermal junction. **Intra-epidermal** blisters break easily to form erosions, while **sub-epidermal** ones can persist for several days and may contain blood.

Pustules (≤1 cm) contain opaque fluid (pus). Prick the lesion and pus comes out.

Loss of some or all of the epidermis results in an **erosion**, which will heal without scarring. Erosions can be due to:
● a blister that has burst
● trauma.

Loss of dermis (from any cause) will result in an **ulcer**, which will heal with scar tissue formation. There will be surface exudate, crust or slough.

Splitting of the skin (**fissure**) is due to abnormal keratin (usually secondary to eczema or psoriasis).

e. Other terms used

Weal Fig. 1.35 Urticaria

Transient swelling (i.e. papule or plaque) due to dermal oedema – should last for less than 24 hours; usually synonymous with urticaria.

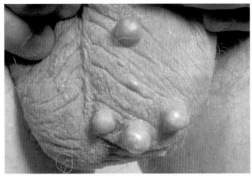

Cyst Fig. 1.36 Scrotal epidermoid cysts

A fluctuant papule or nodule lined by epithelium containing fluid, pus or keratin.

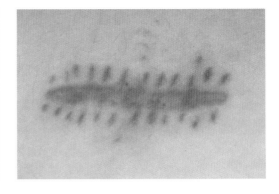

Scar Fig. 1.37 Surgical scar

A healed dermal lesion (macule, papule, plaque, nodule) secondary to trauma, surgery, infection or loss of blood supply.

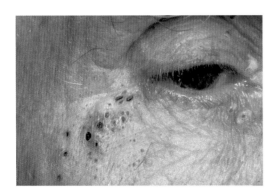

Comedone Fig. 1.38 Solar elastosis

Papule due to a plugged sebaceous follicle containing altered sebum and keratin.

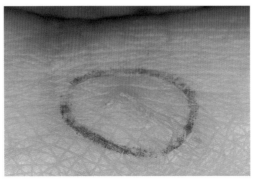

Burrow Fig. 1.39 Scabies

Linear S-shaped papule 3–5 mm long found on the hands and fingers of a patient with scabies.

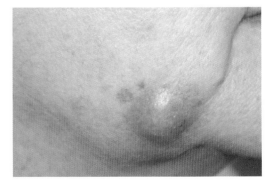

Abscess Fig. 1.40 Boil on angle of jaw

A large collection of pus.

8. SURFACE FEATURES AND TEXTURE

b. Abnormal keratinisation

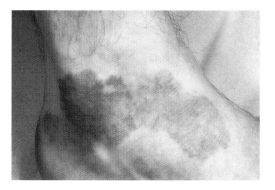

a. Normal Fig. 1.41 Granuloma annulare

Surface not different from surrounding skin and feels smooth. Change in elevation and/or colour only.

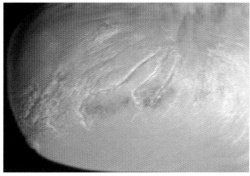

Hyperkeratotic Fig. 1.42 Foot psoriasis

Rough, uneven surface due to increased formation of keratin. Seen usually on palms and soles.

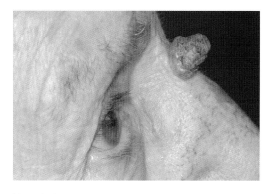

Keratin horn Fig. 1.43 Keratoacanthoma

Accumulation of compact keratin on the surface. Feels rough and is adherent so difficult to pick off.

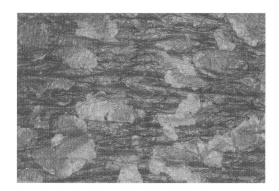

Scale Fig. 1.44 Erythrodermic psoriasis

Dry/flaky surface due to abnormal stratum corneum with increased shedding of keratinocytes.

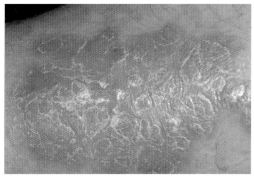

Scratch test – before Fig. 1.45 Psoriasis

If surface is scaly, scratch surface of scale vigorously with fingernail.

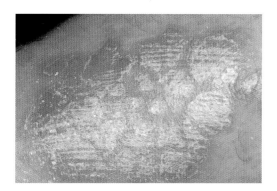

Scratch test – after Fig. 1.46 Psoriasis

Profuse silver scale indicates that the diagnosis is psoriasis.

c. Broken surface

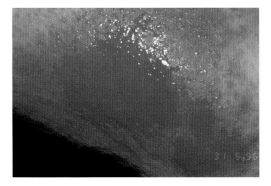

Exudate Fig. 1.47 Acute eczema
Serum, blood or pus that has accumulated on the surface.

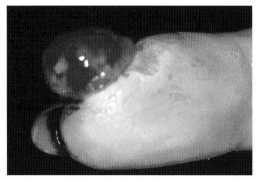

Friable Fig. 1.48 Pyogenic granuloma
Surface bleeds easily after minor trauma.

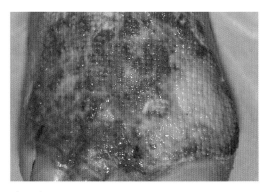

Slough Fig. 1.49 Foot ulcer
A combination of exudate and necrotic tissue.

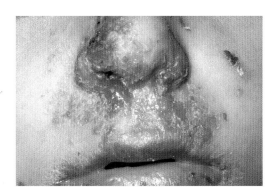

Crust Fig. 1.50 Impetigo
Dried exudate. There should be a history of weeping, pus or bleeding.

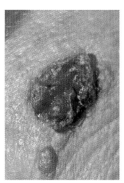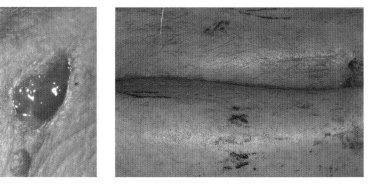

Fig. 1.51 Basal cell carcinoma   Fig. 1.52
To find the cause of a crust, pick it off to see what is underneath. There will be either an ulcer or an erosion. Under the crust in Fig. 1.51 there is an ulcer due to a basal cell carcinoma (Fig. 1.52).

Excoriation Fig. 1.53 Atopic eczema
Localised damage to the skin due to scratching – linear erosions and crusts.

d. Change in thickness

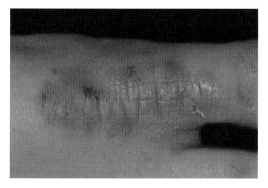

Lichenification   Fig. 1.54 Lichen simplex

Thickening of the epidermis with increased skin markings due to persistent scratching (found in atopic eczema or lichen simplex).

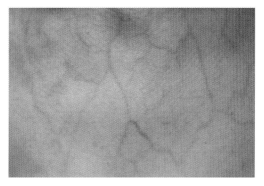

Dermal atrophy   Fig. 1.55 Due to topical steroids

Depression of the surface due to thinning of the dermis. Blood vessels are easily seen under the skin.

Epidermal atrophy   Fig. 1.56 Lichen sclerosus

Fine surface wrinkling like 'cigarette paper'.

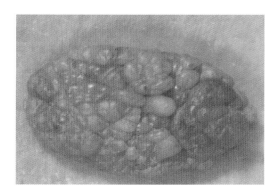

Papillomatous   Fig. 1.57 Congential naevus

Surface consisting of minute, finger-like or round projections.

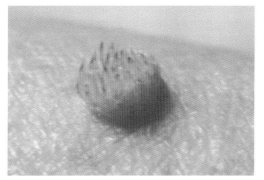

Warty   Fig. 1.58 Filiform wart

Surface consisting of rough, finger-like projections.

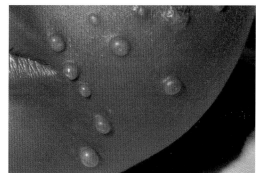

Umbilicated   Fig. 1.59 Molluscum contagiosum

Papule with central depression. Characteristically seen in molluscum contagiosum.

9. COLOUR OF LESION

a. Red, pink or purple

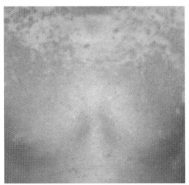 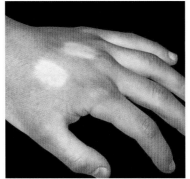

Erythema   Fig. 1.60 Psoriasis   Fig. 1.61 Chilblains

Redness due to dilated blood vessels that blanche (become white) on pressure. It is the result of inflammation and is seen most easily in white-skinned individuals.

b. Brown

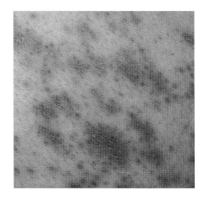 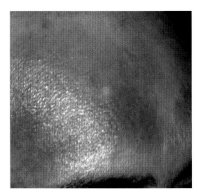

Hyperpigmentation   Fig. 1.65 Lichen planus   Fig. 1.66 Atopic eczema

Increase in melanin pigmentation. It usually follows inflammation in the epidermis. In pigmented skin it can be the first sign of inflammation.

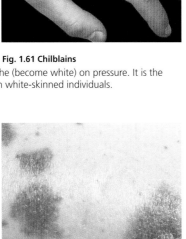 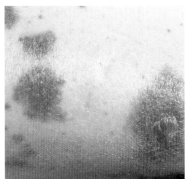

Telangiectasia   Fig. 1.62

Redness due to individually visible dilated blood vessels.

Purpura   Fig. 1.63   Fig. 1.64

Red, purple or orange colour due to blood that has leaked out of blood vessels. Purpura does not blanche on pressure and remains the same colour.

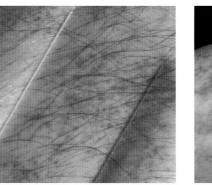 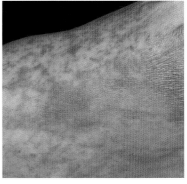

Haemosiderin pigment   Fig. 1.67

Orange-brown due to breakdown of haemoglobin following purpura.

c. Blue-black

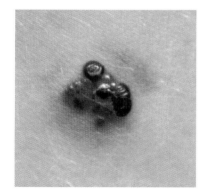

Melanin   Fig. 1.68 Blue naevus
Melanin pigment situated deep within dermis, seen in malignant melanoma and blue naevus.

d. White

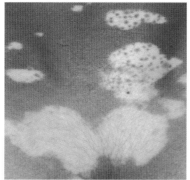

Depigmentation   Fig. 1.69 Vitiligo
Complete loss of melanin due to loss of melanocytes in the epidermis.

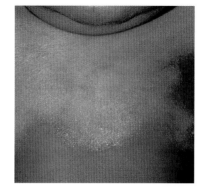

Hypopigmentation   Fig. 1.70 Eczema
Partial loss of melanin secondary to inflammation in the epidermis.

Reduced blood supply
Fig. 1.71 Naevus anaemicus
White colour due to reduced blood supply.

e. Black-purple

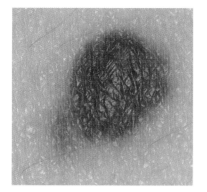

Stagnant blood   Fig. 1.72 Angioma
Black-purple colour from dilated blood vessels within the skin.

f. Yellow

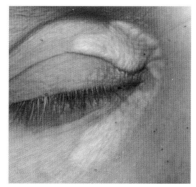

Lipid deposition   Fig. 1.73 Xanthelasma
Yellow colour seen in xanthelasma on inner eyelids.

g. Blue-grey

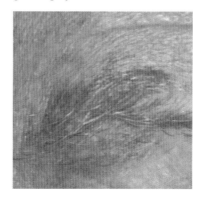

Minocycline pigmentation   Fig. 1.74
Grey-blue colour on eyebrow due to deposition of iron.

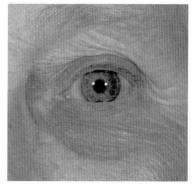

Gold pigment   Fig. 1.75 Chrysiasis
Grey-blue colour seen in patients on gold therapy.

10. BORDER OF LESION OR RASH

a. Well defined or circumscribed
Able to draw a line around the lesion with confidence

b. Poorly defined
Lesions have a border that merges into normal skin

c. Accentuated edge
Border of lesion shows increased scaling with relative clearing in the centre

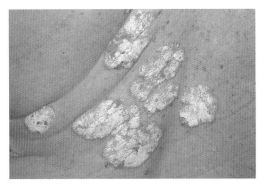

Psoriasis: well-defined plaques   Fig. 1.76

Eczema: poorly defined plaques   Fig. 1.77

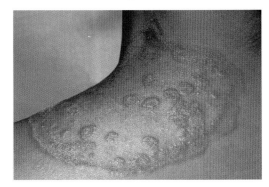

Tinea corporis with accentuated border   Fig. 1.78

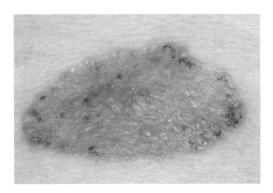

Superficial basal cell carcinoma: single well-defined plaque   Fig. 1.79

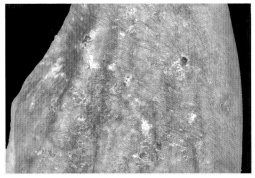

Solar keratoses: poorly defined papules   Fig. 1.80

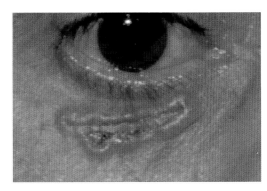

Basal cell carcinoma with raised rolled edge   Fig. 1.81

11. SHAPE OF LESION

a. From above

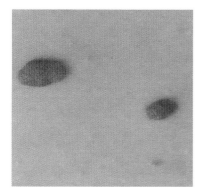

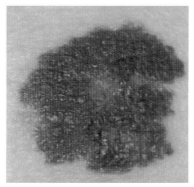

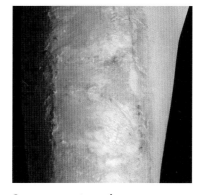

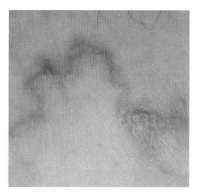

Round or oval   Fig. 1.82 Benign moles

Irregular   Fig. 1.83 Malignant melanoma

Square or rectangular
Fig. 1.84 Straight sides – dermatitis artefacta

Serpiginous   Fig. 1.85 'S' shaped – larva migrans

b. In profile

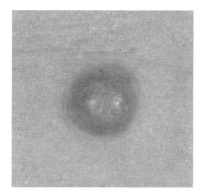

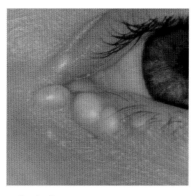

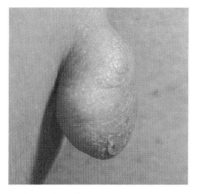

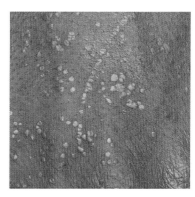

Dome shaped   Fig. 1.86 Benign intradermal naevus

Spherical   Fig. 1.87 Epidermoid cysts/ milia

Pedunculated   Fig. 1.88 Fibroepithelial polyp – skin tag

Flat topped   Fig. 1.89 Plane warts

SPECIAL INVESTIGATIONS

WOOD'S LIGHT

This is a source of ultraviolet light where visible light is excluded by a nickel oxide filter. It is useful in identifying scalp ringworm due to *Microsporum* species, which fluoresce green (*see* Fig. 3.12, p. 77), and erythrasma, which fluoresces bright pink (*see* Fig. 10.27, p. 348). Porphyrins in urine and faeces also fluoresce a bright-pink colour.

In pigmentary disorders, the Wood's light will help distinguish complete loss of pigment in vitiligo (the skin is completely white) from hypopigmentation in pityriasis versicolor or post-inflammatory hypopigmentation (the skin is paler than normal).

DERMOSCOPY

Applying oil to the surface of a skin lesion and looking through the magnifying lens of a dermatoscope (*see* Fig. 1.90) is a useful tool for the diagnosis of pigmented lesions and distinguishing them from vascular lesions. The dermatoscope is useful also for identifying scabetic burrows (*see* p. 249), and distinguishing between scale and crust.

Vascular lesions are easily distinguished from melanocytic lesions because they are red not brown, and you may see individual dilated blood vessels.

Seborrhoeic keratoses have white or black keratin cysts on the surface, and a regular edge.

Pigmented lesions. The main thing you want help with from a dermatoscope is deciding whether a lesion is benign or malignant. The majority of pigmented lesions seen in general practice will be benign. The pigment in a **benign naevus** may appear as a reticular network, as dots/globules or be amorphous. Two shades of brown is acceptable providing there is overall symmetry and the absence of malignant features.

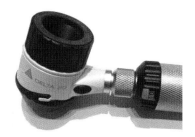

Fig.1.90 Dermatoscope

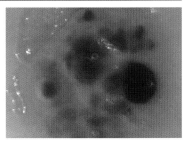

Fig. 1.91 Angioma: dilated vascular spaces with red-black colour

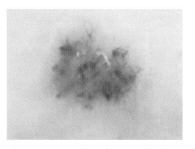

Fig. 1.92 Hereditary haemorrhagic telangiectasia

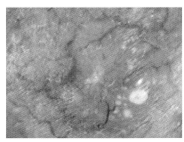

Fig. 1.93 Basal cell carcinoma: blood vessels over the edge

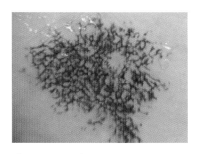

Fig. 1.94 Lentigo

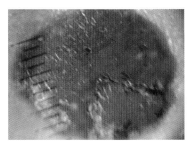

Fig. 1.95 Seborrhoeic keratosis

The things that would make you suspicious of a **malignant melanoma** are:

- asymmetry
- multiple colours within the lesion (dark brown, light brown, black, red, grey, blue, white)
- multiple patterns (reticular network, streaks, globules of varying size, distribution and colour, blue-grey veil, amorphous)
- an irregular edge (i.e. streaks)
- a blue-grey veil, where one or more parts of the lesion is bluish/grey/white.

For further images see the International Dermoscopy Society website (dermoscopy-ids.org).

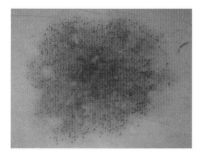

Fig. 1.96 Junctional naevus: two colours of light brown, symmetrical reticular pattern

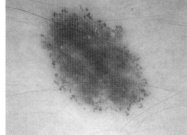

Fig. 1.97 Junctional naevus with central amorphous area and regular peripheral dots

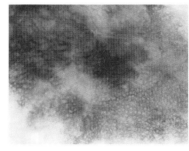

Fig. 1.100 Abnormal network top left of image, and normal network at bottom right in superficial spreading melanoma

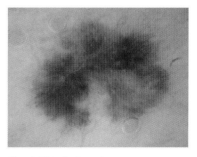

Fig. 1.101 Early melanoma: asymmetry, multiple colours and patterns

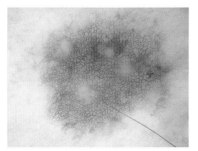

Fig. 1.98 Junctional naevus with multifocal hypopigmentation, minor colour variation and normal network pattern

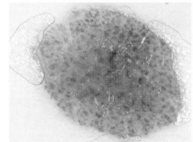

Fig. 1.99 Compound naevus with symmetrical shape, globules and regular border

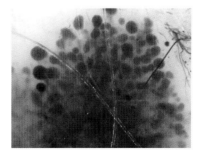

Fig. 1.102 Superficial spreading malignant melanoma: irregular globules of varying size, no pigment network visible

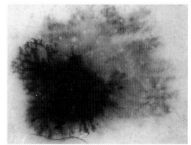

Fig. 1.103 Nodular malignant melanoma: blue-grey veil and linear streaks, multiple patterns and colours

BACTERIOLOGY

Swabs can be taken from vesicles, pustules, erosions or ulcers to identify the causative bacteria by Gram stain and culture. Viruses can be identified by electron microscopy or culture. If you suspect herpes simplex or zoster you can do a Papanicolaou (PAP) stain on blister fluid and see multinucleate giant cells.

MYCOLOGY

Superficial fungal infections caused by dermatophytes (ringworm/tinea) and yeasts (candidiasis and pityriasis versicolor) all live on keratin and can be identified in scales taken from the edge of a scaly lesion. Use a blunt scalpel blade (e.g. banana-shaped – Swann Major shape 'U', obtainable from Swann-Morton.com). If the scales are too dry and do not stick to the blade, moistening the skin with surgical spirit helps. The scales can be mixed with 20% KOH (potassium hydroxide) solution; to dissolve the keratin, gently heat the mixture on a glass slide until the solution bubbles. You can examine immediately under the microscope to see the fungal hyphae or yeast spores (*see* Fig. 10.03, p. 337, and Fig. 10.15, p. 342).

Alternatively the skin scales may be sent to the mycology laboratory in special envelopes (Dermapak.com, PO Box 841, Bedford, MK45 4WG; Mycotrans.com, PO Box 1172, Biggar, ML12 6NN, Scotland) where direct microscopy and culture can be performed.

SKIN BIOPSY

If the diagnosis is in doubt, an ellipse of skin can be taken through the edge of the lesion, so that both normal and abnormal skin is included in the specimen. It should include epidermis, dermis and fat.

Immune complexes can be identified by immunofluorescence. The sample needs to be sent to the laboratory in Michel's medium. In some instances a 'punch biopsy' can be used, which takes a 3–6 mm core of tissue, but this technique produces only a limited sample, which may be inadequate for proper histological examination.

If a skin tumour is present, the whole lesion should be excised as an ellipse so that the wound can be sewn up in a straight line.

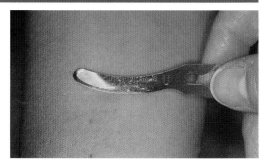

Fig. 1.104 Taking skin scraping using a Swann major U blade

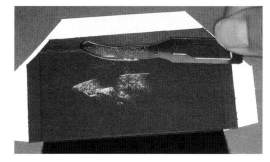

Fig. 1.105 Putting scales into a Dermapak envelope (black paper so scales show up), which can be sent to the mycology laboratory through the post

PRICK TESTING

This identifies an immediate hypersensitivity reaction in asthma, hay fever or allergic urticaria (contact urticaria to fragrances is done by short contact patch testing). It is not of any use in the diagnosis of atopic eczema or idiopathic urticaria. It is useful in identifying natural rubber latex allergy. A drop of latex protein is placed on the forearm and the surface of the skin is broken by pricking. A weal indicates a positive reaction. A saline (negative) and histamine (positive) control should also be used. The risk of anaphylaxis is low but resuscitation drugs and equipment should be available. If latex prick testing and a RAST test are negative, then a 'use test' wearing a finger of a latex glove on wet skin for 15 minutes, with a finger of a vinyl glove as control, will confirm the diagnosis.

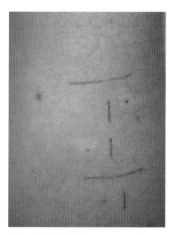

Fig. 1.106 Prick test: a positive result shows a weal around the needle prick after a few minutes

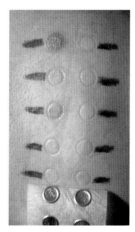

Fig. 1.107 Patch test: 48-hour reading – the patches have just been removed and a single test (top left) is positive (erythema and vesicles = eczema)

PATCH TESTING

This is used to identify a type IV hypersensitivity reaction in the skin, i.e. allergic contact dermatitis. The allergens are suspended in white soft paraffin or aqueous solution and placed on aluminium discs – 10 mounted on Scanpor tape (Finn Chambers). These are applied to the back and left in place for 48 hours. The tapes are removed and a small circular plaque of eczema at the site of the aluminium disc at 48 and 96 hours indicates an allergic response to a specific allergen. The relevance of the positive allergen(s) (*see* Table 1.02) is then determined, and if relevant the patient is advised on avoidance.

Table 1.02 Standard battery of allergens and their source

Allergen	Source of allergen
Prescription creams	
Budesonide	A marker of steroid allergy and suggests the need for further assessment of possible reactions to other steroids
Caine mix	Local anaesthetic ointments
Ethylenediamine	Found in *Tri-Adcortyl* cream, topical antihistamines
Fucidic acid	Antibiotic cream – *Fucidin* and *Fucidin H*
Neomycin	Antibiotic ointment
Quinoline mix	Antiseptic agent in steroid creams with letter C or word vioform
Tixocortol pivalate	All hydrocortisone creams and ointments
Wool alcohols (lanolin)	Oily cream, E45 cream, other ointments with lanolin as the base
Cosmetic products	
Propolis	Resin found in beehives, used in cosmetics, herbal remedies
Balsam of Peru	Fragrances, citrus fruit peel
Fragrance mix	Cosmetics with fragrances
Cetyl/stearyl alcohol	Moisturiser and lubricant, prescribed creams and soap substitutes, sunblocks

Allergen	Source of allergen
Benzalkonium chloride	Antiseptic found in creams
Paraphenylenediamine (PPD)	Permanent hair dyes, temporary tattoos, black rubber
Disperse Blue mix	Dark blue dyes in synthetic materials
Preservatives in creams	
Formaldehyde	Fabrics that are treated with formaldehyde resins to make them crease resistant Preservative in household and industrial products, e.g. cosmetics, shampoos, cleaners, disinfectants
Parabens	Preservative in creams and paste bandages
Quaternium–15	Cosmetics: foundation, eye make up, blushers, moisturisers, shampoos and floor waxes and polishes
Kathon CG Isothiazolinone	Preservative in hair products, wet wipes, detergents, washing powders and liquids
Methylisothiazolinone (MI)	Preservative in cosmetics, shampoos and baby wipes
Chlorocresol (PCMC)	Preservative in creams, ointments, moisturisers, (not cosmetics and shampoos)
2-Bromo-2-nitropropane-1-3 diol	Preservative in shampoos, cosmetics, washing detergents and fabric softeners
Imidazolidinyl urea (Germal 115)	Preservative in cosmetics and hair gels
Diazolidinyl urea (Germal II)	Preservative in cosmetics, shampoos, sunscreens, deodorants
Methyldibromoglutaronitrile	Preservative in cosmetics, shampoos, baby wipes, sunscreens; now banned in the European Union
Chloroxylenol (PCMX)	Mainly in Dettol; preservative in steroid creams, soaps, deodorants, cosmetics, topical antiseptics and industrial liquids
Sodium metabisulphate	Antioxidant and preservative in creams and ointments, and some foods, beer and wine

Allergen	Source of allergen
Rubber chemicals	
Black rubber IPPD (isopropyl-phenyl-PPD)	Industrial black rubbers, car tyres, boots, hoses, face masks, squash balls, black rubber clothing
Thiuram mix	Rubber gloves but also condoms, elasticated bandages, stockings, elastic in underwear
Mercapto mix	Rubber shoe soles and insoles, rubber in bandages, clothing, swimwear, condoms
Mercaptobenzothiazole	
Carba mix	Rubber especially gloves, insoles of shoes, some bandages, condoms
Glues	
Colophony (rosin)	Elastoplast, glues and adhesives, chewing gum, paper products, rosin used on violin bows
PTBPF resin (Para-tertiary butyl phenol formaldehyde)	Glues used to stick two layers of leather together in watch straps, shoes, handbags and belts DIY glues, wood, rubber items
Epoxy resin	Glues and adhesives (Araldite), particularly used in boat building, some dental bonding agents
Plants	
Primin	Indoor *Primula obconica* plant
Sesquiterpene Lactone mix	Plants of the Compositae family: yarrow, tansy, arnica, chrysanthemum, chamomile, feverfew, etc.
Compositae Mix II	
Metals	
Nickel	Most non-rusting metals except silver and gold, especially watch and belt buckles and cheap jewellery
Cobalt	
Potassium dichromate	Cement, leather gloves, leather shoes

Introduction to dermatological treatment

2

GENERAL PRINCIPLES OF TREATMENT

Make a diagnosis before embarking on treatment. Never think of treating a patient without first making a diagnosis or putting in hand the necessary investigations so that a diagnosis can be reached.

Be realistic about what is possible. Because skin disease is visible, the patient will often assume that it must be easy to cure. Generally speaking, skin disease can be put into three groups with regard to this.

1. Those diseases that have a specific cause and hence a specific treatment. Once this has been given correctly, this should be the end of the problem. Such conditions include:
   - allergic contact dermatitis
   - fungal and bacterial infections
   - infestations such as scabies and lice
   - skin tumours.
2. Those diseases where no cure is possible, but spontaneous remissions and exacerbations occur. These may be helped considerably by treatment, but a cure is not possible and should not be sought. Examples include:
   - atopic eczema
   - pemphigus and pemphigoid
   - psoriasis
   - rosacea.
3. Those diseases that persist for a limited period of time and then disappear on their own. This group may require symptomatic treatment, but not always, and the patient should be reassured of their benign nature. Examples of these are:
   - alopecia areata
   - lichen planus
   - guttate psoriasis.
   - erythema multiforme
   - pityriasis rosea

The patient should be made aware of which of these categories their skin disease fits in, so that they have a better idea of response to treatment and prognosis.

Look at the whole person and not just at his or her rash. Often the problem that presents itself is quite straightforward but at the same time there may be deeper needs shouting for attention. Body language speaks louder than words.

Patients with widespread skin disease often feel dirty, ashamed or guilty, thinking that somehow it is their own fault that they are ill. They may be afraid that their skin disease is contagious, or that they have cancer or a sexually transmitted infection; women with hirsutism may fear that they are turning into men; teenagers with acne lose their self-confidence.

Patients may also be embarrassed about having a rash because:
- It is on a part of the body that shows, such as the face or the hands. They will notice people looking at it and assume that people will think it is contagious, or that they have cancer or a sexually transmitted infection. They will often wear clothes that will hide it and limit their activities so that others will not see it (e.g. not going swimming or to the beach on holiday).
- The treatment makes a mess. Grease on the clothes and bedding, and the smell and mess of tar preparations are not popular with patients or their families.
- The shedding of scales makes a mess, particularly in psoriasis.
- It smells, especially in patients with ulcerated legs.
- It is present on the genital area. It may interfere with sexual activity because of embarrassment and the patient may be afraid that his or her partner will think that it is catching.

It is important that you understand how the patient feels about having a skin problem as well as what to do about it.

Listen to what the patient has to say. Very often the patient will tell you what is wrong if you give him or her the opportunity.

Understand that not everyone wants to get well. Some patients get a lot of attention because of their illness and do not want to give it up by getting well. For others it is somehow respectable to have a rash (which will not go away) but not to own up to guilt about some person or event, a poor self-image or conflict in the family. Using one ointment or pill after another will not resolve any of these and it is better to face up to reality sooner rather than later.

Treatment of acute rashes. Resting the skin is important in any acute or extensive skin disease. Going to bed is a helpful treatment in its own right. It is the basis for most inpatient treatments but can often be done just as well at home (by this we mean actually going to bed and not just lying down on the sofa, as the latter will not stop the patient from pottering about). Sedating antihistamines (promethazine or alimemazine) may be needed to keep the patient resting in bed.

Localised acute rashes should also be rested. If the patient has an acute blistering rash on the feet, it will not get better unless he or she stops walking around. A patient with an acute hand eczema is unlikely to get better while continuing to do the washing up.

The more acute the rash, the more bland the treatment needs to be. If in doubt, white soft paraffin is unlikely to do any harm and will keep the patient comfortable.

Explain to the patient what is going on. It is important to explain to the patient what is wrong with him or her, what the treatment is and how to use it. Time spent at the first consultation explaining the nature of the problem and the correct use of the treatment will be time well spent.

TOPICAL TREATMENT

Any applied agent contains two components:
1. the vehicle or base
2. the active constituent.

Both are equally important, but often the right type of vehicle is not taken into consideration when prescribing a treatment. The function of the base is to transport the active constituent into the skin so that it is delivered to where it is needed. Generally speaking the base is determined by the hydration of the skin at the particular site, while the active constituent is determined by the pathological process.

THE BASE

All bases are made up from one or more of the following:
- powders, e.g. zinc oxide, starch, calamine (zinc carbonate and ferric oxide)
- liquids, e.g. water, alcohol, propylene glycol
- oils and greases (ointments), e.g. liquid paraffin, yellow and white soft paraffin[UK]/petrolatum[USA], lanolin (wool alcohols), polyethylene glycols (synthetic waxes).

These may be used singly or mixed together to produce shake lotions, creams and pastes.

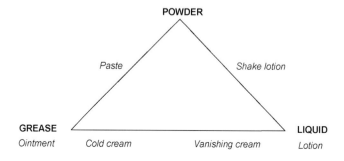

Table 2.01a Emollient products: how and when to use

Type	Class	Oil (%)	Examples (this list is not exhaustive)	Definition	Usage	Patient groups
Leave-on emollients Use as routine moisturiser anywhere	Ointment (no water) Aerosol spray	100	White soft paraffin (Vaseline), 50/50 white soft/liquid paraffin, Diprobase ointment, Epaderm/Hydromol/Emulsifying oints, Dermamist, Emollin spray	100% paraffin base (no preservative required)	Very dry skin Use twice a day Useful at night-time Greasy – may put off some patients	Severe atopic eczema Ichthyosis Sprays useful in the elderly and in hard-to-reach areas
	Occlusive cream	30–70	Oily cream/hydrous ointment (lanolin), QV intensive, Unguentum M, Lipobase (used as a diluent in Lipocream).	Water-in-oil emulsion (oily/cold creams) and 100% lipid ointments	Dry skin Trunk and limbs 2–3 times a day	Moderate atopic eczema or psoriasis
	Emollient gel containing *glycerol*	30	Doublebase gel, Doublebase Dayleve gel	Water and oil emulsion with humectant Water held in stratum corneum by humectant (glycerol or urea)	Very dry skin Use 3–4× a day, or 2× a day for Dayleve	Very dry skin Psoriasis, Ichthyosis
	Emollient cream containing *urea*	5–10% urea	Aquadrate, Balneum cream, Calmurid, E45 Itch Relief, Eucerin intensive, Hydromol intensive, Nutraplus.		Dry skin Use twice a day	Useful in older patients and in psoriasis
	Emollient cream (others without urea)	11–30	Aquamax, Aquamol, Aveeno cream (colloidal oatmeal), Cetraben, Diprobase cream, Epaderm cream, E45 cream (lanolin), Hydromol cream, Oilatum cream QV cream (contains glycerol), Ultrabase Zerocream, Zerobase cream, Zeroguent	Oil-in-water emulsion (vanishing cream) (*Note: tubs can become contaminated – prescribe pumps*)	Normal to dry skin conditions Face and flexures Good patient compliance 3–4x a day	Mild/moderate atopic eczema Other dry skin conditions such as psoriasis and endogenous eczema
	with antimicrobial		Dermol cream, Eczmol cream	Product contains benzalkonium chloride, and/or chlorhexidine	Useful in preventing flares of atopic eczema Use lotions as a soap substitute	Infected/colonised atopic eczema Healthcare workers Folliculitis
	Emollient lotion *with antimicrobial*	5–14	Dermol lotion			
	without antimicrobial		Aveeno lotion (colloidal oatmeal), E45 lotion (lanolin), QV lotion	Oil-in-water emulsion with low oil content Lighter than creams	Easy to apply 4x day Hairy areas (e.g. trunk, scalp) Summertime use	Poor compliers (teenagers, men)
	Antipruritic emollient		Balneum Plus cream, E45 Itch Relief cream	Product contains antipruritic agents (lauromacrogols)	Pruritus, especially if due to dry skin	First-line therapy for itching (especially in the elderly)

Adapted from Moncrieff G, Cork M, Lawton S, *et al.* Use of emollients in dry-skin conditions: consensus statement. *Clin Exp Dermatol.* 2013; **38**: 231–8.

Table 2.01b Wash and bath emollient products: how and when to use

Type	Class	Oil (%)	Examples	Definition	When to use	Patient groups
Wash products Use only for washing, do not leave on the skin	Emollient wash products	15–30	Aquamax cream wash, Doublebase shower gel, E45 wash cream, Hydromol bath and shower emollient, QV gentle wash, Oilatum shower emollient.	Products contain emulsifiers Should NOT contain harsh detergents such as sodium lauryl sulphate (e.g. aqueous cream)	Instead of soap, which is an irritant and therefore should be avoided in any dry skin conditions	Atopic eczema Hand dermatitis and psoriasis
	Antimicrobial wash products	2–50	Dermol shower/wash/lotion, Eczmol cream.	Emollient wash product containing topically active antimicrobial agents (such as benzalkonium chloride and/ or chlorhexidine)	Useful in managing and preventing flares of atopic eczema	Recurrent infections or relapses in atopic eczema and hand dermatitis
Bath emollients Add to bath water, can be used to wash with	Bath oil: Semi-dispersible oil or dispersible emulsion	50–91	Aveeno (colloidal oatmeal), Balneum, Cetraben, Dermalo, Diprobath, Doublebase bath additive. E45 bath oil, LPL 63.4, Oilatum, QV bath oil, Zerolatum, Zeroneum	Deposits a layer of oil on the surface of the water that leaves a slick around the bath; non-foaming and fragrance free / Oil disperses evenly through the bath water	All patient with moderate-very dry skin (atopic eczema, ichthyosis) Bathing in water alone is drying; bath oils should not be rinsed off	Use as part of complete emollient therapy in all dry skin conditions (*see* p. xx)
	Antimicrobiol bath oil	50–55	Dermol bath, Emulsiderm, Oilatum Plus, Zerolatum Plus	Bath oil containing topical antiseptic agent	Prevention of infection.	Atopic eczema with recurrent infections
	Antipruritic bath oil	85	Balneum Plus bath oil (soya oil)	Bath oil containing topical antipruritic agent	Protection of the skin barrier during bathing if pruritus is a problem	Should be used in conjunction with an antipruritic emollient

Ointments

Ointments contain little or no water and consist of organic hydrocarbons, alcohols and acids. These are greasy and form an impermeable layer over the skin, which prevents evaporation of water. Examples include:

- white soft paraffin[UK]/petrolatum[USA] (Vaseline)
- emulsifying ointment[UK]
- lanolin (wool fat purified from sheep wool 6%, paraffins 94%).

Organic hydrocarbons are subdivided by their melting points:

- liquid paraffin[UK]/liquid petrolatum[USA] is liquid at room temperature and is used in bath oils
- white soft paraffin[UK]/petrolatum[USA] is semi-solid at room temperature, but melts at body temperature, so rubs in easily; a mixture comprising equal parts of liquid paraffin and white soft paraffin is useful for covering large areas of the body with grease
- waxes have high melting points and are useful for stiffening up an ointment base.

Some ointments may be water-soluble and consist of polyethylene glycols such as fatty acid propylene glycol (used as the base for *Metosyn* cream). These compounds are semi-solids similar to white soft paraffin, so they spread well on the skin and wash off with water.

Creams

Creams are a mixture (emulsion) of an ointment with water. In order to prevent the two elements separating from one another, stabilisers and emulsifiers have to be added. Sodium lauryl sulphate (SLS) was first produced in 1958 as one of the first emulsifiers, but now *should not be used in eczema*, as it has been shown to damage the natural moisturising factor found in the stratum corneum. There are two types of cream:

1. An **oil-in-water emulsion** (like milk and cream). These are the vanishing creams. They rub into the skin easily and mix readily with water so they are more cosmetically acceptable than oily creams or ointments. They contain a high proportion of water and the oil component is kept in solution by using an emulsifying agent such as glycerol or sodium lauryl sulphate. Examples of oil-in-water creams are:
   - aqueous cream[UK] – **not to be used as a leave-on emollient because it contains SLS**
   - cetomacrogol A is used as a diluent for many steroid creams
   - hydrophilic ointment[USA].

One of the main disadvantages of creams is that they tend to make dry skin even drier because the water in them evaporates. If the skin is dry (e.g. in atopic eczema) a vanishing cream may make the condition worse; a cold cream or ointment will be better A further disadvantage is that they must contain preservatives, such as parahydroxybenzoic acid esters (parabens), chlorocresol, propylene glycol or ethylenediamine to prevent the cream from becoming contaminated by bacteria. All these preservatives can act as sensitisers and cause an allergic contact dermatitis in some patients.

2. A **water-in-oil emulsion** (like butter). These are the cold creams. They behave like oils in that they do not mix with any exudate from the skin. They are easier to apply than ointments, and more cosmetically acceptable, although they are greasier than the vanishing creams. Many of them contain lanolin as the oil, which can cause an allergic contact dermatitis in some patients. Examples include:
   - oily cream/hydrous ointment[UK] (lanolin 50%, water 50%)
   - Pond's Dry Skin cream[USA].

Humectants (substances that retain water, such as glycerol, propylene glycol and urea) can be added to creams to reduce the amount of oil in the base without losing the moisturising effect.

Lotions

A lotion is any liquid such as normal saline or potassium permanganate solution. A **shake lotion** is a suspension of an insoluble powder in a liquid, such as calamine lotion (15% calamine, 5% zinc oxide, 5% glycerine, 75% water). This has a cooling effect because the liquid evaporates leaving the inert powder on the skin. In practice these are hardly ever used except to cool sunburn.

Emollient lotions contain a low concentration of oil (5%) in water. They spread easily and are useful as moisturisers for hairy areas such as the chest and back of men (*see* Table 2.01a).

Pastes

Pastes are a mixture of a powder in an ointment. They stay where you put them and they do not spread away from that site like creams and ointments do as the skin warms up. Examples include:

- Lassar's paste^{UK} – this contains 2% salicylic acid, 24% zinc oxide, 24% starch and 50% white soft paraffin
- zinc oxide paste^{USA} is the one most commonly used – it contains 25% starch, 25% zinc oxide and 50% white soft paraffin.

Cooling pastes are preparations that contain a powder (zinc oxide), water (lime water) and an oil (arachis oil). They are called creams rather than pastes in the United Kingdom. For example:

- zinc cream BP (zinc oxide 32 g, oleic acid 0.5 mL, arachis oil 32 mL, wool fat 8 g, calcium hydroxide 45 mg, water to 100 g).

Gels

Traditionally, gels are two-component semi-solid systems of natural or synthetic polymers (e.g. methylcellulose, agar, carbomer or gelatine) in a liquid (e.g. water). These polymers build a three-dimensional matrix throughout a hydrophilic liquid, from which the active ingredients diffuse relatively freely. They have the property of being semi-solid in the cold and becoming liquid on warming up (e.g. when rubbed into the skin).

Emollient gels (Doublebase) are a water and oil emulsion with a jelly feel. Salts in the skin induce separation of the water and oil. The water is held in the stratum corneum by a humectant (glycerol), which is sealed in by a lipid layer.

When to use which kind of vehicle

Ointments and creams are used most of the time. Which you use depends mainly on the patient's preference and the hydration of the skin. Start with a cream on normal or moist skin and an ointment on dry skin.

Creams are much more cosmetically acceptable, particularly on the face (patients do not like walking around with a shiny face), in the flexures and when the medicament has to be applied all over (so that the clothes are not covered with grease), but may be too drying if the skin is itself dry (e.g. in patients with atopic eczema and ichthyosis). In general, ointments are more effective than creams, as they are occlusive and do not contain potential allergens. You may have to try both to see which suits the patient best. Because creams contain water, they must also contain preservatives to prevent contamination by bacteria and fungi; these preservatives can cause an allergic contact dermatitis. In patients with an acute eczema or contact allergic dermatitis where you do not know the cause, always use an ointment (and one that does not contain lanolin) rather than a cream until you have discovered the cause.

Gels are used as alternatives to ointments on the body and lotions on hairy parts of the body. For instance, since all topical steroid lotions are in an alcoholic base they are not suitable for applying to excoriated eczematous skin, because they will sting. A steroid gel (which does not contain alcohol) can be rubbed into the scalp without causing stinging. It becomes liquid when it is rubbed in and is therefore cosmetically acceptable (like a lotion).

Due to the lightweight feel and the absence of an oily phase, gels are also popular as a moisturiser (Doublebase), or for delivering the active ingredients in the treatment of acne vulgaris, and psoriasis (Dovobet gel).

Lotions are used on wet surfaces and on hairy areas, for example:
- in the mouth as a mouthwash
- on the scalp so that it does not make a mess
- on wet rashes (e.g. weeping eczema).

For wet rashes, use an astringent that will coagulate protein and dry up the exudate. The two that are commonly used are as follows.

1. **Potassium permanganate (KMnO$_4$)**: this is dispensed as crystals, as a tablet (Permitabs^{UK} – *see* Fig. 2.01) or a made-up solution. The affected area can be bathed in this solution to dry up exudate. If the solution used is too strong (i.e. purple), the skin and nails will be stained brown (*see* Fig. 2.02).

2. **Aluminium acetate (Burow's solution)**: it is made by mixing five parts of a 13% solution of aluminium acetate in 100 parts of sterile water, or by dissolving a packet or tablet of Domeboro or Bluboro in 1 pint of water. This is used as a soak. The neat 13% solution may be used as ear drops to treat exudative otitis externa.

Pastes are used where you want to apply a noxious chemical to a particular part of the skin without getting it onto the surrounding normal skin, e.g. dithranol^{UK} (anthralin^{USA}) in psoriasis. They are rarely used except in hospital because they are unsightly. They have to be applied with a gloved hand or a spatula and they have to be cleaned off with oil (e.g. arachis oil) rather than soap and water.

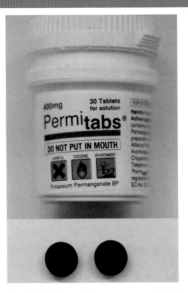
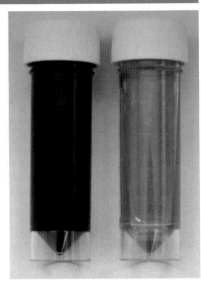

Fig. 2.01 Permitabs: place two tablets of potassium permanganate (above left) in a universal container, add water and shake to produce a dark-purple solution (left tube above right); add a few drops of this solution to a bowl of water to produce a light-pink colour, which is how it should be used (right tube)

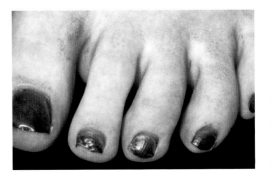

Fig. 2.02 Staining of toenails and feet from soaking in potassium permanganate solution that is too strong (purple colour); if the pink colour is used, this will not occur

ACTIVE INGREDIENTS

Topical steroids

Topical steroids are extremely useful in inflammatory conditions of the skin, particularly in eczema, but they are not the treatment for everything (they are contraindicated in acne, rosacea, all infections [bacterial, viral and fungal] and infestations).

Topical steroids are divided into four groups in the United Kingdom and seven groups in the United States according to their potency (*see* Table 2.02).

There are a very large number to choose from and it is best to become familiar with a few (perhaps one or two from each group) rather than all of them. Relative potencies of the different groups compared with the potency of 1% hydrocortisone are important in deciding on which topical steroid to use. As a general rule, use the weakest possible steroid that is effective.

We would recommend that you only use 1% hydrocortisone or equivalent (weak[UK]/group 6–7[USA]) topical steroid on the face. For eczema on the trunk and limbs you can use a moderately potent[UK]/group 4–5[USA] steroid. The potent[UK]/group 2–3[USA] is useful for localised persistent eczema. Remember that in the flexures absorption of the steroid will be increased because of occlusion.

There is little place for very potent[UK]/group 1[USA] steroids in general practice, and where you might be considering their use, systemic steroids might be safer. As little as 50 g of 0.05% clobetasol propionate (Dermovate[UK]/Temovate[USA]) per week will suppress the patient's adrenal glands. Hydrocortisone is 50 times weaker so is obviously a lot safer; in theory a patient could use up to 2.5 kg/week before getting the same side effects.

Absorption of topical steroids

The potency of the steroid molecule can be enhanced by the base used, e.g. an ointment base makes the steroid more potent than a cream or lotion. Occlusion over the site of application increases the steroid potency 50-fold. Occlusion causes over-hydration of the stratum corneum, reducing the skin's natural barrier. It induces a reservoir effect so that the steroid can persist in the skin for several days. The site and degree of inflammation also affects absorption. The relative ability to be absorbed at various sites is:

back < forearm < scalp < forehead < cheeks < axilla < scrotum normal skin < inflamed skin < erythrodermic skin.

Application of topical steroids

Although topical steroids are traditionally applied twice a day, there is no evidence that this is the best way to use them. Since the steroid molecule persists in the stratum corneum and is slowly absorbed, it may be that a single application at night would work just as well. Using a moisturiser frequently in the daytime might be more effective than increasing the number of applications of a topical steroid.

Repeated application of potent topical steroids can result in a diminished effect (tachyphylaxis). Recovery of response returns within a week of stopping. To prevent this happening, use potent steroids for 3–5 days at a time followed by a moisturiser for the next 3 days.

One 15 g tube of ointment or cream is enough to cover the adult body surface once; daily application for a week will require over 100 g. If a patient has widespread eczema, *adequate amounts* of topical steroid should be prescribed or he or she is likely to relapse. A useful guide is the **fingertip unit**, which is the amount that is squeezed onto the index finger from tip to the distal interphalangeal joint.

Table 2.02 Classification of topical steroids by potency

Group	UK brands	USA brands	Clinical indication
Weak[UK] Group 6–7[USA] Potency = 1% hydrocortisone	Hydrocortisone 0.5%, 1.0%, 2.5% (*Dioderm, Mildison*) Fluocinolone 0.0025% (*Synalar 1:10*) cream	Hydrocortisone 0.5%, 1.0%, 2.5% (numerous products) Alclometasone 0.05% (*Aclovate*) Desonide 0.05% (*Desowen/Tridesilon*)	Eczema on the face Eczema at any site in infants
Medium potent[UK] Group 4–5[USA] Potency = 2.5 (×1% hydrocortisone)	Betamethasone valerate 0.025% (*Betnovate RD*) Clobetasone butyrate 0.05% (*Eumovate*) Fluocinolone .00625% (*Synalar 1:4*) Fluocortolone 0.25% (*Ultralanum plain*) Fludroxycortide 0.0125% (*Haelan*) Hydrocortisone 17-butyrate 0.1% (*Locoid*)	Clocortolone pivalate 0.1% Desoximetasone 0.05% (*Topicort LP*) Fluocinolone 0.025%* Fluticasone 0.005% (*Cutivate*) Flurandrenolide 0.05% Hydrocortisone butyrate 0.1% (*Locoid*) Hydrocortisone valerate 0.2%* Hydrocortisone probutate 0.1% Prednicarbate 0.1% Triamcinolone 0.025%* (*Kenalog*)	Eczema (atopic) on the trunk and limbs, or flexures (both adult or children) Seborrhoeic eczema on trunk Flexural psoriasis
Potent[UK] Group 2–3[USA] Potency = 10 (×1% hydrocortisone)	Betamethasone dipropionate 0.05% (*Diprosone*) Betamethasone valerate 0.1% (*Betnovate*) Diflucortolone valerate 0.1% (*Nerisone*) Fluocinolone acetonide 0.025% (*Synalar*) Fluocinonide 0.05% (*Metosyn*) Fluticasone propionate 0.05% (*Cutivate*) Mometasone furoate 0.1% (*Elocon*)	Amcinonide 0.1% (*Cyclocort*) Betamethasone dipropionate 0.05% (*Diprolene*) Betamethasone valerate 0.1% (*Beta-Val*) Desoximetasone 0.05% (*Topicort*) Diflorasone diacetate 0.05% (*Apexicon*) Fluocinonide 0.05% (*Lidex*) Halcinonide 0.1% (*Halog*) Mometasone furoate 0.1%* (*Elocon*) Triamcinolone 0.5%, 0.1%*	Lichenified atopic eczema Discoid eczema Varicose eczema Scalp eczema Hand and foot eczema or psoriasis Lichen planus
Very potent[UK] Group 1[USA] Potency = 50 (×1% hydrocortisone)	Clobetasol propionate 0.05% (*Dermovate*) Diflucortolone valerate 0.3 (*Nerisone forte*)	Clobetasol propionate 0.05% (*Temovate*) Fluocinonide 0.1% (*Vanos*) Halbetasol propionate 0.05% (*Ultravate*)	Lichen simplex Resistant discoid eczema Discoid lupus erythematosus Lichen sclerosus et atrophicus

Note: *cream in a lower potency group; the ointment and cream base may result in differing groups for same molecule.

Table 2.03 Fingertip units as a guide to quantities needed to cover body surfaces

No units	Quantity g	Area of skin to cover
1	0.5	Both palms
2.5	1.25	Face and neck
3	1.5	Arm
6	3	Leg
7	3.5	Trunk front or back

Infants <1 year = ¼ of above; 1–3 years = ½ of above

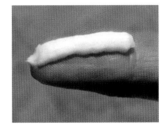

Fig. 2.03 Fingertip unit

Side effects of topical steroids

- Skin atrophy (Fig. 2.04) and striae (p. 212) from loss of collagen
- Tearing of the skin leading to odd-shaped scars (stellate scars) due to loss of dermal collagen (Fig. 2.05)
- Easy bruising due to loss of collagen support of the blood vessels in the dermis (Fig. 2.05)
- Perioral dermatitis (*see* p. 115) when steroids stronger than 1% hydrocortisone are applied to the face of young adults
- Telangiectasia on the face when steroids stronger than 1% hydrocortisone are applied to the face in middle and old age (*see* Fig. 5.21, p. 122)
- Rebound phenomenon causing worsening of the skin condition when the steroid is stopped
- Susceptibility to infection (bacterial, viral and fungal)
- Tachyphylaxis: repeated use results in loss of effect
- Allergic contact dermatitis: about 2% of patients being treated with topical steroids become allergic to the steroid itself (rather than the base)
- Cushing's syndrome when large amounts of potent or very potent[UK]/groups 1–3[USA] steroids are used; this includes a moon face and buffalo hump and all the systemic effects that you get with oral steroids (*see* p. 51)

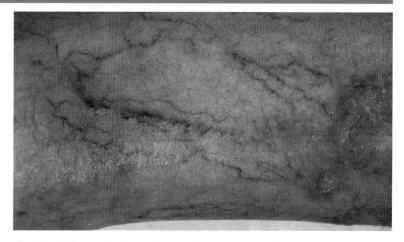

Fig. 2.04 Skin atrophy in a patient with atopic eczema from long-term application of topical steroids – note patch of eczema on right

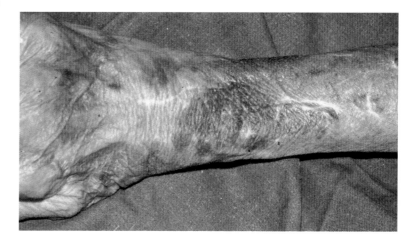

Fig. 2.05 Stellate scars and bruising due to loss of dermal collagen following long-term use of topical steroids

Topical immune modulators

Calcineurin inhibitors

These are macrolide lactones isolated from *Streptomyces tsukubaensis*. They block the activity of calcineurin and inhibit T-cell activation. Their action is very similar to that of ciclosporin, but because of their lower molecular weight they are absorbed through the skin.

Two agents are currently available:
1. 0.03% and 0.1% tacrolimus (Protopic) ointment
2. 1% pimecrolimus (Elidel) cream.

Their main use is in atopic eczema. Tacrolimus is as effective as a moderately potent[UK]/group 4–5[USA] steroid, while pimecrolimus is more equivalent to 1% hydrocortisone in potency. Because they have no effect on collagen synthesis, there is no thinning or bruising of the skin from long-term use. The only important side effect is itching and burning of the skin in up to 50% of patients when they are first applied. This lasts for 15–20 minutes but stops after the first few days.

The standard regimen for their use is twice a day for 2 weeks, then once a day for a month or so. They are useful as a prophylactic in eczema – applied twice weekly to at-risk sites. There are theoretical concerns about their use since they reduce the skin's ability to repair sun damage. Sun protection should be recommended. Stop using it prior to sunny holidays or if light therapy is to be used. There is no firm evidence that they can lead to cutaneous lymphoma.

Toll-like receptor 7 activators

Imiquimod (Aldara) cream is the first of a new group of compounds that stimulate the production of interferon and other cytokines by activation of the TLR7 (Toll-like receptor) on monocytes, macrophages and dendritic cells. It has both anti-viral and anti-tumour activity.

The following treatment regimens are used:
- genital warts: three times a week for up to 16 weeks
- solar keratoses: three times a week for 4 weeks
- Bowen's disease: five times a week for 6 weeks*
- superficial basal cell carcinomas: five times a week for 6 weeks*
- lentigo maligna five times a week for 12 weeks*

(*Stop and reduce to three times a week if a severe reaction occurs.)

It produces a marked inflammatory reaction (*see* Fig. 9.72b, p. 291) that although dramatic is non-scarring. Assess the efficacy when the inflammatory response has subsided.

Tar

Tar is not used very much these days because it is brown and smelly and patients do not like it. It is still used occasionally in both eczema and psoriasis. There are basically three types of tar available.
1. **Wood tars**, which are produced by the destructive distillation of beech, birch, pine or juniper. Oil of Cade can be used to treat psoriasis of the scalp.
2. **Bituminous tars** were originally obtained from the distillation of shale deposits containing fossilised fish, hence the name ichthyol. They are mainly used today in paste bandages (e.g. ichthammol bandages, Ichthopaste[UK]) to soothe chronic eczema.
3. **Coal tars** are a mixture of about 10 000 different compounds, mainly aromatic hydrocarbons such as benzol, naphthalene and anthracene. Crude coal tar is what remains when coal

is heated without air, originally to produce coal gas. Which compounds in tar actually work is not known. They reduce DNA synthesis and therefore epidermal proliferation and they are useful for stopping itching. Crude coal tar can be refined by boiling and then alcoholic extraction to produce coal tar solution (liquor picis carbonis[UK]/liquor carbonis detergens[USA]).

Crude coal tar is now only used for treating psoriasis and eczema as an inpatient or in a treatment centre. It is usually prescribed as coal tar and salicylic acid ointment BP[UK] (2% crude coal tar and 2% salicylic acid), White's tar ointment[USA] (5%), or various strengths (2%–10%) in white soft paraffin or Lassar's paste.

Coal tar solution is less messy but also less effective. The messier the tar preparation the more effective it is, but less cosmetically acceptable for the patient. Coal tar solution can be dispensed as an ointment (2%–10% coal tar solution in white soft paraffin) or as numerous proprietary creams, lotions, scalp applications or bath oils.

Side effects of tar and problems with using it
- It is brown, smelly, and it will stain the clothes and bedding.
- It can cause an irritant reaction on the skin.
- Occasionally it will cause an allergic contact dermatitis.
- It may cause a photosensitivity reaction.
- It can cause a folliculitis on hairy areas and is best avoided in hairy patients.

Dithranol[UK]/anthralin[USA]

This is a synthetic anthracene derivative which can be very effective in the treatment of stable plaque psoriasis. It is a yellow powder that can be made up into a cream, ointment, stick or paste. The major problems with dithranol are:
- irritation and burning of normal skin
- brown discoloration of the skin and a mauve/purple staining of the patient's clothes that will not wash out.

For these reasons it is rarely prescribed, as patients find it difficult to use at home. It is best applied in Lassar's paste at a dermatology department by trained nurses.

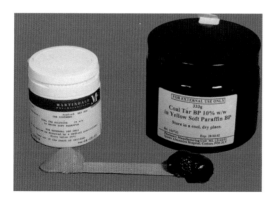

Fig. 2.06 Coal tar solution in WSP (left) and crude coal tar ointment (right)

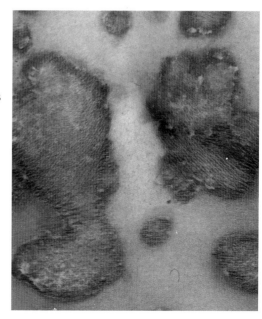

Fig. 2.07 Dithranol stain over treated psoriatic plaques

Vitamin D₃ analogues

Calcitriol (Silkis), calcipotriol (Dovonex), and tacalcitol (Curatoderm) are vitamin D_3 analogues that are the first-line treatment for psoriasis (*see* p. 228). They decrease epidermal proliferation and are effective in flattening the psoriatic plaques and removing the scale but not so good at getting rid of the redness. Only calcitriol and tacalcitol can be used on the face and flexures. Calcipotriol can cause redness and irritation at these sites and occasionally elsewhere. They do not cause hypercalcaemia and hypercalcuria, since less than 1% applied to the skin is absorbed.

They can be used in conjunction with a potent[UK]/group 2–3[USA] topical steroid for a limited time only (not more than 1 month).

Retinoids

Topical retinoids act by increasing epidermal turnover and differentiation of corneocytes. Clinically they are useful for treatment of comedones in acne (*see* p. 119). They can occasionally be useful in psoriasis (*see* p. 228). Retinoic acid also has an effect on the dermis whereby solar damage and solar elastosis may be reversed. The irritant effects of retinoic acid – inflammation and skin peeling – limit its usefulness.

The topical retinoids available for acne are:

- 0.1% adapalene (Differin) cream and gel – a synthetic retinoid that avoids the irritancy of the retinoic acids
- 0.05% isotretinoin (13-cis-retinoic acid) as Isotrex gel.

The topical retinoid used for psoriasis is:

- tazarotene 0.05% gel (Zorac). This can cause irritation if applied to the normal skin around the psoriasis.

Keratolytic agents

These are used to remove hyperkeratosis in a whole variety of skin conditions including warts, hyperkeratotic eczema on the palms and soles, psoriasis and palmoplantar keratoderma. The ones most commonly used include the following.

1. **α-hydroxy acids**
   - **Salicylic acid** ointment applied twice a day is useful for treating hyperkeratosis of the palms and soles or plane warts. The 2% ointment BP is readily available, but higher strengths (5%, 10%, 20%) need to be made up by a pharmacy (and can be expensive). It can be mixed with coal tar (coal tar and salicylic acid ointment BP) for treating psoriasis, or with a topical steroid ointment (Diprosalic) for treating hyperkeratotic eczema.
   - **Lactic acid** is a useful moisturiser, either in over-the-counter products or combined with urea (Aquadrate[UK], Calmurid[UK]). It is also combined with salicylic acid in proprietary wart paints (*see* p. 434).
   - **Benzoic acid** is combined with salicylic acid (in Whitfield's ointment) for treating superficial fungal infections (*see* p. 37).

2. **Propylene glycol** is included in over-the-counter products and acts as a humectant (absorbs and retains water) and keratolytic agent. For hyperkeratotic eczema of the hands and feet 50% propylene glycol in water can be used under polythene occlusion at night to reduce the excess keratin.

3. **Urea**, like propylene glycol, is both a humectant and a keratolytic agent. 10% urea cream (multiple brands) can be used for keratosis pilaris (*see* p. 324) or mixed with 1% hydrocortisone cream (Alphaderm[UK], Calmurid HC[UK], Carmol HC[USA]) to treat atopic eczema. It can be combined with lactic acid as a moisturiser (Aquadrate[UK], Calmurid[UK], Ureacin[USA]).

Antibiotics

As a general rule, topical antibiotics should not be used on the skin because most of them are potent skin sensitisers and will cause an allergic contact dermatitis. You do not want to sensitise someone to a drug that may at some future date be life-saving. It is much easier to become allergic to an antibiotic applied to the skin than to one taken by mouth or given parenterally.

Virtually everyone will become sensitised to penicillin so this should never be used topically. Tetracyclines rarely cause problems and would be safe to use, but in practice they are not much use because the common skin pathogens, *Staphylococcus aureus* and *Streptococcus pyogenes* are not sensitive to tetracycline. Mupirocin (Bactroban), fusidic acid (Fucidin) and retapamulin (Altargo) are the ones most commonly used.

Topical antibiotics should only be used in very superficial infections that will clear up in a matter of days, i.e. impetigo. They should not be used in infected eczema, as skin bacterial carriage is never cleared and antibacterial resistant strains are promoted. Also, the patient may well become sensitised after using it several times. The same is true for chronically infected leg ulcers (almost all patients with chronic venous ulceration are allergic to a number of antibiotics on patch testing because they have been used inappropriately in the past).

Do not be tempted to use steroid–antibiotic mixtures (e.g. Fucibet), because if the patient becomes allergic to the antibiotic in the mixture, the topical steroid will damp down the local reaction and you will only realise what has happened when the patient develops a widespread eczema. Most bacterial infections of the skin are more appropriately treated with systemic antibiotics.

Antiseptics

Chlorhexidine and benzalkonium chloride are combined with moisturisers as soap substitutes (Dermol[UK], Eczmol[UK]). Aqueous cream contains 1% phenoxyethanol. These can all be irritant, especially in patients with atopic eczema.

Nasal and flexural carriage of *S. aureus* can result in recurrent skin infections. A 4% chlorhexidine wash to the body once daily for 5 days can reduce infected episodes. Octenilin is an alternative to the irritant chlorhexidine-containing body washes in patients with atopic eczema.

Antiviral agents

The only topical antiviral agents currently available are 5% aciclovir (Zovirax) cream and 1% penciclovir (Vectavir[UK] / Denavir[USA]) cream. They are used for the treatment of herpes simplex (*see* p. 108). They inhibit phosphorylation of viral thymidine kinase, which prevents viral DNA synthesis and virus replication. There must be active viral replication to be effective so they need to be used immediately the first symptoms are noticed (usually tingling or paraesthesia). They are applied five times a day for 2–3 days until crusting has occurred.

Antifungal agents

Those active against dermatophyte fungi (tinea).

- **Keratolytic agents** act differently to all other antifungal agents. They remove the keratin on which the fungus lives rather than killing the fungus itself. The one most commonly used is Whitfield's ointment, a mixture of 6% benzoic and 3% salicylic acid in emulsifying ointment.

The others all interfere with the synthesis of ergosterol in the fungal cell membrane.

- **Undecanoate** as the acid zinc salt in Mycota[UK], or Desenex[USA] powder: these proprietary powders can be bought over the counter.
- **Tolnaftate** (Mycil[UK], Tinactin[UK], Tinaderm[UK]) is fungistatic. It is sold over the counter as a powder or cream.
- **Amorolfine** (Loceryl) is fungistatic. It is available as a nail lacquer or cream. The nail lacquer needs to be applied weekly after filing the surface of the nail. In the nails it also works against saprophytic moulds (such as *Hendersonula* or *Scopulariopsis*).
- **Imidazoles**: there are a large number of drugs in this group available as creams (clotrimazole, econazole, ketoconazole, miconazole, oxiconazole[USA], sulconazole). Tioconazole (Trosyl[UK]) is another used as a nail lacquer. They are all fungistatic rather than fungicidal and of more or less equal efficacy. A number of imidazole–hydrocortisone mixtures are also made; these generally are not a good idea, because it encourages treatment without first making a diagnosis on the mistaken belief that they will work for both fungal infections and eczema.
- **Allylamines**: terbinafine (Lamisil) and naftifine[USA] are fungicidal and more effective than any of the other topical antifungal agents.

Those active against yeasts such as *Candida* and *Pityrosporum* species.

- **Imidazoles** are broad-spectrum antifungal agents that work for yeasts as well as dermatophytes (*see* previous list).

- **Polyenes**: nystatin (named after the New York State Department of Health) is only effective against *Candida* – it is cheaper than the imidazoles but has the disadvantage that it stains everything it comes into contact with yellow; amphotericin B is a broad-spectrum polyene antifungal agent used as lozenges for treating *Candida* infections in the mouth.
- **Clioquinol** is effective against *Candida* and various bacteria but not against dermatophytes. It is usually combined with a topical steroid (e.g. Ala-Quin[USA], Betnovate C[UK], Locoid C[UK], Vioform HC[UK]). It stains the skin and clothing yellow.
- **Rosaniline dyes**: gentian violet is effective against yeasts and Gram-positive organisms. It is used as a 0.5% aqueous solution but stains everything it comes into contact with purple. It is useful in wet areas, e.g. toe webs and flexures.

LOCAL ANAESTHETICS

Topical local anaesthetics are useful in children when applied before giving an injection of local anaesthetic, or for providing anaesthesia to large areas of skin, e.g. before cautery of comedones or laser treatment.

The one most commonly used is EMLA cream (a eutectic mixture of local anaesthetics), which contains 2.5% lignocaine and 2.5% prilocaine in an oil-in-water cream base. This combination allows penetration of local anaesthetic through the stratum corneum. It is applied under occlusion (i.e. a film dressing) and left on for 90 minutes for maximum effect. Both are amides so do not cause contact sensitisation.

Tetracaine (amethocaine, Ametop) gel is an alternative and needs to be applied for only 45 minutes. Occlusion is not necessary but it can cause some local vasodilation and irritation.

SUNSCREENS

Sunscreens work either by absorbing or reflecting ultraviolet light.

Absorbent sunscreens contain chemicals that absorb ultraviolet light.

1. Those that protect the skin from **UVB (290–320 nm)**. They are useful in protecting against sunburn, preventing solar urticaria or polymorphic light eruption (*see* p. 100). Examples include:
   - PABA (para-aminobenzoic acid) esters, e.g. Padimate O (octyldimethyl PABA) – only gives partial protection against UVB, but penetrates into the stratum corneum after ½ to 2 hours, so not easily removed by water
   - cinnamates – these have tended to replace PABA esters but are a less effective screen, e.g. octinoxate (octyl methoxycinnamate), octocrylene, amiloxate (isoamyl p-methoxycinnamate)
   - salicylates are less effective but are water-resistant and safe at higher concentrations, e.g. octisalate (octyl salicylate)
   - ensulizole (phenylbenzimidazole sulphonic acid) is water-soluble so used in lighter, less oily cosmetics for routine cosmetic use.
2. Those that protect primarily against **UVA (320–400 nm)**. These are needed for patients with porphyria, photosensitive eczema or photosensitivity due to drugs:
   - avobenzone (butyl methoxydibenzoylmethane) has excellent protection in the whole of the UVA range, but it needs to be carefully combined with other sunscreens.
3. Those that protect against **UVB and UVA up to 350 nm**:
   - oxybenzone (benzophenone-3)
   - anthranilates, e.g. meradimate (methyl anthranilate)
   - bisoctrizole (methylene bis-benzotriazolyl tetramethylbutylphenol) is produced as microfine organic

particles that will scatter as well as absorb ultraviolet light (not available in the United States)
   - bemotrizinol (bis-ethylhexyloxyphenol methoxyphenyltriazine) is highly photostable and helps prevent the photodegradation of other compounds, especially avobenzone (not available in the United States).

Reflectant sunscreens contain inert mineral pigments, either titanium dioxide or zinc oxide, which put an opaque barrier between the sun and the skin. They protect against both UVB and UVA but are unsightly for the patient because they are white. Newer, microsized particles of titanium dioxide to some extent overcome this problem, but most high-factor sunscreens contain a mixture of organic filters and an inorganic reflectant (TiO_2).

The efficacy of sunscreens in protecting against **UVB** is measured by the sun protection factor (SPF). The higher the number, the greater the protection. An SPF of 10, for example, allows a person to remain in the sun 10 times longer than he or she normally would before burning. Anything above SPF 30 is probably adequate. A sunscreen should be applied quite thickly and reapplied every 2 hours. This is probably more important than the actual SPF value. If UVA protection is required, make sure the sunscreen contains either avobenzone or titanium dioxide.

SKIN CAMOUFLAGE AGENTS

These are used to cover up birthmarks, scars and pigmentary disorders. They are ointments with a high pigment content set with a finishing powder that makes them waterproof. They are smudge proof but not rub proof; they need to be touched up or removed (on the face) after 8–16 hours. To get the right skin match they need to be applied initially by a skilled professional. In the United Kingdom the Red Cross run private clinics. Patients with hyperpigmentation may need an 'undercoat' before the skin match is applied. Topical treatments and sunscreens can be applied before the camouflage. Make-up should be applied afterwards. Multiple products are available on prescription.

TOPICAL AGENTS FOR WOUND CARE

Wound healing occurs in three stages:

1. an influx of inflammatory cells to aid reabsorption of necrotic cells and prevent infection – this causes erythema and exudate
2. the formation of granulation tissue and revascularisation – at this stage there is a reduction in exudate
3. migration of epidermal cells to cover the wound and growth of new connective tissue underneath.

Wound healing takes place most rapidly when:

- there is a moist environment (not too wet, not too dry) and any excess fluid is able to evaporate
- the wound is warm – a drop in temperature of 2°C significantly reduces healing
- there is good blood perfusion; dressings do not affect this, but topical negative pressure (suction pump) may.

Management of chronic wounds

Successful treatment of leg ulcers and other chronic wounds therefore depends on the following.

1. **Dealing with the underlying cause**: e.g. compression bandages for venous hypertension, taking the weight off pressure sores etc.
2. **Attention to nutrition and correction of any deficiencies**.
3. **Management of the wound itself** (*see* Tables 2.04a & b):
   - **Removal of dead and necrotic tissue** (*see* Table 2.05). Wound cleansing for its own sake is not a good thing. The wound bed is disturbed and any new epithelium ripped off. Any necrotic material should be removed – this can be done by using a debriding agent or surgically with a pair of scissors or a scalpel by a competent practitioner.
   - **Reduction of bacterial counts** and **treatment of clinical infection** (*see* Table 2.06). All wounds left open will become colonised by bacteria. Taking swabs is not usually helpful. Clinical signs of infection are cellulitis of the surrounding skin, a foul odour, or *increasing* levels of pain, exudate or capillary bleeding with pitted/spongy granulation tissue. The organisms that matter are:
     (i) a group A β-haemolytic streptococcus that causes cellulitis (*see* p. 373) – this should be treated with high dose flucloxacillin, clindamycin or clarithromycin (*see* p. 374).
     (ii) *Pseudomonas*, which causes a green discoloration and has a distinctive foul smell – this can be treated with 0.75% metronidazole (Anabact) gel applied directly to the wound, acetic acid (apply as household vinegar diluted 50:50 in water, soaked onto a swab and left on for 5 minutes) or silver dressings (*see* Table 2.06).

Do not use antibiotic impregnated tulle dressings because patients frequently become allergic to them.

Wounds being treated for infection should be reviewed within 14 days; by that time treatment will have worked, if it is going to.

- **Reduction of excessive exudate** (*see* Table 2.07). Venous ulcers produce serous exudate because of the high hydrostatic pressure. Exudate is a problem because it soaks through bandages and makes a mess of clothing and bedding. Drawing the exudate away from the wound surface will allow better healing.
- **Covering the wound** (*see* Table 2.08). This helps to maintain the temperature and prevent drying out of the wound.

Table 2.04a Summary of types of wound and what dressings to use

Wound type	Dry adherent slough	Dirty superficial yellow slough – low exudate	Necrotic slough – moderate/ high exudate	Local infection – low exudate	Local infection – high exudate
Primary objective	Debride	Debride	Absorb exudate and debride	Reduce bacterial counts and debride	Reduce bacterial counts
Primary/wound contact	Hydrogel/ Hydrocolloid/ Viscopaste PB7	Hydrogel	Hydrocolloid/Hydrofiber (Aquacel) Capillary action	Honey/Iodine/Silver Flamazine, PHMB (polyhexamethylene biguanide)	Alginate + silver Hydrofiber + silver Cadexomer iodine
Secondary/surface	Light foam or gauze	Hydrocolloid or Bordered foam	Super-absorbent dressing	Light foam/ Low adherent	Super-absorbent dressing
Alternative	Surgical debridement	Maggots	Maggots	Maggots/ Surgical debridement	Potassium permanganate soaks

Table 2.04b Summary of types of wound and what dressings to use

Wound type	Smelly fungating wound	Granulating – low exudate	Granulating – high exudate	Epithelialising – low exudate	Epithelialising – high exudate
Primary objective	Reduce smell and bacterial counts	Protect wound	Reduce exudate	Protect wound	Reduce exudate
Primary/wound contact	Activated charcoal Metronidazole (Anabact) gel	Bordered Foam/ Hydrocolloid Low adherent dressing	Hydrofiber/Alginate	Low adherent/Film	Hydrofiber
Secondary/surface	Super-absorbent dressing	Gauze	Super absorbent	Gauze	Super absorbent
Alternative	Surgical debridement	Film		White soft paraffin	Potassium permanganate soak

Table 2.05 Debriding agents

Type	Brand names	Available	Used on	How to use	Comments and contraindications
Hydrogel A three-dimensional polymer that absorbs water	ActivHeal hydrogel, Aquaform, Askina, Cutimed, Flexigran, GranuGel, Intrasite, Nu-Gel, Purilon	Gel	Dry Sloughy or necrotic wounds	Squeeze gel onto wound and cover with a secondary dressing	Do not use on wet wounds Provides a moist environment for autolytic debridement
	Actiform cool, Aquaflo, Gel FX, Geliperm, Hydrosorb, Intrasite conformable, Novogel, Vacunet	Sheets		Apply sheet and cover with secondary dressing	
Hydrocolloid Comprising carboxymethyl cellulose backed with waterproof polyurethane foam or vapour-permeable film	ActivHeal hydrocolloid, Alione, Askina, Comfeel plus, Duoderm, Flexigran, Granuflex, Hydrocoll, NuDerm, Tegaderm hydrocolloid, Ultec Pro	Sheets	Low to moderate exudate Clean, granulating or sloughy wounds	Apply with a 2 cm overlap to hold in the exudate that is produced; the dressing is changed as soon as it begins to leak (approximately once or twice a week); there is a tendency for the exudate, as it accumulates, to force its way out of the dressing and run down the patient's leg, particularly when walking about; emollient ointment (see Table 2.01a) can be used to protect the skin	The hydrocolloid interacts with the ulcer exudate to form a soft moist gel that provides an acid environment allowing autolytic digestion of any necrotic material Aerobic and anaerobic bacteria will flourish in this environment producing an unpleasant smell
Maggots	*LarvE* from BioMonde, Bridgend, CF31 3BG Wales	Sterile maggots in small container or bag	Very sloughy wounds with mild to moderate exudate	Add saline to the maggots and tip them onto the fine mesh net provided; place this with the maggots in contact with the ulcer inside a hydrocolloid sheet cut to the size of the ulcer; cover the outside of the net with moistened swabs, a non-adherent dressing and Sleek adhesive tape; the maggots should be left in place for 48–72 hours and then washed out with saline or potassium permanganate	Maggots are extremely efficient debriding agents, feeding on necrotic tissue without affecting normal skin Do not use if blood clotting is inhibited – either naturally or by drugs

Table 2.06 Reducing bacterial counts and odour

Type	Brand names	Available	Used on	How to use	Comments and contraindications
PHMB (polyhexamethylene biguanide) Kendall AMD, Suprasorb, Telfa AMD		Gauze dressing Foam, Pad	Low exudate	As wound contact	Can be used as a prophylactic dressing
DACC (dialkyl carbamoyl chloride) Cutimed		Swab Pad	Low-moderate exudate	As wound contact	Novel anti-microbiological agent
Silver	Flamazine (silver sulphadiazine)	Cream	Infected wounds with low exudate	Apply direct onto wound or mix with a hydrogel	Silver is effective against pseudomonas but needs moisture to activate it
	Multiple products (see BNF)	Sheet only + alginate + foam + hydrofibre + hydrocolloid	High exudate	Direct to wound. Compound dressings available to aid absorption of increased exudate	Silver products are expensive and some question their efficacy; silver ion Ag⁺ is the active agent – some question the availability of the ion and its efficacy
Manuka honey	Activon, Algivon, Manuka pli, Medihoney, Melladerm Plus, Mesitran	Paste/ointment + alginate + hydroactive gel as dressing	Infected sloughy wounds	Need covering with film dressing	Works by osmotic action, and by altering the pH to make the wound inhospitable for bacteria; it reduces inflammation (and pain) and provides a good environment for debridement and granulation
Iodine Cadexomer iodine	Inodine Iodoflex, Iodosorb	Fabric dressing Paste, ointment	Low exudate High exudate	Apply direct to wound	May cause allergic contact dermatitis; wide spectrum, quickly deactivated by exudate
	Iodozyme, Oxyzyme	Hydrogel sheet	Low-moderate exudate	Apply direct to wound	Two component dressing where glucose oxidase and iodine ions release free iodine
Metronidazole	Anabact 0.75%	Gel	Smelly wounds	Apply direct to wound	Needs secondary dressing
Activated charcoal	Askina Carbosorb, Carbopad VC, CliniSorb	Non-absorbent cloth	Smelly wounds	Needs absorbent pad + secondary dressing	Charcoal absorbs odour but has no antibacterial activity; not effective if wet
	CarboFlex, Lyofoam C Sorbsan Plus Carbon	Absorbent sheet	Smelly wounds with high exudate	Apply direct and change when necessary	5 layers including alginate and hydrocolloid Activated charcoal cloth with outer layer of polyurethane foam Alginate fibre pad with absorbent backing

Table 2.07 Absorption of exudate

Type	Brand names	Available	Used on	How to use	Comments and contraindications
Alginate (naturally occurring polysaccharides found only in brown seaweeds [*Phaeophyceae*])	ActivHeal, Algisite M, Algosteril, Kaltostat, Melgisorb, Seasorb soft, Sorbalgon, Sorbsan, Suprasorb A, Tegaderm, UrgoSorb	Sheet or ribbon	Moderately exuding wounds	Cut to the exact size and shape of the ulcer; they expand laterally when wet so can cause maceration of the surrounding skin; leave in place for several days or up to a week at a time; removed by irrigation or by lifting off with a pair of forceps A secondary dressing is required	On contact with exudate, calcium ions in the alginate are exchanged for sodium, which turns the fibres into a gel, consisting of mannuronic or guluronic acid residues; the ratio of these determines whether a soft flexible gel forms (e.g. Sorbsan), which can be removed by irrigation, or a firm gel, which keeps its shape but needs to be removed with forceps (e.g. Kaltostat)
Hydrofibre	Aquacel Extra Aquacel Foam (foam backing)	Sheet	Heavily exuding wounds	Change according to the amount of exudate being produced (daily to weekly) The solid gel needs to be removed before a new sheet is applied	The fibres absorb fluid and the material is drawn down into the ulcer to form a gel. The advantage over alginates is that it will lock in moisture, as well as absorbing five times the amount of exudate that alginates do
Capillary action	Advadraw, Cerdak Basic, Sumar, Vacutex	Sheet or sachets	Exuding and sloughy wounds	Apply to surface, or cut to shape in deep wounds	A polyester and cotton sheet with its fibres arranged in such a way that fluid is drawn away from the wound Avoid in bleeding wounds
Polyurethane matrix	Cutinova hydro	Sheet	Moderately exuding wounds	Place over the wound or cut into strips to pack a deep wound; cover with a secondary dressing. Change every 2–3 days initially; leave on longer as exudate diminishes	Highly absorbent dressings made from a polyurethane matrix that absorbs water but leaves other molecules within the wound
Super absorbent	Cutisorb Ultra, DryMax Extra, KerraMax, Sorbion, Zetuvit Plus	Sheet Pad	Heavily exuding wounds	Available either as a pad or sheet to absorb excess fluid	These contain super-absorbent polymers and cellulose with a polyethylene wound contact layer

Table 2.08 Wound and ulcer dressings

Type	Brand names	Available as	Used on	Comments and contraindications
Low-adherent primary dressings	Atrauman, Urgotul, N-A dressing and others	Woven acrylic mesh dressing	Clean open wounds, low exudate	Will need retention bandage or skin adhesive to hold dressing in place
	Jelonet and multiple other brands	Paraffin gauze	Clean open wounds, low exudate	Large mesh allows epidermis to grow through resulting in trauma on removal; needs a secondary dressing *NICE no longer recommends these*
	Mepitel, N-A Ultra and multiple other brands Mepilex (+ foam backing)	Woven silicon mesh dressing	Clean open wounds, low exudate	These are more expensive but less adherent, so are less likely to damage the wound surface Will need a secondary dressing
Island dressings	Mepore and multiple other brands	Adhesive woven cloth with central pad	For protection of dry surgical wounds	Absorbs moisture but vapour permeable
Film dressings	Opsite, Tegaderm and multiple other brands (*see BNF*)	Transparent film ± absorbent pad	Clean wounds with low exudate	Waterproof and adhesive but lets vapour/air through; have no insulating properties so wounds become cooled and heal more slowly
	Cavilon, SuperSkin	Silicon liquid or spray	Protects normal skin around stomas	Useful for skin in contact with faeces or urine
Cream/ointment	Cavilon Vaseline (*see* Table 2.01a)	Cream Ointment and gel	Protects normal skin around stomas etc.	Useful for skin in contact with faeces or urine and skin around leg ulcers
Foam dressings	Allevyn, Aquacel foam, Biatain and multiple other brands Mepilix (+Silicon weave contact)	Sheet (various thicknesses) with or without adhesive border	As a secondary dressing As a pressure pad For insulation For over granulation	Polyurethane hydrophilic layer which absorbs limited amounts of exudate, and a thicker spongy outer hydrophobic breathable foamy layer, which keeps wound moist, warm and protected from trauma, while allowing some evaporation
Collagen & cellulose dressing	Promogran	Sheet	Clean, low exudate, no infection or bleeding	Derived from pig small intestine mucosa and containing collagen and regenerated cellulose

SYSTEMIC TREATMENT

ANTIBIOTICS

Systemic antibiotics are used for the following.

1. **Staphylococcal infections**
   a. Staphylococcal infections in the skin, e.g. boils, carbuncles, ecthyma, staphylococcal scalded skin syndrome, sycosis barbae, and infected eczema and scabies. Flucloxacillin 500 mg every 6 hours (double this for severe infections will also cover streptococcal infection) is the drug of choice. For patients who are allergic to penicillin, erythromycin 500 mg every 6 hours is an alternative. With this dose, gastro-intestinal upsets occur in about 20% of patients. The cephalosporins are not as good as flucloxacillin against *S. aureus* so should not be used as the first line of treatment. Nasal and flexural carriage of *S. aureus* can result in recurrent skin infections. Take swabs from the nose, groin and open wounds. If positive, decolonise the skin with 4% chlorhexidine body wash daily for 5 days and mupirocin ointment applied three times daily to the anterior nares. Octenilin is an alternative to the irritant chlorhexidine-containing washes in patients with eczema.
   b. **MRSA (methicillin-resistant *S. aureus*)** infected wounds may need treatment with oral doxycycline or intravenous vancomycin. It is best to liaise with your local microbiologist or infection control team to check current sensitivities. Again chronic carriage as for *S. aureus* may warrant decolonisation as outlined in previous point.
   c. **Panton–Valentine leukocidin (PVL) toxin-positive** *S. aureus* skin infections can be acquired in the community and lead to recurrent and potentially serious infections of the skin (as per staphylococcal infections above) and necrotising pneumonia. It is not easily eradicated from the skin with conventional courses of flucloxacillin or erythromycin. Its prevalence is increasing and PVL-positive *S. aureus* is associated with higher morbidity and mortality, and is more transmissible, when compared with PVL-negative *S. aureus*. Send microbiology samples specifically requesting PVL gene detection, as well as microscopy, culture and sensitivity. The UK Health Protection Agency advises treating PVL-positive MRSA isolates with rifampicin and one other agent (clindamycin, doxycycline, sodium fusidate, or trimethoprim). All patients plus their close contacts should be treated with topical decolonisation (*see* 1a on left).

2. **Streptococcal infections** in the skin, e.g. erysipelas and cellulitis. Streptococci are always sensitive to penicillin, so intravenous benzyl penicillin 1200 mg every 6 hours is the treatment of choice. Alternatively use high dose flucloxacillin 1 g every 6 hours. Erythromycin or clarithromycin 500 mg every 6 hours orally is useful in patients who are allergic to penicillin. Streptococcal ecthyma, or eczema and scabies that are secondarily infected with *Streptococcus pyogenes*, can be treated with phenoxymethyl penicillin 500 mg every 6 hours.

3. **Acne, perioral dermatitis and rosacea**: these are not due to infection with bacteria but nevertheless respond well to low doses of broad-spectrum antibiotics (*see* pp. 119, 116, 124). How they work is not fully understood.

ANTIFUNGAL AGENTS

Normally superficial fungal infections of the skin are treated with topical antifungal agents. The exceptions are when the hair and nails are involved when it is not possible to get the antifungal agent to the site where it is needed. Four groups of antifungal agents are available for systemic use.

1. **Antibiotics – griseofulvin**: this is the cheapest of the options and works well for tinea capitis; it is not very effective for nail infections. It is long-acting so only has to be given once a day but it has to be taken with food because it is absorbed with fat. Side effects are unusual – headache, irritability and nausea are the most common. Occasionally it can cause photosensitivity or a drug-induced lupus erythematosus. If the patient is on warfarin, the INR will need to be checked because the anticoagulant effect will be diminished. Do not use in patients with acute intermittent or variegate porphyria because it can induce acute attacks.

2. **Allylamines – terbinafine**: this is a fungicidal drug that is much more effective than griseofulvin and also much more expensive. It works well for any kind of dermatophyte infection (but not candida), but is particularly useful for tinea of the nails. It is taken once a day for 3 months for nail infections or for 2 weeks for infections on the skin. It occasionally causes mild gastro-intestinal upsets – anorexia, nausea, diarrhoea, abdominal fullness and a morbilliform rash. Check liver function if given for more than 2 months. Do not use during pregnancy and lactation.

3. **Imidazoles – ketoconazole**: this is very effective for treating pityriasis versicolor, where it is given as a single 400 mg dose. It should not be used for longer periods of time because there is a small risk of liver toxicity. It is a potent inhibitor of cytochrome P450 (*see* side effects of triazoles).

4. **Triazoles – itraconazole and fluconazole**: they are used for infections with *Candida albicans*, cryptococcosis or histoplasmosis in patients who are immunosuppressed (those with malignant disease, HIV or those on cytotoxic drugs), and in patients with myeloma.

Side effects of itraconazole include nausea, abdominal pain, dyspepsia and headache. Do not use in patients with ventricular dysfunction or risk of heart failure. Check liver function if given for more than 1 month. As it is a potent inhibitor of cytochrome P450 enzymes it may elevate the blood levels of other drugs being taken concurrently such as statins, midazolam, ciclosporin, warfarin and oral hypoglycaemics (check *BNF* before prescribing). Fluconazole rarely causes hepatotoxicity.

Nystatin is not absorbed when given by mouth so the only reason for using it is if you want to clear the gut of *C. albicans*, e.g. when a patient is getting recurrent perianal infection.

ANTIVIRAL AGENTS

Aciclovir, famciclovir and valaciclovir are the systemic antiviral agents in current use for both herpes simplex and herpes zoster infections. They all inhibit phosphorylation of viral thymidine kinase, which prevents viral DNA synthesis and virus replication. They are only effective while there is active viral replication and must therefore be given within 48 hours of the onset of vesicles. They can be used for treating:

- herpes simplex if the patient has disseminated disease, frequent recurrences, eczema herpeticum or recurrent erythema multiforme (*see* pp. 108, 109, 175)
- herpes zoster – this is much less sensitive to these drugs than herpes simplex, so bigger doses need to be given (*see* p. 180).

Ganciclovir is active against herpes simplex but also cytomegalovirus and human herpes-like viruses that are thought to play a role in late deteriorating drug hypersensitivity eruptions such as DRESS (drug reaction with eosinophilia and systemic symptoms, p. 168). It is given by intravenous infusion and needs close monitoring.

ANTIHISTAMINES

Antihistamines act as competitive blockers of histamine receptors. They have a close structural resemblance to histamine. As there are two types of histamine receptor, H_1 and H_2, there are two types of antihistamines. Cutaneous blood vessels have both H_1 and H_2 receptors, but for skin disease H_1 antihistamines are the most effective.

- **Non-sedative antihistamines** are the most useful drugs in urticaria and angioedema. Cetirizine, levocetirizine, fexofenadine, loratadine, desloratadine, mizolastine and rupatadine are the ones most commonly used. They are *not useful in eczema*, as histamine is not the cause of the itching in this condition. High doses (off-licence) are often required in urticaria and four times the standard hay fever dose is accepted practice, e.g. cetirizine 20 mg bid.
- **Sedative antihistamines** are useful for sedating children with atopic eczema to ensure that they and their parents get a good night's sleep. It is essential to give a big enough dose (administered 2 hours before bedtime) to ensure the child sleeps through the night. They are also useful for adults with very widespread rashes who need to rest the skin, e.g. patients with erythrodermic eczema or psoriasis, and patients with acute blistering conditions on the feet who would otherwise find it difficult to rest in bed. Hydroxyzine (Atarax), promethazine (Phenergan) and alimemazine are the most useful. Chlorphenamine (Piriton) is no good for treating any of the above because it is short acting (4 hours). It can be used in acute urticaria and in patients with photosensitive eczema who may be allergic to the others. Warn the patients about the sedating and hangover effect (driving, operating machinery etc.).
- **H_2 antihistamines.** Ranitidine (Zantac) can be worth trying in patients with urticaria where H_1 antihistamines alone have not been effective. Cimetidine (Tagamet) can also be given to reduce haemolysis and methaemoglobinaemia in patients taking dapsone (*see* p. 246).

RETINOIDS

Retinoids are derivatives of vitamin A. Their exact mode of action is unknown but they have many effects, including:

- induction of differentiation of epidermal cells – this may be how they work in psoriasis, solar keratoses and Bowen's disease; in patients who have had organ transplants they may suppress the development of epithelial tumours (e.g. basal cell carcinomas and squamous cell carcinomas), but they do not make established tumours go away
- shrinking of sebaceous glands causing decreased production of sebum
- anti-inflammatory effects by reducing prostaglandins and leukotrienes
- modulation of the immune response by enhancing T helper cells and stimulating interleukin 1.

There are four retinoids in current use.

1. **Isotretinoin**, the 13-cis isomer of retinoic acid (Roaccutane[UK]/Accutane[USA]), is used for the treatment of severe acne (*see* p. 120) at a dose of 0.5–1.0 mg/kg/day for 4–6 months to achieve a total dose of 120 mg/kg body weight. Lower total dose regimens are associated with an increased recurrence rate in both the long and short term.
2. **Acitretin** (Neotigason) is used to treat psoriasis and disorders of keratinisation [Darier's disease (*see* p. 247), pityriasis rubra pilaris (*see* p. 244), severe types of ichthyosis (*see* p. 323)]. It can also be used in conjunction with PUVA (RePUVA) in a patient with psoriasis to decrease the amount of ultraviolet light that the patient is exposed to (*see* p. 61). Acitretin may

help prevent the development of epithelial tumours (basal cell carcinomas and squamous cell carcinomas) in patients who are immunosuppressed, especially those who have had renal transplants. It is given at a dose of 10–50 mg/day. Female patients must not become pregnant while taking it or for 2 years after stopping because some of it is converted to etretinate (an ester of acitretin), which has a long half life of 2 years.

3. **Alitretinoin** (Toctino), the 9-cis-retinoic acid, is used for treating severe chronic hand eczema. Due to the cost of the drug it should only be used by dermatologists for patients who have not responded to standard treatments (such as potent topical corticosteroids) and when their eczema is severe and affecting their quality of life. Alitretinoin treatment should be stopped as soon as the eczema has clearly improved or if unresponsive to 12 weeks of treatment. The standard dose is 30 mg/day unless it is not tolerated or there is a medical history of hyperlipidaemia, diabetes or significant risk factors for ischaemic heart disease when 10 mg/day is used.

4. **Bexarotene** (Targretin) is a retinoid specifically selective for retinoid X receptors. It is an oral antineoplastic agent indicated for the treatment of cutaneous manifestations of cutaneous T-cell lymphoma in people who are refractory to at least one prior systemic therapy. Its side effects are similar to the other retinoids but it has a greater tendency to produce a rise in triglycerides and can cause hypothyroidism.

Side effects of retinoids

- Teratogenic (no effect on sperm). They must *not* be given to women of childbearing age unless on adequate contraception (two concurrent forms ideal including either the oral contraceptive pill or an implantable device).
- Dryness of the lips: this always occurs and you can tell whether a patient is taking the drug from this sign. *Vaseline* or a lip salve applied frequently will be necessary.
- Dryness of the nasal mucosa, which can lead to nose bleeds.
- Musculoskeletal aches and pains especially after exercise: those on long-term acitretin therapy can develop ossification of ligaments. Monitor by yearly X-ray of the lumbar spine.
- Conjunctivitis and dry eyes are usually not a problem unless the patient wears contact lenses. Hypromellose eye drops may help.
- Itching of the skin with or without an eczematous rash may need treatment with a moisturiser or 1% hydrocortisone ointment.
- Rise in serum triglycerides due to decreased extra-hepatic breakdown and increased secretion by the liver.
- Increase in liver enzymes which will resolve on stopping treatment.

Specific side effects of isotretinoin:

- Suicide risk and depression. Research indicates that acne itself confers an increased risk of suicide, and any association with isotretinoin may be related to the fact that the severest cases receive this treatment. There seems to be no way of predicting this and in practice it is very uncommon (1:8000). Many patients who are already depressed benefit from the drug as this improves their acne, and it does not result in worsening of their depression. Any preceding affective disorder should be treated and stabilised before considering systemic retinoids. If there are any concerns a psychiatrist should be involved in the patient's care. Regular assessment of mood should be documented and any concerns (your own, the patient's or that of family/friends) should be acted on.
- Irregularity or cessation of periods in women.
- Possible association with inflammatory bowel disease.

Specific side effects of acitretin:

- Peeling of palms and soles occurs at the beginning of treatment; they may also feel sticky or clammy.
- Increased sweating does not usually cause problems.
- Poor wound healing. The skin easily bruises and cuts take longer to heal.
- Hair loss bad enough to be noticeable only occurs in a few patients and is reversible on stopping treatment.
- Paronychia. Painful swelling around finger- and toenails occurs in a minority of patients.
- Nausea, vomiting and abdominal pain are unusual complaints.

Long-term treatment requires monitoring of blood for liver function and lipids, and X-ray of the spine for ossification of ligaments.

SYSTEMIC STEROIDS

Systemic steroids have a very limited use in the treatment of skin disease and are best restricted to use by a dermatologist. They should not be used in eczema or urticaria because, although the response may initially be dramatic, the disease is likely to flare badly when the tablets are stopped and it is then very difficult to get the patient off them. It is better to refer such a patient for an urgent dermatological opinion than to start him on prednisone.

Systemic steroids are essential and may be life-saving in:
- pemphigus (*see* p. 259)
- pemphigoid (*see* p. 256)
- systemic lupus erythematosus (*see* p. 131)
- dermatomyositis (*see* p. 132).

High doses are needed in all of these conditions and the risk of side effects is considerable. Interestingly such patients often do not show the typical steroid facies until the disease comes under control. For example, a patient can be on prednisolone 60 mg for several weeks without any evidence of a moon face, but as soon as the disease comes under control the face fattens up.

EQUIVALENT DOSES OF DIFFERENT SYSTEMIC STEROIDS	
Cortisone	100 mg
Hydrocortisone	80 mg
Prednisone or prednisolone	20 mg
Dexamethasone	2–4 mg

Side effects of systemic steroids:
- increased fat deposition on the face, shoulders and abdomen causing a moon face, buffalo hump and enlarged abdomen
- acne and hirsutism
- easy bruising and tearing of the skin
- striae (*see* Fig. 8.38, p. 212)
- delayed tissue healing
- increased susceptibility to infections (bacterial, fungal and viral)
- salt and water retention leading to oedema, hypertension and congestive cardiac failure
- diabetes
- peptic ulceration leading to bleeding and perforation
- proximal muscle weakness
- osteoporosis leading to fractures particularly of the vertebrae and ribs
- aseptic necrosis of the femoral head
- cataracts and glaucoma
- depression or euphoria (steroid psychosis)
- growth retardation in young children; this is not usually a problem unless steroids are given for more than 6 months

- suppression of the pituitary-adrenal axis leading to adrenal insufficiency on withdrawal or if the patient has some intercurrent illness or needs surgery.

To prevent complications

1. Patients will need regular checking of:
   - weight – to pick up fluid gain (monthly)
   - blood pressure – looking for hypertension (monthly)
   - urinalysis – looking for glycosuria (monthly)
   - DEXA scan (yearly) if patient is on steroids for more than 3 months), though pragmatically all female patients should be started on preventive treatment regardless if postmenopausal
   - chest X-ray – looking for reactivation of tuberculosis (yearly).
2. Patients should carry a **steroid card** or **medical alert tag** with them all the time. If they have an accident or have some other illness extra steroids can be given to prevent an Addisonian crisis.
3. To prevent stomach ulceration either use enteric coated prednisolone (expensive), or prescribe a proton pump inhibitor (e.g. omeprazole 10 mg day) in addition to the steroid.
4. To prevent osteoporosis give lifestyle advice – regular exercise, stop smoking, reduce alcohol intake. Start the patient on Calcichew D$_3$ forte, two tablets a day. Patients over the age of 45 (or postmenopausal women) or at risk of osteoporosis should also be on a bisphosphonate to reduce bone turnover e.g. alendronate (Fosamax) 70 mg/week. If intolerant to this (or there are contraindications to this drug) alternatives should be discussed with a rheumatologist.

IMMUNOSUPPRESSIVE AGENTS

A number of different immunosuppressive agents are used for severe skin disease, either in their own right or as steroid-sparing agents. They are all potentially dangerous and should only be initiated by a dermatologist.

Methotrexate

Methotrexate is used for psoriasis, eczema, the autoimmune bullous disorders, Hailey–Hailey disease (chronic benign familial pemphigus, *see* p. 340) and dermatomyositis (*see* p. 132). It inhibits dihydrofolate reductase and therefore cell division. It is probably the most effective of the systemic agents in use for the treatment of psoriasis and it works very quickly (within 48 hours).

Following routine blood tests (*see* under bone marrow suppression on p. 53), a 5 mg test dose is given and provided no adverse reaction has occurred it is given as a single dose of 10–25 mg orally, subcutaneously or intramuscularly *once a week*. It is excreted unchanged principally through the kidneys, so the dose needs to be reduced if renal function is impaired or the patient elderly. It can be continued long term at the lowest dose that keeps the psoriasis under control.

Methotrexate is available in 2.5 mg and 10 mg tablets that look identical. Most reports of acute toxicity have been related to inadvertent switching between tablet size and mistaken daily instead of weekly dosing. It is therefore advised that only 2.5 mg tablets ever be supplied (with close liaison with local prescribing chemists to facilitate this) and that all patients receive and carry a patient booklet where all doses, side effects and monitoring results are recorded.

Serious side effects:

- **Teratogenic** so must not be used in women who might become pregnant. In men it causes reversible oligospermia.
- **Bone marrow suppression**: check full blood count before starting, then weekly for 1 month and then every 2–3 months. If the mean corpuscular volume becomes elevated (over 100), reduce the dose.
- **Fibrosis of the liver** can occur after several years of treatment, so do not give to a patient with pre-existing liver disease or anyone who has a history of alcohol abuse. Patients on methotrexate should not drink any alcohol. Measuring blood levels of type III procollagen (P3NP) every 6 months can monitor the development of liver fibrosis. This is a non-specific marker of fibrosis and can be raised by other causes of fibrosis rendering it less useful, e.g. in patients with psoriatic arthritis. In the psoriatic population other causes of liver fibrosis are also commoner such as alcoholic and non-alcoholic fatty liver disease.

P3NP LEVELS

<4.2 mg/L	normal
>8.0 mg/L	consider liver biopsy
>10.0 mg/L	stop methotrexate

Less serious side effects:

- nausea, vomiting, diarrhoea and abdominal discomfort – these effects can often be avoided by changing from oral to intramuscular methotrexate
- stomatitis and ulceration of the mouth
- general malaise – patients frequently feel generally unwell

(headache, lethargy, irritability and depression) for about 24 hours after a dose of methotrexate

- extensive ulceration of the skin – this usually occurs at the same time as a profound fall in the white blood cell count
- hair loss – theoretically this is possible but is extremely rare
- lung problems such as acute pneumonitis or diffuse interstitial fibrosis can occur when methotrexate is used for treating neoplastic disease; with the lower doses used for treating psoriasis, these changes do not seem to happen.

Most side effects can be prevented by giving 5 mg folic acid once a week (3–4 days after the methotrexate) without stopping the therapeutic effect.

Patients on methotrexate must not take aspirin, diuretics, hypoglycaemics, non-steroidal anti-inflammatory drugs, phenytoin, probenecid, sulphonamides or trimethoprim. These all increase the risk of pancytopenia.

Ciclosporin

Ciclosporin is an immunosuppressive drug that is useful in the treatment of severe atopic eczema and psoriasis. The starting dose is 3–5 mg/kg/day. Its effect is rapid (within 2 weeks). Once the disease is under control the dose can be reduced and replaced by a safer agent long term, as its continuous use beyond 1 to 2 years is associated with oncogenesis. It is not teratogenic so it can be useful in severe skin disease in pregnancy.

The bioavailability and pharmacodynamics of different ciclosporin formulations varies significantly and it is advised to stick to a single available agent from a single manufacturer in a prescribing region, as loss of efficacy as well as toxicity has been described on inadvertent brand switching.

Side effects:

- **nephrotoxicity** (this is most important side effect) – ciclosporin reduces renal blood flow and causes a rise in urea and creatinine; keeping the maximum dose below 5 mg/kg/day reduces toxicity; if the blood creatinine levels increase by 30% over baseline, the dose should be reduced
- **hypertension** secondary to reduced kidney blood flow; if blood pressure increases above 160/95 use a calcium channel blocker, e.g. amlodipine (5–10 mg od) to reduce it
- increased liver enzymes, serum uric acid and cholesterol
- nausea and vomiting
- gingival hyperplasia in patients with poor dental hygiene
- tiredness, headaches, parasthesiae, tremor and convulsions are rare and reversible on reduction of the dose
- hypertrichosis (particularly a problem in women; may not be noticed in men)
- increased risk of lymphoma and non-melanoma skin cancer.

To prevent complications

Ideally measure the GFR (glomerular filtration rate) before starting treatment. Always check blood pressure, potassium, blood creatinine, liver function and lipids before treatment. Monitor these fortnightly for 6 weeks, monthly for 3 months and then every 2–3 months. Repeat GFR if creatinine levels increase more than 30% above baseline.

Azathioprine

Azathioprine is used for atopic and photosensitive eczema, and as a steroid-sparing drug in pemphigus, pemphigoid, dermatomyositis and systemic lupus erythematosus. It is given at a dose of 1–3 mg/kg/day, usually 50–100 mg bid. Before starting, check the thiopurine methyltransferase (TPMT) level (normal 25–50, carrier 10–25, deficiency <10 pmole/L/mg Hb), since if it is low, there is an increased risk of myelosuppression. It takes 6–8 weeks before there is any effect so it is no good as a first line treatment in patients with pemphigus and pemphigoid. The patient is often started on azathioprine as well as the steroids; after 6–8 weeks, when the azathioprine will have begun to work, the dose of steroid is gradually reduced.

Side effects:

- nausea, vomiting and diarrhoea, particularly in the elderly – if this is going to occur it usually does so in the first week; it may be so severe that the drug must be stopped
- bone marrow depression – a full blood count should be measured regularly (once a week for the first month and then every 2–3 months)
- teratogenicity – do not give to pregnant women; safe in men
- mild cholestasis – not usually a problem, unlike methotrexate
- long term (> 10 years) there an increased risk of lymphoma and non melanoma skin cancer especially squamous cell carcinoma.

Mycophenolate mofetil

Mycophenolate mofetil is a drug normally used to prevent rejection of organ transplants. It is used for treating recalcitrant eczema and autoimmune bullous conditions in conjunction with prednisolone, as well as for pyoderma gangrenosum. It takes about 8 weeks to work. The usual dose is 1.0 g bid (maximum 1.5 g bid).

Side effects are gastro-intestinal upsets (nausea, vomiting, diarrhoea), bone marrow suppression (check full blood count weekly for 1 month and then monthly) and an increased risk of infection, particularly in the elderly.

Cyclophosphamide

Cyclophosphamide is used in mucous membrane pemphigoid where it is the drug of first choice (*see* p. 146). It takes 6–8 weeks to work, given at a dose of 1–3 mg/kg/day (50–100 mg bid).

Side effects:
- pancytopenia – the patient should have a full blood count measured regularly (weekly for a month and then 2 monthly)
- hair loss
- haemorrhagic cystitis – drink plenty of fluids to prevent this.

Hydroxycarbamide (hydroxyurea)

This is an antimetabolite which inhibits DNA synthesis without affecting RNA or protein synthesis. It is used for psoriasis in patients who have not responded to methotrexate but it takes 8–12 weeks to work. It is given at a dose of 500 mg bid.

Side effects are mainly on the bone marrow. It causes a macrocytic anaemia or pancytopenia. Patients should have a full blood count measured regularly (once a week for the first month and then every 2 months).

Fumaric acid esters

The fumaric acid esters are used to treat psoriasis, and have been used and marketed for over 30 years in Germany. They have to be imported and used on a named patient basis, which makes them expensive. Fumarates are thought to work by shifting a Th1-type cytokine response to a Th2-type pattern (*see* p. 225). They comes in two strengths: initial (30 mg) and high strength (120 mg).

Side effects:
- gastro-intestinal complaints including diarrhoea, stomach cramps and tenesmus occur in up to 60% of patients
- flushing with headaches in 30% of patients; both are greatest at the onset of therapy and decrease with time
- lymphopenia seen in 75% of patients which is usually mild; transient eosinophilia is occasionally observed; liver enzymes are frequently raised (25% of patients); check full blood count and liver function monthly.

In about 7% of patients these side effects lead to drug withdrawal. This can be minimised by using a slow incremental dose regimen, which will delay the response to around 8–12 weeks.

There are no reports of severe long-term toxicity, development of cancers or a higher susceptibility to bacterial infections. This makes fumaric acid esters a safe regimen, compared to other agents. Dosing starts at 30 mg daily, increasing weekly to a maximum of 240 mg three times a day.

BIOLOGIC AGENTS

Toxic epidermal necrolysis

Human immunoglobulin from purified plasma of multiple donors has been available since the 1980s, and is given by slow intravenous infusion usually at 1 g/kg body weight for 3–4 days in severe cases of toxic epidermal necrosis, although its effectiveness is vigorously debated. It may cause hypersensitivity reactions, acute renal tubular necrosis and thromboembolic episodes (due to the volume infused and hydration status of the patient). The potential transmission of unknown infective agents is also of concern.

Psoriasis

Biologics are antibodies that target specific cells, mediators or molecules. Their number and uses are expanding rapidly, and are revolutionising the care of many medical conditions. Five new agents – efalizumab, etanercept, infliximab, adalimumab and ustekinumab – have been released in Europe and the United States for the treatment of severe psoriasis. However, the first, efalizumab, which inhibits T-cell activation, has already been withdrawn due to JC virus reactivation and subsequent progressive multifocal leukoencephalopathy (incidence 1 in 500).

Infliximab (Remicade), adalimumab (Humira) and etanercept (Enbrel), inhibit the cytokine TNF-α (tumour necrosis factor-α). **Infliximab** is a modified mouse monoclonal antibody and is given by intravenous infusion fortnightly (5 mg/kg) for 6 weeks and then every 8 weeks. It seems to have the most rapid onset of action. **Adalimumab** is a human monoclonal antibody and is better tolerated than infliximab. It is given on alternate weeks subcutaneously (40 mg). **Etanercept** is a receptor blocker to TNF-α and is also given subcutaneously (50 mg) weekly. **Ustekinumab** (Stelara), is directed against interleukin 12 and 23 (IL-12/23), and is given subcutaneously (45 mg) at 0, 4 and 12 weeks and then every 12 weeks.

They are very useful in severe cases of psoriasis unresponsive to immunosuppressives and seem to have a good side effect profile, not affecting either the liver or kidneys. Etanercept or adalimumab should be used first for stable plaque psoriasis; patients requiring rapid disease control may benefit from infliximab. In patients who fail to respond to one of these, another TNF-α antagonist should be tried next. As it is the newest antipsoriatic biologic with the shortest long-term safety data, ustekinumab should only be used when anti TNF-α therapy has failed or is contraindicated.

All these drugs lose efficacy over time probably due to the development of antibodies. Continuous treatment is recommended as infusion reactions may occur on retreatment. Efficacy can be enhanced by the addition of methotrexate, which may prevent the development of antibodies; this is an area of ongoing research. Additionally monoclonal antibodies to IL17 and small molecules (which have the benefit in being oral formulations) which inhibit enzymes such as phosphodiesterase 4 and the JAK/STAT pathway, are all approaching licensing for use in psoriasis.

Screening of patients with psoriasis before starting biologics

- Patient meets NICE criteria for use:
  — failure of topical and systemic therapy
  — PASI > 10, DLQI > 10 or involved body surface area >10%
- Tuberculosis screen – history, chest X-ray, Mantoux
- Baseline bloods – full blood count, liver function tests, urea and electrolytes, lupus autoantibodies
- History of cardiac disease, malignancy, demyelination
- Screening for hepatitis B and C antibodies

If there is no effect after 12–16 weeks, the drug should be stopped.

Complications

- Infection – especially reactivation of tuberculosis, but also other bacterial, viral and fungal infections
- Constitutional symptoms
- Injection site reaction
- Hepatitis (infliximab)
- Rarer possible side effects:
  i. deterioration of psoriasis (with acral and pustular pattern seen)
  ii. malignancy (lymphoma, non-melanoma skin cancers)
  iii. drug-induced lupus (usually subacute cutaneous lupus type) with possible anti-histone antibodies
  iv. aplastic anaemia, pancytopenia
  v. demyelination
  vi. cardiac – increase in ischaemic heart disease, arrhythmias, cardiomyopathy and heart failure.

For all these drugs, registration with BADBIR (the British Association of Dermatologists Biologic Interventions Register) is recommended for monitoring long-term safety and effectiveness.

Biologics for other conditions

Omalizumab (*Xolair*) is a recombinant human monoclonal antibody that binds to immunoglobulin E (IgE), so inhibiting IgE-FCRI receptors present on mast cells and basophils. It is licensed for severe asthma but can also be used for difficult cases of chronic urticaria.

Off licence the anti-CD20 (B-cell) molecule rituximab (MabThera) is used in severe bullous disorders and the anti-TNFs in pyoderma gangrenosum and hidradenitis suppurativa. Sometimes they work, sometimes they do not.

Biologics in skin cancer

- **Vismodegib**, an oral inhibitor of the 'hedgehog signalling pathway', has been licensed for inoperable basal cell carcinomas, as well as basal cell carcinomas occurring in Gorlin's syndrome (where huge numbers of disfiguring basal cell carcinomas can occur). It offers response rates of 30%–60%.
- **Vemurafenib and ipilimumab** have recently both been approved by NICE for clinical use in inoperable malignant melanoma. They are the first really promising treatments available for metastatic melanoma. They improve life expectancy and disease-free survival by months in many patients and years in some, but they are extremely expensive (£2000 a week).
- **Vemurafenib** is an oral inhibitor of mutant BRAF, a cell signalling defect found in around 50% of melanoma cases. Blocking this pathway prevents melanoma cell proliferation. Unfortunately escape pathways exist which accounts for its loss of efficacy over time. Blocking this pathway also selectively induces an alternate MEK pathway, which induces multiple keratoacanthomas and squamous cell carcinomas in treated patients. Photosensitivity and other skin rashes occasionally require a reduction in the dose. Trials of combination BRAF and MEK inhibitors are underway in an attempt to improve efficacy and reduce the cutaneous side effects.
- **Ipilimumab** as an infusion is useful in melanomas that do not have the BRAF mutation. It is a monoclonal antibody to CTLA-4, which dampens down the activity of cytotoxic T-cells. Blocking this increases the body's own immune response to melanoma. It is currently licensed for use after standard chemotherapy has failed. Ten per cent of patients are unable to tolerate it due to side effects on the gastro-intestinal tract, skin, eyes, liver and endocrine systems.

- **Nivolumab** blocks proteins in tumour cells that protect them from the immune system, which can then recognise and destroy such tumours (e.g. metastatic melanoma).

PHYSICAL TREATMENTS

CRYOTHERAPY WITH LIQUID NITROGEN

The indications for using cryotherapy are limited. It is not a treatment to be used on any skin lesion that you think is probably benign. Do not use it on dermal lesions (e.g. melanocytic naevi) and malignant lesions (except Bowen's disease).

It is essential to make an accurate diagnosis before treatment. If there is any doubt, do a biopsy first, as once a lesions has been frozen the histology is much more difficult to interpret. We would recommend that in general practice it is only used for treating viral warts, seborrhoeic warts and solar keratoses.

Freezing the skin produces changes similar to those caused by a burn:
- erythema
- a blister at the dermo-epidermal junction
- necrosis of the skin

} depending on how long you freeze for.

For most skin lesions for which freezing is an appropriate treatment (viral and seborrhoeic warts, solar keratoses) you will want to cause a blister at the dermo-epidermal junction so that the abnormal tissue (in the epidermis) is lifted off in the blister roof.

For pre-malignant lesions, necrosis of the abnormal cells is required. Cell death occurs at a skin temperature of −40°C. At this temperature ice crystals form within the cells and disrupt the cells as they are rewarmed. Maximum damage occurs if the skin is frozen rapidly and allowed to thaw slowly. The thaw time should be at least three times as long as the freezing time. Repeated freeze–thaw cycles are more effective than a single long freeze.

Table 2.09 Freeze times for various lesions treated with liquid nitrogen

Skin condition	Approximate freeze time
Viral warts	
filiform	5 seconds
common	10 seconds
periungual	15–20 seconds
genital	10–30 seconds (depends on size)
Molluscum contagiosum	5 seconds
Seborrhoeic warts	5–10 seconds
Solar keratoses	5–10 seconds
Bowen's disease	15 seconds × 2
Lentigo maligna	15–30 seconds × 2

Note: on lower legs cut the freeze time by half.

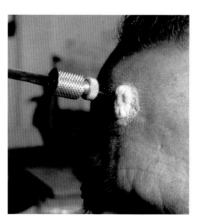

Fig. 2.08 Cryotherapy using a Cry-Ac spray gun

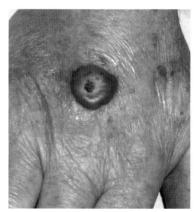

Fig. 2.09 Blister after cryotherapy to a solar keratosis

Freezing can most easily be done using a Cry-Ac or Cryo-Pro spray gun (*see* Fig. 2.08). This is a stainless steel insulated vacuum flask with a side arm and a spray tip. Different tips are available depending on the size of lesion to be frozen. Spray liquid nitrogen onto the middle of the lesion to be treated. A white ball of ice will form and gradually expand. Keep freezing until it is 2 mm outside the margin of the lesion you are treating. At that stage, stop freezing and give short, sharp squirts of liquid nitrogen to hold the ice ball at a constant size for the period of time given in Table 2.09. After a time you will become experienced at estimating the amount of freeze that is necessary for treating a particular type of lesion. Do not freeze over-enthusiastically at first, and *when freezing the lower legs, halve the freeze time recommended* in Table 2.09 (excessive freezing on the lower legs can lead to ulceration).

Cryotherapy with dimethyl ether/propane

Dimethyl ether/propane gas can be obtained in an aerosol can (Histofreezer or Wartner). The gas is discharged through a cotton bud or directly onto the skin and can freeze the skin to –50°C. This is a useful method of freezing if you only wish to freeze warts very occasionally. There are reports of patients self-treating what has turned out to be squamous cell carcinomas or melanoma (thought to be a viral wart or seborrhoeic keratosis).

IONTOPHORESIS

Iontophoresis involves passing a low electric current into the skin. Skin resistance is lower through the sweat ducts than the skin so the current passes preferentially down them. This is a useful treatment for **hyperhidrosis of the hands and feet** and with a new attachment for the axillae. It is available in most dermatology or physiotherapy departments, where the first course of treatment should be given. If this is beneficial, then mains and battery-operated units are commercially available from STD

Pharmaceutical (Plough Lane, Hereford HR4 0EL, England, tel. 01432 373555) or IontoCentre (Unit 19 Mahoney Green Ind Park, Green Lane West, Rackheath NR13 6JY, England, tel. 0800 472 5461) for treatment at home.

The hand or foot to be treated is placed in a container with only enough tap water to cover the palmar or plantar surface. A solution of an anticholinergic agent (0.05% glycopyrronium bromide in distilled water) works better but is expensive to make up. This is connected to the positive terminal of a DC unit producing up to 50 milliamps. The opposite foot or hand (not

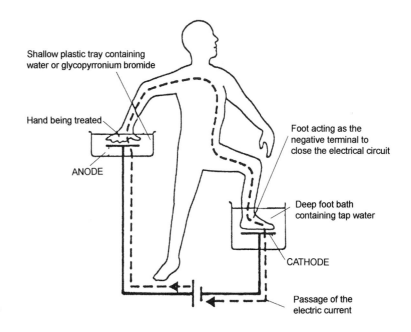

Shallow plastic tray containing water or glycopyrronium bromide

Hand being treated

ANODE

Foot acting as the negative terminal to close the electrical circuit

Deep foot bath containing tap water

CATHODE

Passage of the electric current

Fig. 2.10 Iontophoresis

being treated) is placed in a deep bath of tap water connected to the negative terminal (*see* Fig. 2.10). A current of 10 milliamps is given for 10 minutes three times (first week), two times (second week) and then weekly until the sweating stops. The current and time can be increased if the treatment is not effective, and pulsed current machines can allow greater currents to be used if required. The sweating will gradually return after weeks to months, when the treatment can be repeated. Treatment response tends to be variable; not all patients respond well.

ULTRAVIOLET LIGHT

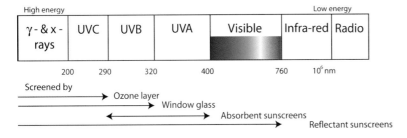

Fig. 2.11 The electromagnetic spectrum

Many skin diseases improve in the summer and particularly on sun exposure. For some of these, treatment with artificial ultraviolet light can be beneficial. The light is produced by banks of fluorescent lamps in stand-up booths (*see* Fig. 2.12) or lie-down units. The lamps (whether UVB or UVA) must be of sufficient intensity (watts = joules/sec) to deliver a therapeutic dose (joules/cm^2) within a short period of time and it must also be possible to measure accurately the dose given.

UVC radiation (200–290 nm), UVC from the sun is filtered out by the ozone in the atmosphere. It is not used therapeutically.

UVB radiation (290–320 nm) is responsible for tanning and sunburn. UVB is present in sunlight but is filtered out by window glass. For treating psoriasis UVB (especially at 311–313 nm) works much better than UVA. As a treatment UVB is given either by tubes emitting the whole UVB spectrum (broadband UVB) or by special TL01 tubes emitting at 311–313 nm (narrowband UVB). Narrowband UVB is theoretically safer than broadband UVB because it is less carcinogenic and more effective for psoriasis. Narrowband UVB is given three times a week and is the ultraviolet light treatment of choice in psoriasis. Pregnant women can have UVB but not PUVA. Medical UV light sources can be purchased on-line. This is not recommended until the patient has undergone supervised treatment through a dermatology department. They are obtained from skinmattersbristol.com or androv-medical.com.

Although **tar** has traditionally been used in conjunction with UVB the reason for its apparent benefit is not clear. It has been assumed that the phototoxic agents in tar potentiate the effect of the radiation. In practice, if erythemogenic doses of UVB are used, there is no evidence that the topical application of tar is any better than using a simple lubricant (e.g. white soft paraffin). If a suberythema dose of UVB is used, tar is helpful.

UVA radiation (320–400 nm) is ineffective on its own. Sunbeds bought commercially produce mainly UVA, although a low dose of UVB also is emitted, which probably produces the tan. Addition of a psoralen followed by UVA (**PUVA therapy**) has been found to be an effective treatment for several conditions (*see* Table 2.10).

PUVA therapy (P = psoralen + UVA)

Psoralens are three-ringed compounds that can cross link DNA (through thymidine or cytosine in one chain of the double helix and pyrimidine in the other) in the presence of UVA light. The cross linking of DNA chains prevents cell division which is how it works in psoriasis. There may also be an effect on the immune system and increased production of melanin.

Either 8-methoxypsoralen (8-MOP) or 5-methoxypsoralen (5-MOP) can be used. Maximum photosensitivity occurs 2–3 hours after ingestion and exposure to the UVA is timed to coincide with this. UVA penetrates further into the dermis than UVB, and combined with the psoralen is more effective. The psoralen is taken 2 hours before irradiation at a dose dependent on weight (8-MOP tablets – 0.6 mg/kg body weight; 5-MOP tablets – 1.2 mg/kg body weight). Alternatively the 8-MOP can be put in a bath and the patient soaks in the solution for 15 minutes immediately before UVA exposure (bath PUVA), or applied directly to the skin as a gel (usually for hands and feet). Treatment is given twice weekly for 6–12 weeks until the skin is clear.

Determining the patient's sensitivity to UVB or PUVA

The dose of UVA or UVB is worked out in terms of light energy (joules/cm^2), and depending on the output of the machine (measured by an internal ultraviolet light meter), the time of exposure is calculated. The reaction on the patient's skin induced by PUVA or UVB is a phototoxic one, i.e. erythema, oedema and as a maximum response, blistering. The erythema caused by PUVA differs from that produced by UVB in that it appears later, lasts longer and is more intense. It does not peak until 48–72 hours (and sometimes not until 96 hours). The aim of UVB or PUVA therapy is to deliver to the patient as much ultraviolet light as possible without producing more than a barely perceptible erythema,

the **minimal erythematous dose** (MED). The MED for UVB or the **minimal phototoxic dose** (MPD) for PUVA are measured by applying a template with a number of 1 cm^2 cut-outs to the patient's skin (*see* Fig. 2.13) and irradiating them with increasing doses of ultraviolet light (the rest of the patient's skin being completely covered up). This is done in the same treatment booth that will be used for the treatment. For PUVA it is done 2 hours after the ingestion of 8-MOP. The tests are read at 72 hours and a barely perceptible erythema is the end point that you are looking for. The dose of ultraviolet light (joules/cm^2) needed to produce this amount of erythema is the MED or MPD. The starting dose for treatment is 75% of the MED/MPD. Each dose is increased by 25% of the previous dose given until the disease is clear. Alternatively, the starting dose can be assessed according to skin type (*see* p. 3).

It is recommended that the lifetime exposure to PUVA should be limited to 1000 joules/cm^2 or 200 treatments to reduce the long-term risk of skin cancer. No limit has been established as yet for narrowband UVB, although every effort is made to keep the amount of radiation to a minimum.

In an ultraviolet light machine the patient must protect his eyes against damage from ultraviolet light during and with PUVA for 24 hours after the treatment by wearing glasses that filter out both UVB and UVA.

RePUVA therapy

Some patients with psoriasis who do not respond to either PUVA or oral retinoids (*see* p. 49) will respond when they are given together. The retinoid (acitretin 20–50 mg/day) is started 2 weeks before the PUVA therapy. Then both are continued together (the retinoid taken daily, the PUVA given twice a week) until the skin is clear. The PUVA can then be stopped and the retinoid continued long term.

Table 2.10 Diseases that may respond to ultraviolet light treatment

UVB	PUVA
Psoriasis	Psoriasis
Atopic eczema	Severe atopic eczema
Chronic superficial scaly dermatosis	Mycosis fungoides
Acne	Polymorphic light eruption
Pityriasis lichenoides chronica	Pityriasis lichenoides acuta
The itching of AIDS	Urticaria pigmentosum
Vitiligo – in conjunction with a topical steroid	Vitiligo especially in dark-skinned individuals
The itching of chronic renal failure	Alopecia areata

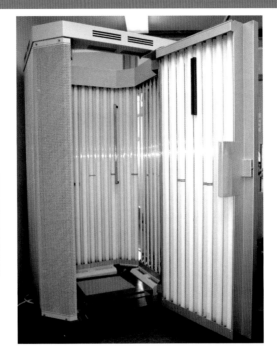

Fig. 2.12 Ultraviolet machine

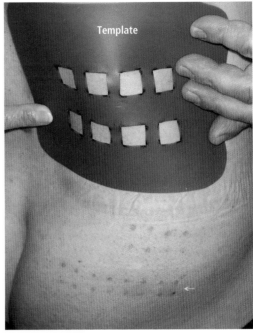

Fig. 2.13 Determining the MED. The MED is where the erythema just fills the square seen on the right of the bottom line (arrowed)

Short-term side effects of PUVA

- Nausea: this can be prevented by taking the 8-MOP tablets with food or a glass of milk. Occasionally an antiemetic is required; we usually give 10 mg metoclopramide hydrochloride (Maxolon) at the same time as the 8-MOP.
- Dryness and itching of the skin: this is very common and may need an antihistamine such as chlorphenamine 4–8 mg given

with the 8-MOP. Rarely severe persistent itching makes the patient stop treatment. It can persist for several days or even weeks after treatment.

- Erythema and tenderness: a few patients will get excessive erythema, oedema and tenderness of the skin 48–72 hours after treatment. This is the main reason why treatment is only given twice a week. If the patient gets burnt, the dose of irradiation is reduced for the next treatment. All patients are at risk of developing a phototoxic reaction after PUVA and should avoid direct sunlight for 8 hours after treatment by using a sunscreen that blocks out both UVB and UVA.

- PUVA pain: severe skin pain is unusual but when it occurs treatment needs to be stopped. It can sometimes persist for several weeks after treatment is stopped.

Long-term side effects of PUVA

- Cataracts: the eyes are protected during treatment and for 24 hours afterwards by wearing sunglasses to prevent cataract formation.
- Skin cancer: there is an acceleration of the ageing process in the skin of patients who have been treated with PUVA and an increase in the incidence of basal and squamous cell carcinomas in the skin after 5–10 years. There have also been some reports of malignant melanoma occurring.
- Men must shield the genitalia during treatment because there is an increased risk of squamous cell carcinoma of the penis.

PHOTODYNAMIC THERAPY

Photodynamic therapy (PDT) is a treatment for pre-malignant lesions (solar keratoses and Bowen's disease) and non-melanoma skin cancers (superficial basal cell carcinomas). Off-licence benefits have also been reported in the acantholytic dermatoses, Hailey–Hailey disease and Darier's disease: treatment during a mildly inflammatory phase seems most beneficial.

A photosensitising chemical, 5-amino-levulinic acid (ALA), is converted to protoporphyrin-9 when irradiated with red light (630 nm). The porphyrin accumulates in the abnormal cells and in the presence of oxygen releases singlet oxygen, which causes cell death. Topical ALA is available as the methyl ester (methyl aminolevulinate, Metvix cream) or the acid (Levulan[USA only]). The methyl ester has the advantage of being taken up preferentially into neoplastic cells (due to their defective stratum corneum).

Lesions to be treated have any scale or crust removed from the surface with saline, forceps or a curette. The Metvix cream is applied to the affected skin in a 1 mm thick layer, covered with a non-adherent dressing and left in place for 3 hours. After this it is removed and the area irradiated with red light (Aktilite produces a continuous spectrum 570–670 nm for

8 minutes at 37 j/cm²). The patient feels a burning sensation, which may last for a few hours. The site is retreated a second time after 7 days.

The affected skin becomes inflamed, crusts after about a week, and heals within 4 weeks. Oedema, pain or redness can occur. Itching, ulceration, infection or pigmentary changes are less likely. In general PDT works very well on the scalp and face, but less well on the limbs. Patients for PDT should be referred to a dermatology department who have a lamp emitting the correct spectrum of light.

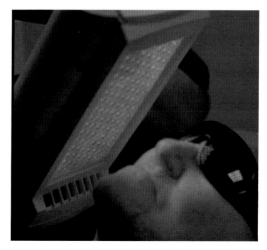

Fig. 2.14 Photodynamic therapy with red light to lesion on face

LASERS

Laser is an acronym for **L**ight **A**mplification by **S**timulated **E**mission of **R**adiation. It is a device that produces coherent, collimated, monochromatic (single wavelength) light: an intense beam of pure monochromatic light that does not diverge (collimated) and in which all the light waves are of the same polarity and travel in step in the same direction (coherent).

How lasers work

Various gases, liquids and solids (laser medium) will emit light when they are suitably stimulated or pumped (excitation source). In a typical gas laser (CO_2 or argon), the gas is contained in a lasing tube that has a fully reflective mirror at one end and a partially reflective mirror at the opposite end (*see* Fig. 2.15). The laser medium is stimulated by means of a high voltage electric current. A stimulated molecule of the gas emits a photon (a light particle), which strikes another stimulated molecule causing it to emit an identical photon (amplification). Emission of photons occurs in all directions but the light waves become aligned by resonance between the mirrors at either end of the laser tube, and the coherent light exits through the partially reflective mirror at one end. The type of gas, liquid or solid in the lasing tube determines the wavelength of the coherent light that is produced.

The objective for any medical laser treatment is to restrict laser-induced injury only to selected sites such as blood vessels or pigment cells with minimal damage to the surrounding adjacent tissues. This effect is called **selective photothermolysis**.

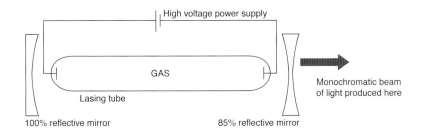

Fig. 2.15 How a gas laser works

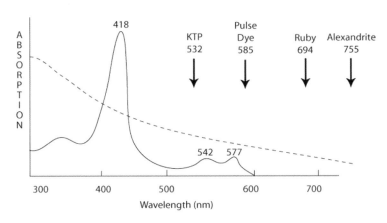

Fig. 2.16 Absorption spectrum of haemoglobin (solid line) and melanin (hatched line)

It is achieved if the laser fulfils three requirements.

1. The laser light emission is at the same wavelength that the target absorbs, e.g. for haemoglobin at 542 or 577 nm (*see* Fig. 2.16).
2. The laser emits sufficient energy to damage the target tissue.
3. The duration of exposure of the tissue is short enough to limit damage mainly to the target without excess heat diffusing outwards and damaging the surrounding tissues. This is determined by the **thermal relaxation time** of the surrounding tissue, which is how long it takes for the target to dissipate half its thermal energy. For a blood vessel in a port wine stain this is 1–10 milliseconds, while for tattoo pigment it is only 1–10 nanoseconds (10^{-9}). The pulse duration of the lasers treating these targets must be of these magnitudes.

The **penetration into the skin** is determined by the wavelength of the light (up to 2000 nm). Longer wavelengths penetrate deeper but tend to have less energy. For hair removal, the laser must penetrate to the root of the hair follicle. The Alexandrite laser with a longer wavelength (755 nm) will be able to reach the dermal papilla at the depth of a follicle (1 mm) with more energy than the Ruby (694 nm). For port wine stains the highest peak of haemoglobin absorption at 418 nm is no good, as light of this wavelength will not penetrate very far. The light of the pulsed dye laser at 585 nm provides a compromise between penetration and energy absorption by haemoglobin.

There are **several groups of skin lasers** (*see* Table 2.11) depending on the target tissue.

- **Vascular lasers** target haemoglobin. Wavelengths selected are around the 577 nm absorption peak (*see* Fig. 2.16) to ensure

adequate penetration. Pulse duration is selected depending on the diameter of the vessel being treated. If it is too long scarring may result; if it is too short it causes purpura without destroying the vessel. The 'V'-beam modification to the pulsed dye laser results in a longer pulse with more energy into the blood vessels. This is meant to produce uniform damage to the vessels and less purpura.

- **Resurfacing or cutting lasers** target the water in the skin using infrared radiation. A short pulse duration and high energy results in vaporisation of tissue with minimal damage to underlying structures (**ablative lasers**). Healing comes from re-epithelisation from hair follicles like a burn. Healing takes about 2 weeks with considerable post-operative pain, redness and swelling. Possible problems include scarring, secondary infection with herpes simplex or bacteria. Redness and tenderness can last several months. About 75% improvement can be expected with a CO_2 laser. The systems used are the CO_2 laser and the Erbium-YAG lasers. The CO_2 laser penetrates into the dermis. The Erbium is more superficial, penetrating only into the epidermis and resulting in less tissue damage, faster healing and fewer side effects; however, it is also less effective.

- **Fractional resurfacing lasers** punch very fine holes into the epidermis and dermis but leave the intervening skin undamaged. This results in faster healing times with less tissue damage. The idea is to promote epidermal and collagen regeneration with less patient morbidity. Four to five treatments are needed at monthly intervals. The improvement of wrinkles is not as good as with conventional resurfacing lasers. The systems used are the CO_2 and Erbium-YAG lasers. Some systems use a combination of these lasers, while others use only a CO_2 laser.

Table 2.11 Types of dermatological laser

Type of laser	λ nm	Pulse time	Function	Comments
Vascular lasers				
Pulsed dye (PDL)	585 (yellow)	0.45 msec	Port wine stain (capillary malformation)	Recommended – causes bruising that lasts 2 weeks; large spot size good for larger lesions, multiple treatments required (*see* p. 127)
	595	1.5 msec	Telangiectasia Spider naevi	Visible lesions on face; no good for erythema
KTP	532 (green)	2–10 msec	Telangiectasia (Port wine stains)	Does not cause bruising, so good for cosmetic lesions; use if PDL not effective, since the longer pulse duration is better for larger vessels
Copper bromide	578 (yellow) 510 (green)	10–50 msec	Telangiectasia, Spider neavi Lentigines and freckles	Small spot size useful for small lesions, impractical for large lesions such as port wine stains
IPL (intense pulsed light)	560 filter		Erythema and telangiectasia of rosacea	Around 50% improvement after four treatments at 3-weekly intervals (*Br J Dermatol.* 2008;**159**: 628–3)
Resurfacing or cutting lasers				
Ablative Carbon dioxide (CO_2)	10 600 (infrared)	10–20 msec	Resurfacing actinic damage and scarring (acne, trauma)	Ablative = tissue vapourisation Thermal damage up to 100 µm deep, which stimulates collagen and elastic tissue regeneration
Erbium-YAG	2940 (infrared)	200–400 msec	Resurfacing and removal of epidermal lesions	Thermal damage only 10 µm deep – no deep damage; quicker recovery time but less effective for marked scarring
Fractional lasers Erbium-YAG Carbon dioxide	2940 10 600	60 nsec	Wrinkles and facial lines	Punch micro-sized holes with normal skin intervening – quicker recovery, less damage but less effective than full ablative lasers; better on neck, chest, hands; CO_2 penetrates deep, Erbium-YAG superficial
Non-ablative Pulsed dye Nd:YAG IPL (intense pulsed light)	1320 1064 550	50 msec	Correction of facial lines and wrinkles	Non-ablative Dermal collagen targeted, epidermis undamaged; low risk with little post-operative effects. Less effective, multiple treatments required; needs skin cooling device to prevent epidermal damage and pain IPL not good for pigmented skin, as light absorbed by melanin

Type of laser	λ nm	Pulse time	Function	Comments
Pigment lasers				
Nd:YAG	532	6 nsec (Q-switched)	Lentigines and freckles	Good response – short wavelength for surface lesions
	1064		Café au lait patches and Becker's naevus	Variable to poor response
			Naevus of Ota/Ito	Variable response – longer wavelength for deeper lesions
Tattoo removal				
Nd:YAG	1064	6 nsec (Q-switched)	Blue-black tattoos	Useful laser as two options in one machine (1064 and 532 nm)
	532		Red, orange, yellow tattoos	Preferred option due to fast repetition rate (10 Hz = shots/sec)
Ruby	694	25–40 nsec	Blue-black, green tattoos	Slower repetition rate (1 Hz), mainly useful for green, more painful
Hair removal				
Alexandrite	755	2–20 msec	Hair needs to be dark but patient's skin type I or II	Preferred laser since penetrates deeper than Ruby
Ruby	694 (red)	270 μsec		Slow repetition rate (1 Hz) = long treatment times
Nd:YAG	1064	50 msec	Skin types IV–VI	Deeper penetration, very painful, better for darker skin types
IPL	700–750		Hair needs to be dark but patient's skin type I or II	Not true coherent laser light; filters used to produce narrow wavelength bands; less effective than true laser
Phototherapy				
Excimer (XeCl)	308 (UVA)	120 nsec	Psoriasis, vitiligo	Same wavelength as ultraviolet light for phototherapy

- **Non-ablative lasers** target the dermis leaving the epidermis unaffected. They are meant to stimulate new collagen formation. They are much safer and provide a rapid recovery time, but are not as effective as the ablative lasers. The systems used are the Nd:YAG, pulsed dye lasers and intense pulsed light (IPL).

- **Pigment lasers** target melanin and tattoo pigment. Between 650 and 1100 nm there is good penetration and preferred absorption by melanin compared with haemoglobin. Tattoo ink will also absorb laser light at a specified wavelength. Very short pulse widths, which are generated by 'Q-switching' produces a shock wave within the pigment which shatters the pigment granule into sufficiently small particles that can be absorbed and removed by macrophages. Hair removal targets melanin also but longer pulse widths and longer wavelengths are needed to reach and damage the follicle.

● **IPL** is a technology used by both the cosmetic industry and medical practitioners to perform various skin treatments including hair removal and photo-rejuvenation. IPL devices are non-laser high-intensity light sources that make use of a high-output flash lamp to produce a broad wavelength output of non-coherent light, usually in the 500–1200 nm range. A range of filters can be used to deliver more specific narrow bands of wavelengths. Modern devices can be used safely and effectively for the cosmetic treatment of many vascular lesions, unwanted hair and pigmented lesions. Newer technologies may give results equal to those of laser treatments. IPL has been shown to be particularly useful for the treatment of telangiectatic erythema of rosacea.

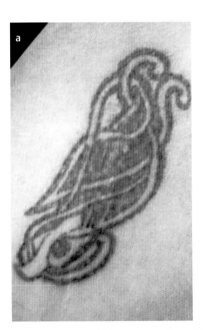 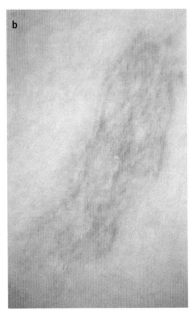

Fig. 2.17 Tattoo: (a) before Q-switched Nd:YAG laser treatment; (b) after five treatments: note 'ghosting' – some pigment still present

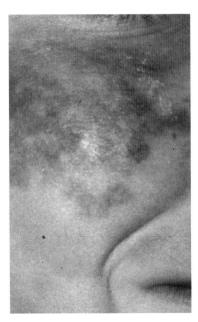

Fig. 2.18 Bruising from the pulsed dye laser on a capillary malformation (port wine stain)

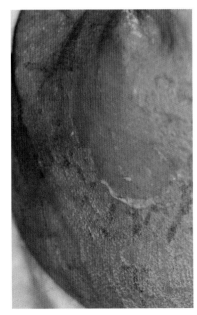

Fig. 2.19 Dermabrasion of the face using a carbon dioxide laser

Hair and hairy scalp

(For bald scalp *see* Chapters 5 and 9)

3

HAIR PHYSIOLOGY
WHAT IS HAIR?

Hair is a modified type of keratin produced by the hair matrix (equivalent to epidermis). On the scalp, apart from its social and cosmetic function, hair protects the underlying skin from sun damage.

Three types of hair occur in humans.
1. Lanugo hair is the soft, silky hair that covers the foetus in utero. It is usually shed before birth.
2. Vellus hair is the short, fine, unpigmented hair that covers the whole skin surface apart from palms and soles.
3. Terminal hair is longer, coarser and pigmented. Before puberty, terminal hair is restricted to the scalp, eyebrows and eyelashes. After puberty, secondary terminal hair develops in response to androgens in the axillae, pubic area and on the front of the chest in men.

HAIR CYCLE

There are between 100 000 and 150 000 hairs on the scalp. The hair cycle (*see* Fig. 3.02) occurs randomly in each follicle over the scalp so that up to 100 hairs are being lost daily, but in normal circumstances moulting does not occur.

The three phases of the hair cycle are:
1. **anagen** (80%–90% of hairs) – this is the growing phase and on the scalp lasts 2–6 years
2. **catagen** – the hair matrix cells stop dividing and hair growth stops; it lasts about 2 weeks
3. **telogen** (10%–20%) – this is the resting phase; the hair shaft moves up in the dermis; it lasts 3 months and at the end of that time the hair is shed.

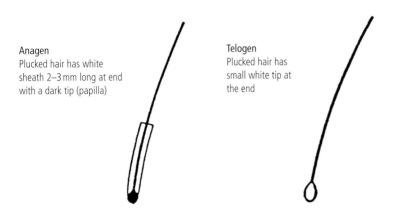

Anagen
Plucked hair has white sheath 2–3 mm long at end with a dark tip (papilla)

Telogen
Plucked hair has small white tip at the end

Fig. 3.01 How to tell the difference between plucked anagen and telogen hairs

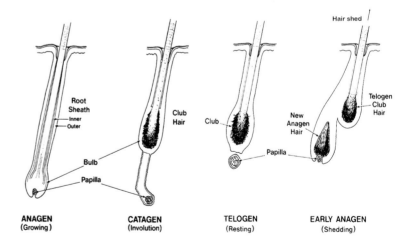

Fig. 3.02 The hair cycle

EXCESS HAIR

Hair in the wrong place or hair that is coarser or longer than is socially acceptable is regarded as excessive. There are two different patterns, hirsutism and hypertrichosis.

HIRSUTISM

Coarse terminal hair in the moustache or beard area for women and on the chest or lower abdomen in the normal pattern for men is known as hirsutism. It is extremely common, the amount of hair being genetically determined. How much facial and body hair is cosmetically acceptable in an individual is dependent on many factors, but particularly the patient's cultural and social background. What is considered normal in many parts of Southern Europe is deemed unacceptable in the United Kingdom or the United States.

The amount of hair on the face, breasts and lower abdomen in women is under androgen control. Testosterone produced by the ovary is converted to dihydrotestosterone in the skin by the action of 5α-reductase and it is this that causes the increase in hair. If the periods are abnormal in any way it is always worth checking the serum testosterone level. If it is more than twice the upper limit of normal, the patient should be referred to an endocrinologist for a full endocrine work-up to exclude a testosterone-secreting tumour. Many such patients have polycystic ovary syndrome with infertility, irregular periods, acne (70%), as well as hirsutism (90%). They are frequently obese with insulin resistance, raised lipids and hypertension (metabolic syndrome). This does not require any specific treatment unless associated with diabetes or ischaemic heart disease.

TREATMENT: HIRSUTISM

By the time the patient seeks help from the doctor she will usually have tried all the simple things that do not require medical advice. If she has not, the following options are available and may be helpful.

- **Bleaching the hairs**. There are a number of bleaching agents available commercially. For patients with very dark hairs, bleaching will often disguise them enough to be acceptable.
- **Depilatory creams**. The common active ingredients are calcium thioglycolate or potasium thioglycolate, which break down the disulfide bonds in keratin and weaken the hair so that it is easily scraped off where it emerges from the hair follicle. In some patients these creams will make the skin sore by a direct irritant effect; they can also cause a contact allergic dermatitis and folliculitis, which will limit their usefulness.
- **Waxing and sugaring**. These are basically methods of mass plucking of hairs. Hot wax or a thick sugar solution is applied to the hairy area of skin; it is allowed to cool and is then peeled off, pulling the hairs out at the same time. Both methods are available from reputable beauticians. This method is suitable for removal of excess hair from the legs and body as well as the face.

(cont.)

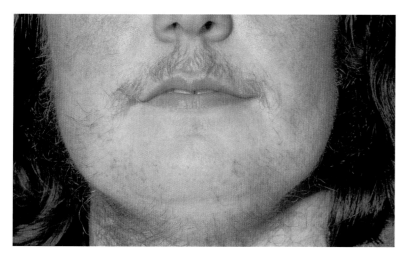

Fig. 3.03 Hirsutism

- **Threading** is another effective method of hair removal also available from some salons.
- **Plucking and shaving**. A surprising number of women still remove unwanted hair by plucking and shaving. Most do not like doing it but have found that other methods make their skin too sore. This does not lead to increased hair growth or thickening of the hair shaft – the cut hair shaft just looks thicker.
- **Electrolysis**. If the amount of unwanted hair is not too extensive, electrolysis and epilation using a short-wave diathermy machine can provide a permanent answer. A fine sterile needle is placed into the hair follicle down to the level of the papilla. A high-frequency alternating current is then passed through the needle for a microsecond. This destroys the papilla permanently and the hair is lifted out without pain. This process works well but is rather time-consuming and expensive. Practitioners should be members of the British Institute and Association of Electrolysis. Side effects may include pain, scarring and pigmentary changes.
- **Lasers** are an effective method of removing hair. The light is absorbed by melanin in the hair shaft and the heat generated damages the follicle. The treatment works best on dark hair in a fair-skinned individual. Dark-skinned patients are at risk of developing hyperpigmentation after treatment. The best laser for hair removal is the Alexandrite (at 755 nm). Tanning should be avoided while undergoing treatment. Intense pulse light is also an effective means of hair removal and works in a similar way to lasers. Shaving is the only method of hair removal permitted while undergoing treatment. Several treatments are necessary, as only follicles in anagen (growth phase) respond. The hair loss is not permanent but a 60% reduction in hair density is seen after about six treatments spread over a year. Twice-yearly 'top-up' treatments will maintain things.
- **Eflornithine** (Vaniqa) cream is an ornithine decarboxylase inhibitor that reduces hair growth over a 2- to 4-month period. It is useful alone or before laser treatment.
- **Anti-androgens** Yasmin or Dianette (co-cyprindiol – contains cyproterone acetate) can be tried in general practice, but risks for thromboembolism need to be assessed. Spironolactone can also be helpful in reducing excess hair.

HYPERTRICHOSIS

Hypertrichosis is excessive hair all over the body. Either the foetal lanugo hair is not lost before birth or it regrows at some later stage. When confined to the lumbosacral area (fawn tail) it may be a marker of an underlying spina bifida.

Some drugs cause hypertrichosis in all patients to a greater or lesser degree:
- ciclosporin
- diazoxide
- minoxidil.

The following drugs occasionally cause hypertrichosis:
- diphenylhydantoin
- minocycline
- penicillamine
- psoralens.

TREATMENT: HYPERTRICHOSIS

There is no good treatment for hypertrichosis. If it is due to a drug and it is possible to stop the drug, the hypertrichosis will be reversible, although it may take up to a year for the hairiness to disappear.

For other methods of hair removal *see* hirsutism.

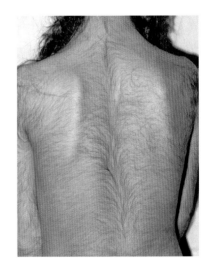

Fig. 3.04 Hypertrichosis

HAIR LOSS

Hairy scalp
Discrete bald patches
Without scarring

BALD PATCHES WITHOUT OBVIOUS SCARRING

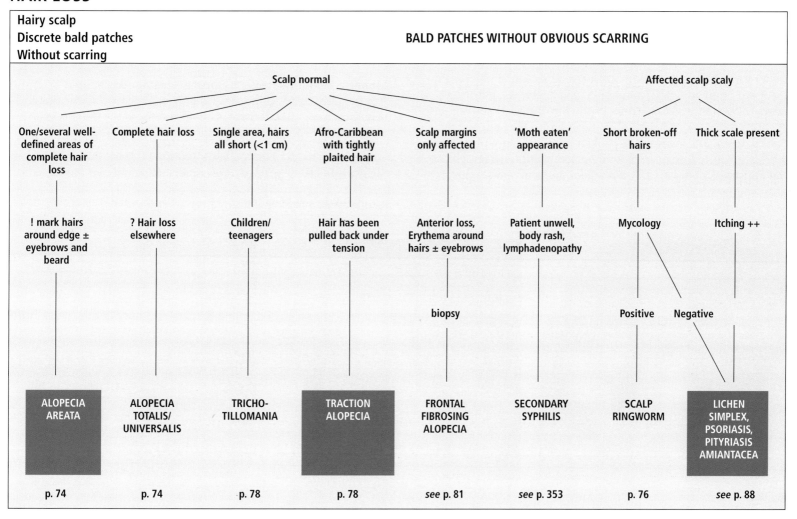

Scalp normal

Affected scalp scaly

| One/several well-defined areas of complete hair loss | Complete hair loss | Single area, hairs all short (<1 cm) | Afro-Caribbean with tightly plaited hair | Scalp margins only affected | 'Moth eaten' appearance | Short broken-off hairs | Thick scale present |

! mark hairs around edge ± eyebrows and beard

? Hair loss elsewhere

Children/ teenagers

Hair has been pulled back under tension

Anterior loss, Erythema around hairs ± eyebrows

Patient unwell, body rash, lymphadenopathy

Mycology

Itching ++

biopsy

Positive   Negative

| **ALOPECIA AREATA** | **ALOPECIA TOTALIS/ UNIVERSALIS** | **TRICHO-TILLOMANIA** | **TRACTION ALOPECIA** | **FRONTAL FIBROSING ALOPECIA** | **SECONDARY SYPHILIS** | **SCALP RINGWORM** | **LICHEN SIMPLEX, PSORIASIS, PITYRIASIS AMIANTACEA** |

p. 74   p. 74   p. 78   p. 78   see p. 81   see p. 353   p. 76   see p. 88

ALOPECIA AREATA

Alopecia areata is the commonest cause of discrete hair loss in both children and adults. The trigger is often a stressful event and alopecia areata itself is often very distressing, especially if it affects a large area. There is no redness or scaling of the underlying scalp. There may be one or several bald patches on the scalp or on any other hairy area (e.g. eyebrows, eyelashes, beard). The hair loss is sudden. While the disease is active, exclamation mark (!) hairs will be seen around the edge of the bald patches. These are short, broken-off hairs. Only pigmented hairs are affected, so normal white or grey hairs will remain in the middle of a bald area. It can take months or years to grow back and new patches may develop.

It will usually regrow white or blonde initially, but it goes back to its original colour after 6–8 weeks. Five per cent of individuals affected will have total scalp hair loss, **alopecia totalis**, and 1% will have **alopecia univeralis**, total loss of both scalp and body hair.

Alopecia incognito (diffuse alopecia areata) causes rapid diffuse thinning of scalp hair and may be confused with telogen effluvium (*see* p. 84). If there is any doubt as to the diagnosis, a scalp biopsy is helpful to distinguish between the two.

Alopecia areata is a common autoimmune disease and spans all ages and ethnic groups. It is worth asking about a family history of autoimmune disease and checking blood sugar and autoimmune profile including thyroid antibodies.

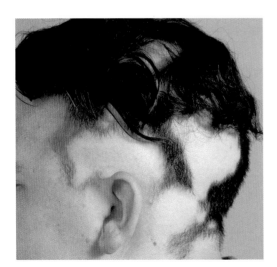

Fig. 3.05 Alopecia areata: discrete bald patches with no evidence of erythema or scaling

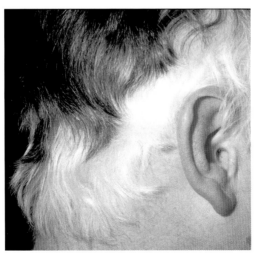

Fig. 3.06 Alopecia areata: regrowth of white hair – this will repigment in due course

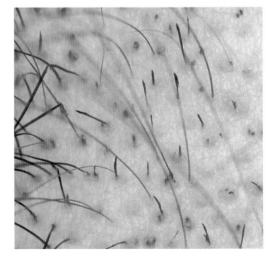

Fig. 3.07 Alopecia areata: ! hairs at edge of bald patch

TREATMENT: ALOPECIA AREATA

Discuss with the patient that hair may take many months to grow back and that there is a risk it may not grow back at all. This is more likely if the hair loss is extensive or occurs in an ophiasis pattern (margin of scalp). Warn the patient that the hair may regrow white or blonde until it is about 1.5 cm long, but that it will go back to its normal colour.

A **wig** may be needed temporarily if the hair loss is extensive.

Treatment currently available is unsatisfactory but includes the following options.

- **Topical steroid**: 0.5% clobetasol proprionate (Dermovate) applied twice daily (not to the face).
- **Intralesional injection of triamcinolone** (10 mg/mL): this is a suitable and often effective treatment for limited areas of hair loss. Side effects include skin atrophy, which is usually temporary, and it may cause hypopigmentation in individuals with darker skin types.
- **Topical minoxidil** (Regaine) lotion or foam. The 5% formulation is unlicensed in women but is likely to be more effective than the 2% preparation. It is expensive but cheaper generics may be found online. It is rubbed into the affected area twice a day. Any hair growth induced will fall out if the treatment is discontinued. Oral minoxidil 2.5 mg is an alternative but there is a risk of downy facial hair growth in women.
- **Topical prostaglandins**: Latisse (0.3% bimatoprost) is available online and may be used to improve eyelash and eyebrow growth.
- **Application of potent skin sensitisers to the bald areas**: Diphencyprone is the drug most commonly used. It is most effective in those whose hair loss has been present for less than 1 year. The scalp skin is sensitised by painting a 2% lotion to the upper inner arm, which becomes eczematised over 2 weeks. The whole scalp is then painted with a diluted solution of the lowest concentration (0.001%–0.1%), which will produce mild erythema. If it works, it is painted on the bald areas once a week until regrowth of hair is well established. Diphencyprone is degraded by light so patients have to keep their heads covered for 24 hours after treatment. Any hair growth may be lost if treatment is stopped, so maintenance is usually required.
- **Oral steroids (e.g. prednisolone 30–40 mg/day)** are effective in a proportion of cases, but over half of those who respond will relapse when the dose is reduced or stopped. There is no standard regimen but treatment should be for a minimum of

12–16 weeks and should be reserved for individuals who have had hair loss within the last year. Potential side effects should be discussed with patients before starting treatment. Continued use of systemic steroids is not justified for alopecia areata because of long-term complications (*see* p. 51).

- Azathioprine may be trialled in steroid-responsive patients (*see* p. 54). Future treatments include abatacept, a drug available for the treatment of rheumatoid arthritis. It inhibits co-stimulation of T-cells. It is currently being trialled in the United States for alopecia totalis and alopecia universalis.

Referral to a clinical psychologist can play an important role in helping patients come to terms with their hair loss.

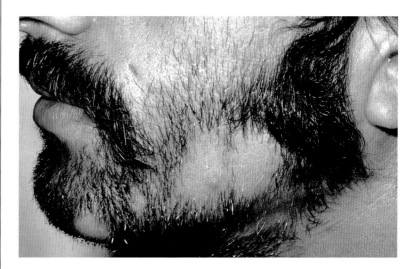

Fig. 3.08 Alopecia areata: bald patches in the beard area

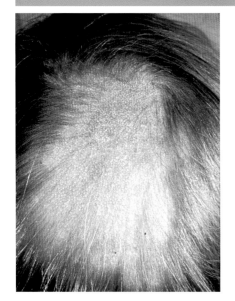

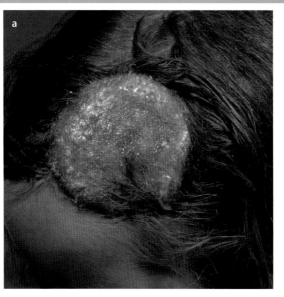

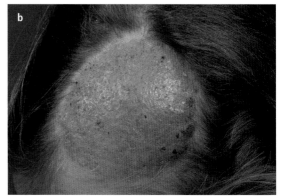

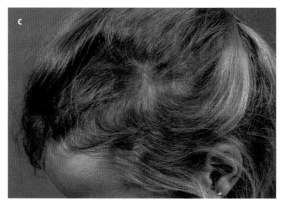

Fig. 3.09 Scalp ringworm: discrete bald patch with scaly surface

Fig. 3.10 Kerion in a 10-year-old child: (a) a red, boggy swelling due to animal ringworm, (b) after treatment and (c) with regrowth of hair

SCALP RINGWORM (TINEA CAPITIS)

Scalp ringworm only occurs in children; it is not a cause of hair loss in adults except those with HIV/AIDS. It is often due to *Trichophyton tonsurans* (caught from other children) or *Microsporum canis* (caught from kittens or puppies). Discrete bald areas occur with short, broken-off hairs in which the underlying skin is scaly and/or red. If the skin is red or if there is associated ringworm on the face or neck, it is more likely to be due to animal ringworm. There will be a history of other children with similar hair loss (in human ringworm), or a new kitten or puppy whose fur is falling out (in animal ringworm). The diagnosis is confirmed by pulling out the short, broken hairs, and sending them for mycology. Scalp ringworm due to *M. canis* fluoresces green under the Wood's light (*see* Fig. 3.12). *T. tonsurans* does not fluoresce.

Animal ringworm of the scalp (due to *M. canis*) can sometimes produce a red, boggy swelling discharging pus; this is called a **kerion** (*see* Fig. 3.10a).

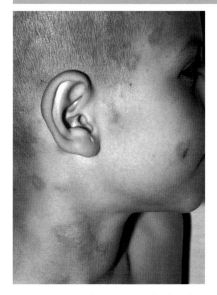

Fig. 3.11 Animal ringworm: child with lesions in scalp and on face and neck

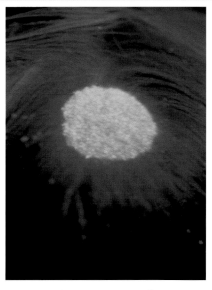

Fig. 3.12 Tinea capitis: green fluorescence of *Microsporum canis* under a Wood's (ultraviolet) light

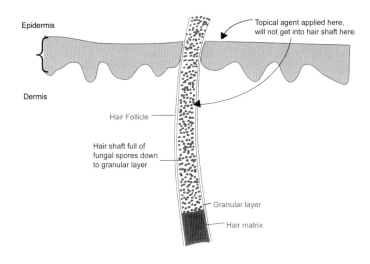

Fig. 3.13 Diagram showing hair shaft invaded by fungal spores that are inaccessible to topical treatment

TREATMENT: TINEA CAPITIS

Treatment is griseofulvin 15–20 mg/kg body weight/day given as a single dose with food daily for 6 weeks. It can be given as tablets (125 mg each) or as a suspension (125 mg/5 mL). Alternatively, it can be given as a single large dose (5 g) in ice cream. There is no need for topical treatment as well, as this is ineffective, since treatment applied to the surface cannot get into the hair shaft (*see* Fig. 3.13).

If it is due to *M. canis*, the affected pet (kitten or puppy) must be treated with griseofulvin too. The pet should be taken to the local vet to get the treatment.

Terbinafine (Lamasil) works well for infections with *Trichophyton* species (*T. tonsurans* is most commonly grown), but is less effective for *Microspsorum* (*M. canis* or *M. audouinii*). The dose depends on the child's weight: 10–20 kg–62.5 mg/day; 21–40 kg–125 mg/day; > 41 kg–250 mg/day, given for 4 weeks.

As human-acquired tinea capitis is contagious, and adults may act as carriers, all family members and possibly classmates should be screened for evidence of infection.

If the child has a **kerion**, the crusts should be softened with arachis oil and then removed. It is worth taking a bacteriology swab from under the crust or from a pustule. If *Staphylococcus aureus* is grown, treat with flucloxacillin as well as with the antifungal.

TRICHOTILLOMANIA

Trichotillomania is a well-defined area of apparent hair loss. Close examination will reveal not a bald area, but an area where all the hairs are short – longer hairs having been pulled out. The remaining hair is just too short to twist around the fingers to pull out. It usually occurs in children as a habit tic or in teenagers who are unhappy.

The only thing likely to be confused with this is alopecia areata. If the diagnosis is in doubt, a biopsy from the abnormal area will show empty anagen follicles and melanin pigment casts.

TREATMENT: TRICHOTILLOMANIA

Most cases in young children are due to a habit tic, but there may be an obvious emotional reason – one of the parents has left home or died, or some other major stress has occurred. Often the parent(s) have not noticed the child twisting the hairs around one of the fingers or pulling them out but will do so once you tell them what is happening. It is best for them not to make a big thing of it, particularly not to punish the child for it, and to give the child as much love and security as they can during the difficult time. Once the time of trauma is over, the child will nearly always stop pulling the hair out and the hair will regrow normally. In teenagers who pull out their hair the cause is often less obvious, but most will need psychiatric help to resolve the problem.

TRACTION ALOPECIA

This is a common condition in races with tight curly hair but much less common in Europeans. It causes hair loss at the temples and sometimes the crown and is due to the hair being tightly pulled back, tied up, plaited, braided or straightened with hot combs. It is important to ask about hair styling practices when Afro-Caribbean or African patients, usually woman, present with hair loss. The hair loss may be reversible if the hair pulling is stopped early. Usually by the time patients present there is significant scarring

and the hair will not regrow. Minoxidil can be helpful in boosting growth where there are still active follicles to improve volume but in many patients the hair loss is so advanced that a wig may be necessary.

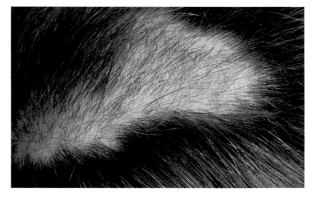

Fig. 3.14 Trichotillomania: looks like a bald patch but in fact short hairs are present

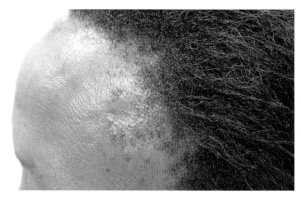

Fig. 3.15 Traction alopecia: note loss of hair on the frontal hairline

Hairy scalp
Discrete bald patches   SCARRING ALOPECIA
With scarring
(All are uncommon; the hair follicle is replaced by scar tissue, so the hair loss is permanent)

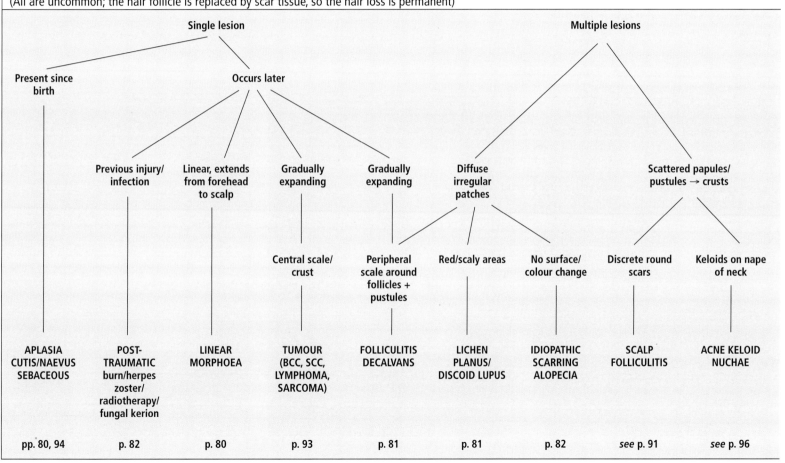

Single lesion

Present since birth

Occurs later

Previous injury/infection

Linear, extends from forehead to scalp

Gradually expanding

Gradually expanding

Multiple lesions

Diffuse irregular patches

Scattered papules/pustules → crusts

Central scale/crust

Peripheral scale around follicles + pustules

Red/scaly areas

No surface/colour change

Discrete round scars

Keloids on nape of neck

APLASIA CUTIS/NAEVUS SEBACEOUS

POST-TRAUMATIC burn/herpes zoster/radiotherapy/fungal kerion

LINEAR MORPHOEA

TUMOUR (BCC, SCC, LYMPHOMA, SARCOMA)

FOLLICULITIS DECALVANS

LICHEN PLANUS/DISCOID LUPUS

IDIOPATHIC SCARRING ALOPECIA

SCALP FOLLICULITIS

ACNE KELOID NUCHAE

pp. 80, 94   p. 82   p. 80   p. 93   p. 81   p. 81   p. 82   see p. 91   see p. 96

APLASIA CUTIS

Aplasia cutis presents at birth as an ulcerated, red area on the scalp. This heals to leave a permanent scar (*see* also naevus sebaceous, p. 94). It is not due to birth trauma.

MORPHOEA

Linear morphoea on the forehead may extend into the scalp resulting in a linear scar (en coup de sabre). It often involves the underlying subcutaneous fat leaving a depression in the skin. It can sometimes be associated with hemifacial atrophy. Aggressive early treatment is required to prevent permanent deformity. Pulsed methyl prednisolone followed by methotrexate or mycophenolate mofetil are preferred. Surgery can improve the appearance once the disease has burnt out.

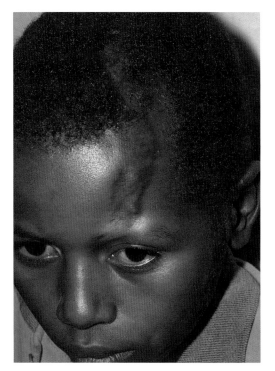

Fig. 3.16 Linear morphoea on scalp and forehead, known as 'en coup de sabre'

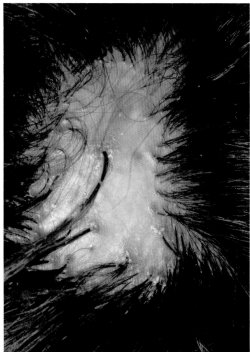

Fig. 3.17 Folliculitis decalvans: bald areas with pustules and crusts around hairs

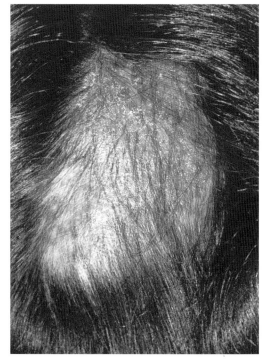

Fig. 3.18 Lichen planus in scalp: note the mauve colour of the underlying skin

FOLLICULITIS DECALVANS

Folliculitis decalvans is a rare condition in which there is an abnormal host reaction to an infection with *S. aureus*. There is a slow progressive scarring alopecia with pustules and crusts around the affected hairs.

TREATMENT: FOLLICULITIS DECALVANS

Once scarring has occurred the hair will not regrow. It is important, therefore, to start treatment as soon as possible to minimise the hair loss. Although due to *S. aureus*, treatment with flucloxacillin does not work. Lymecycline 408 mg bid can be helpful in less severe cases or a combination of rifampicin 300 mg bid with clindamycin 300 mg bid given for 10–12 weeks (up to 2 years if relapse occurs). Isotretinoin 1 mg/kg is an alternative. Patients should be counselled regarding potential side effects of these drugs.

LICHEN PLANUS AND DISCOID LUPUS ERYTHEMATOSUS

Lichen planopilaris (LPP, lichen planus of the scalp) and discoid lupus erythematosus both cause scarring alopecia. In lupus the skin over the bald patches is usually red and scaly and there may be follicular plugging.

Different patterns of LPP are recognised. It may present in an androgenic or female pattern scarring hair loss or as 'footprints in the snow', where small, discrete, scarred areas are seen. Perifollicular erythema and scale may be noted in a more diffuse pattern. **Frontal fibrosing alopecia** is another variant of LPP. It results in a progressive scarring alopecia of the fronto-temporo-parietal hairline. It is usually but not always seen in postmenopausal women. Often the process has been going on for many years before patients notice that their frontal hairline has moved back. Often these patients have associated eyebrow loss and may have also lost hair elsewhere, e.g. axillae. Prominent follicles with perifollicular erythema and scale may be seen along the frontal hairline. Often these patients complain of a burning sensation on their scalp. The cause is not known but it is thought that hormones may play a role, given that the majority of patients affected are postmenopausal women

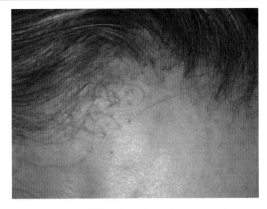

Fig. 3.19 Frontal fibrosing alopecia: progressive scarring of anterior hairline

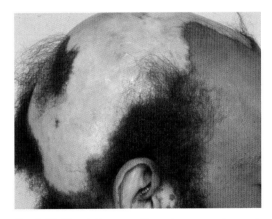

Fig. 3.20 Discoid lupus erythematosus: scarring and loss of pigment on scalp

Sometimes the diagnosis is obvious from the rash elsewhere. If in doubt, a biopsy will confirm the diagnosis. Sometimes nothing is seen histologically except the replacement of hair follicles with scar tissue. This is called idiopathic scarring alopecia or **pseudopelade of Brocq**.

TREATMENT: LICHEN PLANUS AND DISCOID LUPUS ERYTHEMATOSUS

Very potent topical steroids (0.05% clobetasol proprionate) and oral hydroxychloroquine 200 mg bid may be effective if used early enough to prevent scarring in both conditions. Once scarring has occurred, no regrowth is possible. Doxycycline 100 mg daily has been found to be partially effective in lichen planus. Anti-androgens such as finasteride 5 mg weekly and dutasteride 500 µg weekly may help in stabilising, and in some cases improving, frontal fibrosing alopecia. For treatment of lichen planus see p. 198; for discoid lupus erythematosus see p. 137.

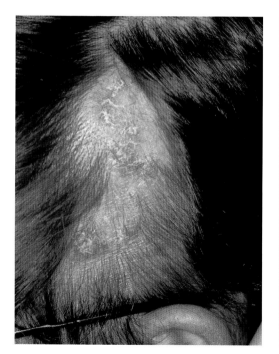

Fig. 3.21 Discoid lupus erythematosus in scalp: note red scaly plaques in bald area

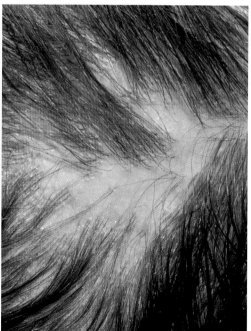

Fig. 3.22 Idiopathic scarring alopecia of the scalp (no cause found on biopsy)

POST-TRAUMATIC ALOPECIA

Any injury or infection resulting in scarring will result in hair loss. Usually the history will make the cause obvious. Before griseofulvin was introduced in 1958, radiotherapy was the usual treatment for scalp ringworm. It caused the anagen hairs to fall out and resulted in cure. If too big a dose was given, the resulting alopecia was permanent. Many of these patients are now developing basal cell and squamous cell carcinomas on their bald scalps.

Hot combing, chemical straightening and hot oil treatments used to straighten black curly hair can all result in permanent hair loss, particularly if aggravated by tight or corn-rolling styling that applies additional traction to hair roots.

Hairy scalp
Diffuse hair loss

DIFFUSE HAIR LOSS

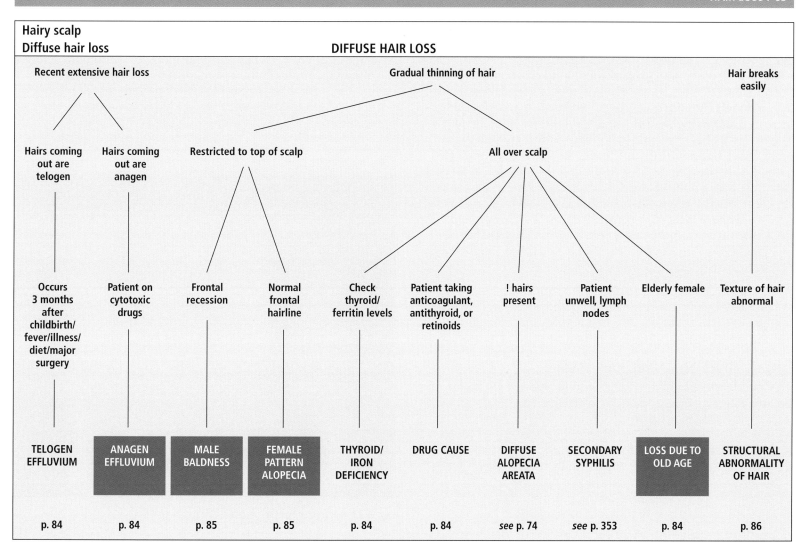

Recent extensive hair loss — Gradual thinning of hair — Hair breaks easily

Hairs coming out are telogen

Hairs coming out are anagen

Restricted to top of scalp

All over scalp

Occurs 3 months after childbirth/fever/illness/diet/major surgery

Patient on cytotoxic drugs

Frontal recession

Normal frontal hairline

Check thyroid/ferritin levels

Patient taking anticoagulant, antithyroid, or retinoids

! hairs present

Patient unwell, lymph nodes

Elderly female

Texture of hair abnormal

| TELOGEN EFFLUVIUM | ANAGEN EFFLUVIUM | MALE BALDNESS | FEMALE PATTERN ALOPECIA | THYROID/ IRON DEFICIENCY | DRUG CAUSE | DIFFUSE ALOPECIA AREATA | SECONDARY SYPHILIS | LOSS DUE TO OLD AGE | STRUCTURAL ABNORMALITY OF HAIR |

p. 84 | p. 84 | p. 85 | p. 85 | p. 84 | p. 84 | see p. 74 | see p. 353 | p. 84 | p. 86

TELOGEN EFFLUVIUM

Telogen effluvium occurs when there is a shift in the normal hair cycle resulting in temporary hair loss. A trigger such as hormonal changes (e.g. post pregnancy or stopping the oral contraceptive pill), extreme dieting, severe illness, stress or certain medications (e.g. retinoids) usually precedes it. Patients may describe noticing increased hair in the shower, on their hairbrush or on the pillow. The hair will often come out in handfuls when you pull gently on the hair. A positive hair pull test is classified as six or more hairs. A false negative result may occur if the patient has washed his or her hair within 48 hours. Telogen hairs have a club-shaped tip (*see* p. 70). Shedding of telogen hairs is followed by regrowth of anagen hairs. Such hair loss peaks after a few months and gradually reverts to normal over 6–9 months. Usually the hair recovers fully but in some cases may be incomplete. Short fronds of hair may be noted at the frontal hairline.

Some patients may notice continued intermittent shedding known as chronic telogen effluvium. They should be reassured that this will not result in baldness, although it may unmask an underlying genetic predisposition to a patterned hair loss.

OTHER CAUSES OF DIFFUSE HAIR LOSS

The hair density gradually decreases with age and the hairs become finer. In younger patients, consider:

- hypothyroidism
- iron deficiency
- diffuse alopecia areata – look for ! hairs
- secondary syphilis – the patient will be unwell with widespread lymphadenopathy and a rash (*see* p. 207)
- systemic lupus erythematosus (*see* p. 131)
- drugs: anticoagulant, antithyroid or retinoids.

ANAGEN EFFLUVIUM

Cytotoxic drugs affect any rapidly dividing cells and the hair matrix is affected, as well as the bone marrow and tumour cells. It is the anagen hairs that are shed, so 90% of all scalp hair will be lost. Once the drug is discontinued, hair will usually regrow normally, although permanent alopecia may sometimes occur, especially after docetaxel for breast cancer (1 in 30 risk).

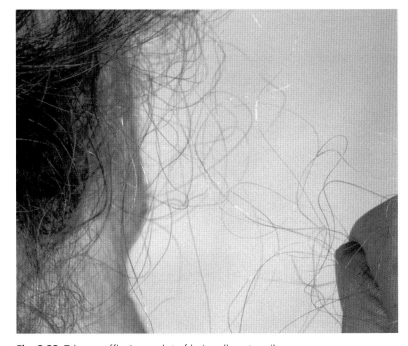

Fig. 3.23 Telogen effluvium: a lot of hair pulls out easily

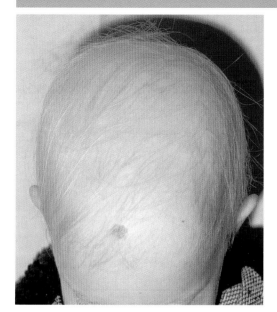

Fig. 3.24 Anagen effluvium in a child on chemotherapy

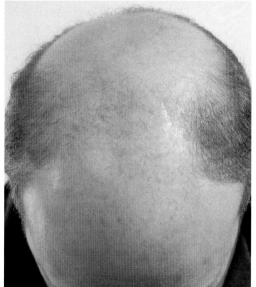

Fig. 3.25 Male pattern baldness: frontal recession with loss on the crown – the sides and occiput are normal

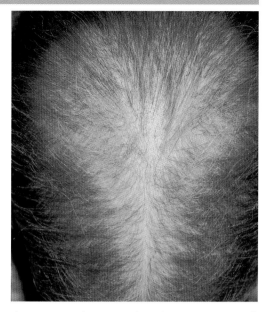

Fig. 3.26 Female pattern alopecia: note retention of the frontal hairline with thinning over the vertex of the scalp

MALE PATTERN BALDNESS

This is hair loss occurring over the temples or on the crown due to androgens (dihydrotestosterone). The hair on the occiput and around the sides of the scalp is never lost (*see* Fig. 3.25). The effect of dihydrotestosterone is a shortening of the anagen growth phase and a corresponding increase in telogen hairs. Gradually the hair follicles get smaller and terminal hairs are replaced by vellus hairs. The amount of hair loss and the age of onset is genetically determined (from mother or father).

FEMALE PATTERN ALOPECIA

This is similar to male pattern baldness but usually without the frontal recession (*see* Fig. 3.26). Decreased hair density from the crown forward with normal hair density at the back and sides occurs. Minor degrees of this are extremely common.

An androgen-secreting tumour should be considered in women with male pattern alopecia if it is very extensive or if there is a change in the menstrual cycle.

TREATMENT: MALE PATTERN BALDNESS

For most men, no treatment is needed or sought since this is a normal physiological process. For a few, who cannot come to terms with their baldness, the following are available (not under the National Health Service).

- A **5% minoxidil** solution or foam: 1 mL is rubbed into the bald scalp twice daily. This does not produce regrowth of normal terminal hair, but of long vellus hair in about a third of those who use it. If treatment is stopped, the longer hair will fall out, so once started it will need to be continued indefinitely. A 2% solution is used for maintenance treatment.
- **Finasteride**: 1 mg orally daily (or 5 mg weekly, which is cheaper!) inhibits type II 5α-reductase, the enzyme that converts testosterone to the more active dihydrotestosterone in scalp follicles. One-third of men will have marked regrowth of hair, one-third will have moderate regrowth and one-third will have little regrowth. Side effects (in about 5% of patients) should be discussed. They include impotence, ejaculatory dysfunction and loss of libido. Patients should be warned that there have been cases of prolonged sexual side effects even after stopping treatment.
- **Hair transplants**: hairs are taken from the occipital area or sides of the scalp by punch biopsy. Follicular units (containing one to four follicles) are transplanted into the bald areas. This is an effective treatment in selected cases.

TREATMENT: FEMALE PATTERN ALOPECIA

For minor degrees of this, no treatment is needed, but if it is noticeable consider one of the following options.

- **Anti-androgens**: Dianette is an option, particularly if there is associated polycystic ovarian syndrome.
- **Spironolactone**: start with 50 mg bid and increase to 100 mg bid depending on side effects. It is worth trying this for 6 months. In younger women it may cause menstrual irregularities and postural hypotension. Premenopausal women should be counselled against becoming pregnant on this treatment. It may be stopped during pregnancy and restarted when breastfeeding has finished. Check renal function and electrolytes (potassium).
- Topical **minoxidil**, as for male pattern baldness.
- **Finasteride** 5 mg weekly is sometimes used in postmenopausal women.
- Other treatments that have been found to be helpful include topical oestrogens, topical prostaglandins (e.g. bimatoprost) and ketoconazole. *Unfortunately, on stopping treatment with any of the drugs listed here, the hair loss will reoccur.*
- **Hair transplants**: although expensive, this is an effective treatment in selected patients.
- A **wig** is another option and is available on the National Health Service.

STRUCTURAL ABNORMALITIES OF HAIR

Some patients notice that their hair breaks easily and will not grow to the desired length. There are numerous structural abnormalities of the hair shaft that cause hair to break off short. All are uncommon. In trichorrhexis nodosa (*see* Fig. 3.27) the hair shaft looks like two paint brushes pushed together (*see* Fig. 3.28). In pili torti the hair shaft is flattened and twisted. In monilethrix the hair shaft shows elliptical nodules.

More common is a phenomenon known as 'weathering' in which hair becomes more coarse and breaks easily secondary to long-term use of hairstyling techniques such as colouring, perming or straightening of the hair. Various shampoos and conditioners on the market, e.g. Dove repair and Fibrology, claim to improve appearance. Patients should refrain from continuing harsh hairstyling techniques.

RASHES AND LESIONS IN THE HAIRY SCALP

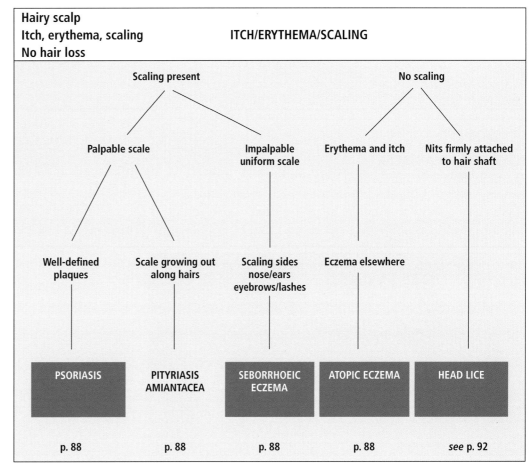

Hairy scalp
Itch, erythema, scaling   ITCH/ERYTHEMA/SCALING
No hair loss

Scaling present — No scaling

Palpable scale — Impalpable uniform scale — Erythema and itch — Nits firmly attached to hair shaft

Well-defined plaques — Scale growing out along hairs — Scaling sides nose/ears eyebrows/lashes — Eczema elsewhere

| PSORIASIS | PITYRIASIS AMIANTACEA | SEBORRHOEIC ECZEMA | ATOPIC ECZEMA | HEAD LICE |

p. 88   p. 88   p. 88   p. 88   *see* p. 92

Fig. 3.27 Trichorrhexis nodosa: hair breaks off easily and is difficult to comb or keep tidy

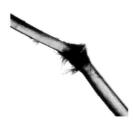

Fig. 3.28 Trichorrhexis nodosa: microscopy showing nodular swelling at which point the hair breaks

PSORIASIS

Psoriasis in the scalp is common, and it may start there. The diagnosis is made by running your hands through the scalp and feeling the thick, heaped-up scales, which are not shed because the scale binds to the hair. When you look, the lesions are identical to those found elsewhere, i.e. discrete, well-defined, red scaly plaques. Hair loss may occur in scalp psoriasis but rarely becomes long-standing. The plaques may extend away from the hairline onto the forehead, neck or around the ears, causing social embarrassment.

PITYRIASIS AMIANTACEA

The term 'pityriasis amiantacea' is used to describe thick scales growing out along the hair shaft. It can be due to either psoriasis or eczema. It is seen more commonly in children than in adults.

ECZEMA

Eczema is differentiated from psoriasis on the scalp because it usually covers all the hairy scalp and is more easily seen than felt. Wherever you look it is red and scaly. **Seborrhoeic eczema** typically starts in the scalp, causing fine scaling (dandruff). This is associated with scaling behind and in front of the ears, in the external auditory meatus and on the face (*see* p. 135)

Atopic eczema also commonly affects the scalp but typical changes will be seen elsewhere (*see* p. 236). When acute, eczema on the scalp may exude serum and become crusted.

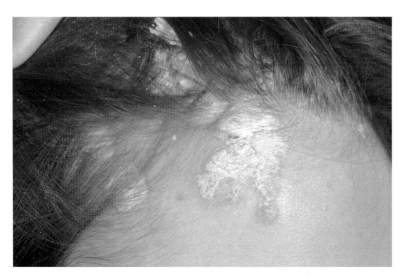

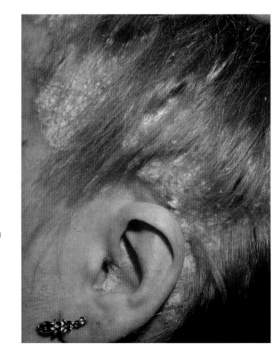

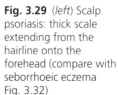

Fig. 3.29 (*left*) Scalp psoriasis: thick scale extending from the hairline onto the forehead (compare with seborrhoeic eczema Fig. 3.32)

Fig. 3.30 (*right*) Scalp psoriasis: thick scaling with some hair loss due to scratching

TREATMENT: SCALP PSORIASIS/PITYRIASIS AMIANTACEA

For **mild scalp psoriasis** where the scales are not very thick, shampooing the scalp twice weekly with a tar-based shampoo such as Capasal[UK], Polytar or T-Gel may be all that is needed. It is useful to alternate with an anti-yeast shampoo, such as ketoconazole (Nizoral) shampoo. Both should be used two to three times a week, left on for 5–10 minutes and then rinsed off. Another alternative is Dermax shampoo.

If that is not enough, or if the **scalp is very itchy**, a topical steroid lotion or gel can be applied every night until it is clear. Calcipotriol lotion may be tried as an alternative twice daily. Topical scalp lotions contain alcohol, so warn the patient that it will sting if the skin is broken. Steroid gels and mousses are water miscible and will not sting. None of these will work if there is thick scaling. Clobetasol shampoo (Etrivex) is a useful alternative for short periods. Apply dry, massage into the scalp and leave on for 10 minutes before rinsing off backwards two to three times a week. Dovobet (calcipotriol/betamethasone) gel can also be applied at night for 4–8 weeks. It. repels water, so it must be removed with dry shampoo before rinsing.

Thick plaques of psoriasis on the scalp or **pityriasis amiantacea** require something to soften up the scale. The most effective treatment is coconut oil compound ointment (unguentum cocois compound [Sebco/Cocois[UK]]) or Dermol lotion (which is less smelly). The hair is parted and the ointment rubbed onto the scalp, it is then parted again a little further along and more ointment applied; this is continued until the whole scalp has been treated. It is done every night before the patient goes to bed and washed off the following morning with a tar-based shampoo (again left for 5–10 minutes and washed off). Because it makes a mess, the head should be covered overnight with a scarf or shower cap to keep the ointment off the pillow. The treatment is repeated each night and washed off each morning until the scalp is clear. This usually takes 7–10 days. Once it is clear, the treatment can be done once a week or once a fortnight to keep it clear.

Seborrhoeic eczema is treated with ketoconazole (Nizoral) shampoo two to three times weekly. It should be left on for 5 minutes and then rinsed off. It should be used for 4 weeks, and then fortnightly to keep it clear. Any thick scaling can be removed (*see* thick plaques of psoriasis).

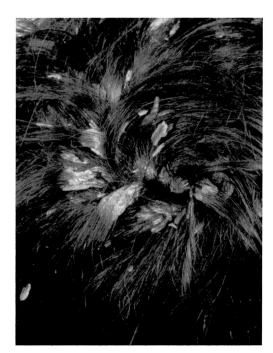

Fig. 3.31 Pityriasis amiantacea: thick plaque with scale growing out along hair

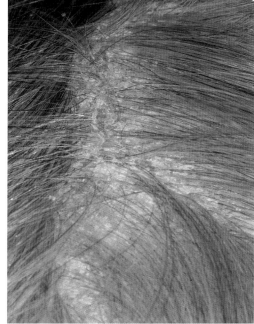

Fig. 3.32 Seborrhoeic eczema: fine impalpable scaling over the whole scalp

Rash in hairy scalp
Pustules, crust, exudate   PUSTULES/CRUST/EXUDATE

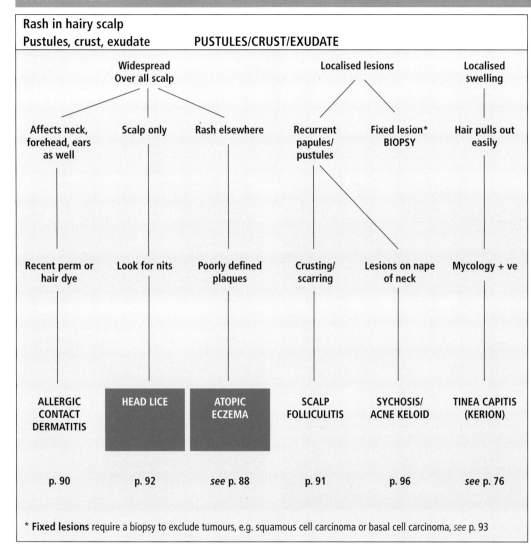

Widespread Over all scalp
Localised lesions
Localised swelling

Affects neck, forehead, ears as well — Scalp only — Rash elsewhere
Recurrent papules/ pustules — Fixed lesion* BIOPSY
Hair pulls out easily

Recent perm or hair dye — Look for nits — Poorly defined plaques
Crusting/ scarring — Lesions on nape of neck
Mycology + ve

ALLERGIC CONTACT DERMATITIS — HEAD LICE — ATOPIC ECZEMA — SCALP FOLLICULITIS — SYCHOSIS/ ACNE KELOID — TINEA CAPITIS (KERION)

p. 90 — p. 92 — see p. 88 — p. 91 — p. 96 — see p. 76

* **Fixed lesions** require a biopsy to exclude tumours, e.g. squamous cell carcinoma or basal cell carcinoma, *see* p. 93

ALLERGIC CONTACT DERMATITIS

Allergic contact dermatitis on the scalp is not common and is usually due to hair dyes (paraphenylenediamine, PPD) or perming solutions (thioglycolates). It usually presents as an acute weeping eczema at the hair margins and on the forehead, face and neck, rather than in the scalp itself. The diagnosis is confirmed once the patient is better by patch testing.

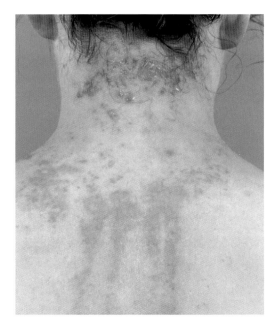

Fig. 3.33 Allergic contact dermatitis to hair dye: acute eczematous reaction affecting neck and back

TREATMENT: ALLERGIC CONTACT DERMATITIS

Stop using hair dyes/perming solutions. If it is very weepy, dry up any exudate by soaking the scalp in a diluted potassium permanganate or aluminium acetate solution (*see* p. 30). Then apply a potent[UK]/group 2–3[USA] steroid ointment. Once it is better, refer to a dermatologist for patch testing to establish the cause.

SCALP FOLLICULITIS

Recurrent pustules on the scalp present a diagnostic and therapeutic difficulty. Sometimes the cause is a staphylococcal folliculitis, which can be confirmed by taking a swab. This is particularly common in African children because of the practice of rubbing petroleum jelly (Vaseline) into the scalp. This is often associated with posterior cervical lymphadenopathy. In Europe and the United States usually no bacteria are grown and it is assumed that the condition is a variant of acne. Some lesions may heal to leave a scar.

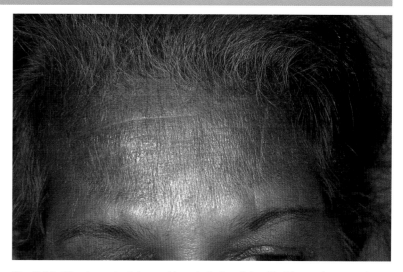

Fig. 3.34 Allergic contact dermatitis to hair dye: lichenified hyperpigmented eczema on forehead

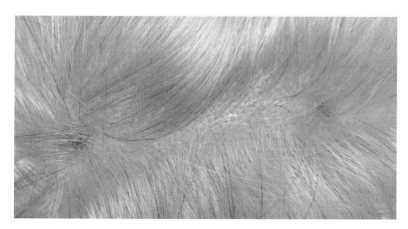

Fig. 3.35 Scalp folliculitis: crusted lesions that may heal to leave a scar

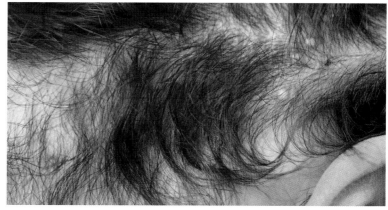

Fig. 3.36 Scalp folliculitis: isolated pustules within the hairy scalp

HEAD LICE (PEDICULOSIS CAPITIS)

Lice are wingless insects that pierce the skin to feed on human blood. The head louse is about 3 mm long. The female lays 7–10 eggs each day during a life span of 1 month. The eggs are firmly attached to the base of the hair, and they hatch in about a week. Head lice are spread by direct contact from head to head, mainly in children. It has nothing to do with poor hygiene. Lice are not transmitted by combs, hats or hairbrushes. Infestation is extremely common and usually asymptomatic. If there are large numbers of lice, itching may be intolerable and result in secondary bacterial infection (impetigo and pustules). Enlarged posterior cervical glands should always make you think of head lice. The diagnosis is made by finding the nits (egg cases), which are white, opalescent oval capsules, firmly attached to hairs (*see* Fig. 3.38), easily distinguished from the scale of seborrhoeic dermatitis (dandruff), which comes off easily (*see* Fig. 3.39).

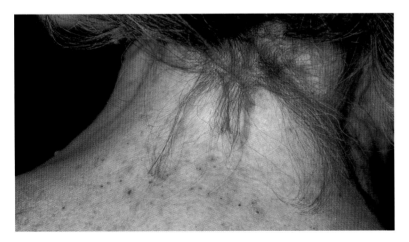

Fig. 3.37 Head lice bites on back of neck

TREATMENT: SCALP FOLLICULITIS

Stop applying greasy ointments on the scalp. Take swabs. If *S. aureus* is grown, treat with flucloxacillin or erythromycin 500 mg qid till clear. If swabs are negative, treat with a tetracycline (e.g. lymecycline 408 mg once to twice daily). Alternatively, rifampicin/clindamycin 300 mg bid may be tried. If these fail, isotretinoin 40 mg daily is usually effective (*see* pp. 120–1) but relapse is common and low-dose maintenance (10 mg day) may be necessary.

TREATMENT: HEAD LICE

There are a number of insecticides available that kill both adult lice and eggs. Dimeticone may be used and acts on the surface of the lice. It should be rubbed into the scalp, left overnight and rinsed off with shampoo in the morning. Two treatments should be given, 7 days apart. Malathion is an alternative but some lice are resistant to this. Permethrin can also be used. Lotions are better than shampoo formulations because the latter have too short a contact time to be effective. The lotion is applied all over the scalp, left on for 12 hours, and then washed off with a normal shampoo. The permethrin cream rinse is used like a conditioner. It coats the lice and eggs with a balsam containing the insecticide, so combining a long contact time with a short treatment time. The egg cases can be removed by combing with a nit comb.

PROBLEMS WITH TREATING HEAD LICE

- Resistance to insecticides is common, and if one treatment fails to cure the infestation, you should try another one. The Bug Buster Kit consists of a nit comb and a conditioner. The wet hair should be combed for 10 minutes every night for about 2 weeks. This is useful if you want to avoid excessive use of insecticides.
- To prevent re-infection, the *whole family* and school friends or contacts should be treated, whether or not they are itching. You may need to involve the health visitor, practice nurse or school nurse.

(cont.)

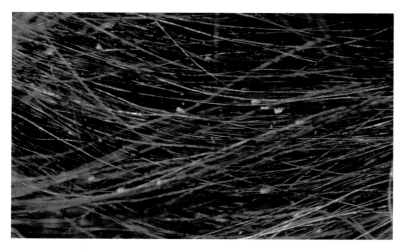

Fig. 3.38 Head lice: nits attached to hair shaft

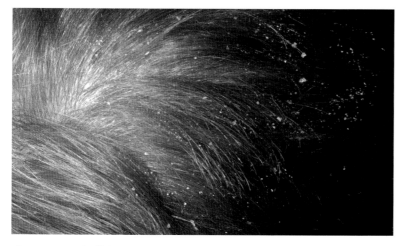

Fig. 3.39 Dandruff: fine scale that is not attached to the hairs

- People are often worried that some of the lice may be missed in children or adults with very long hair. Since the eggs are laid onto the hairs where they leave the scalp, all the viable eggs will be close to the scalp and will be killed, as long as the insecticide has been applied to the scalp (not the hair). In the same way, the adult lice and the immature walking stages have to go to the scalp to feed, so the insecticide will kill them then.
- Only water-based insecticide lotions should be used in patients with eczema, because the alcoholic-based ones will sting excoriated skin.

TUMOURS

Basal cell carcinomas may occur in the hairy scalp as a persistent area of crusting or hair loss. The unusual site results in a misdiagnosis of eczema or 'infection' so that the lesion may become quite large before being recognised.

Squamous cell carcinomas occur in the elderly who have significant hair loss or thinning. They present as an ulcer with an overlying crust that has become matted down with hair (*see* Fig. 9.162, p. 333).

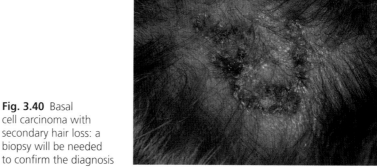

Fig. 3.40 Basal cell carcinoma with secondary hair loss: a biopsy will be needed to confirm the diagnosis

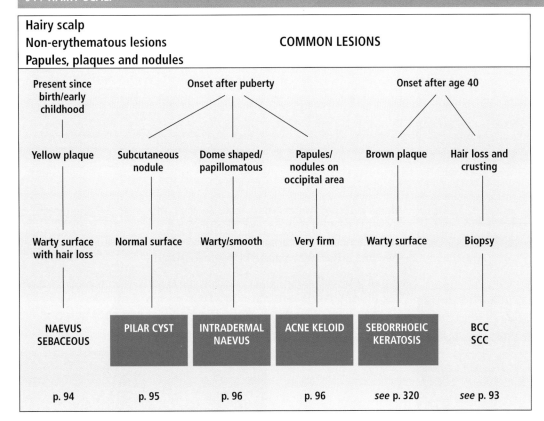

Hairy scalp
Non-erythematous lesions   COMMON LESIONS
Papules, plaques and nodules

Present since birth/early childhood		Onset after puberty			Onset after age 40	
Yellow plaque	Subcutaneous nodule	Dome shaped/ papillomatous	Papules/ nodules on occipital area	Brown plaque	Hair loss and crusting
Warty surface with hair loss	Normal surface	Warty/smooth	Very firm	Warty surface	Biopsy
NAEVUS SEBACEOUS	PILAR CYST	INTRADERMAL NAEVUS	ACNE KELOID	SEBORRHOEIC KERATOSIS	BCC SCC
p. 94	p. 95	p. 96	p. 96	*see* p. 320	*see* p. 93

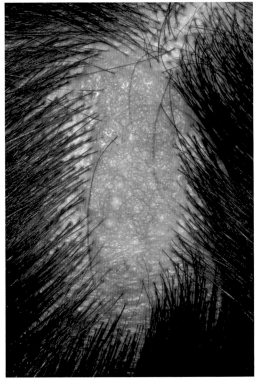

Fig. 3.41 Naevus sebaceous present since birth

NAEVUS SEBACEOUS

This is present from birth or early childhood. It differs from a congenital melanocytic naevus in being yellowish with a flat, warty surface and hair loss. A basal cell carcinoma or other adnexal tumour may develop within it in middle age. If this happens it is obvious, because there will be a lump within the naevus or a discharge from it.

No treatment is necessary. It can be excised to reduce the area of hair loss. If a tumour develops, this will need removing.

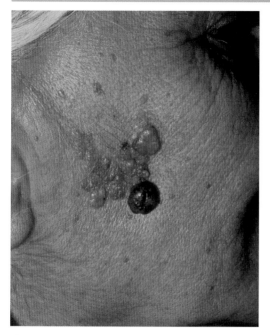

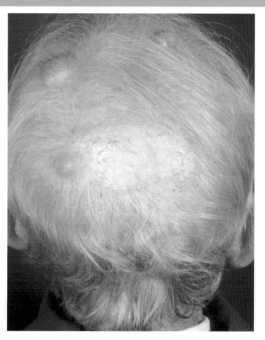

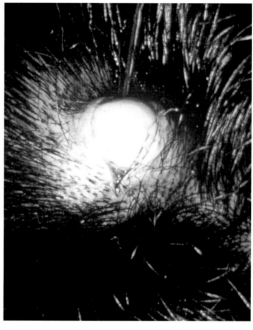

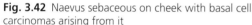

Fig. 3.42 Naevus sebaceous on cheek with basal cell carcinomas arising from it

Fig. 3.43 Multiple pilar cysts in scalp

Fig. 3.44 Excision of overlying skin over a pilar cyst to reveal the right plane for removal

PILAR (TRICHILEMMAL) CYST

Pilar (or trichilemmal) cysts are derived from the external root sheath of hair follicles and occur predominantly on the scalp. They are inherited as an autosomal dominant trait, they appear between the ages of 15 and 30, and present to the doctor because the patient notices a lump when brushing or combing the hair. One or several subcutaneous nodules are present. They do not have a punctum and do not usually become inflamed (compare with epidermoid cysts, *see* p. 273).

TREATMENT: PILAR CYST

First excise the overlying skin with a small ellipse. The top of the cyst will then be visible (*see* Fig. 3.44). It will now shell out very easily, since these cysts have a connective tissue sheath around them. If this is not the case, it is likely that it is an epidermoid cyst.

An alternative method of removal is to cut straight into the cyst with a scalpel, squeeze out the contents and then remove the cyst lining with a pair of artery forceps. It should come out intact and very easily.

INTRADERMAL NAEVUS

Flat, pigmented naevi are not usually recognised on the hairy scalp. Once they become raised they are likely to be caught in combs. Most skin-coloured or light-brown papules on the scalp will be intradermal naevi. They may have a smooth or papillomatous surface (*see* p. 264).

TREATMENT: INTRADERMAL NAEVUS

> Reassure the patient that they are harmless. They can be easily removed by shave and cautery if they become a problem.

ACNE KELOID NUCHALIS

Acne keloid nuchalis is a chronic inflammatory condition of the nape of the neck, most commonly seen in men of African or Afro-Caribbean origin. Itchy follicular pustules develop in the occipital area, which later become keloid scars. In the early stages of the disease (pustules present), long-term, low-dose antibiotics as for scalp folliculitis can be used (*see* p. 92). Once keloid papules, nodules or plaques are present treatment is more difficult. Possibilities include intralesional triamcinolone once a month or wide excision of the affected area down to and including the fat.

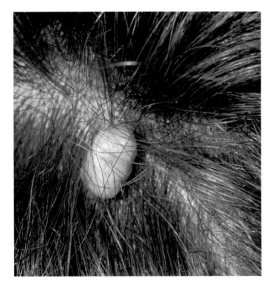

Fig. 3.45 Pedunculated intradermal naevus in scalp

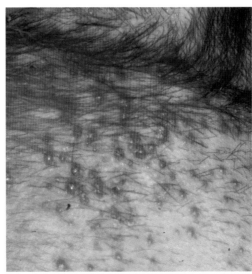

Fig. 3.46 Keloid scars at site of folliculitis on nape of neck

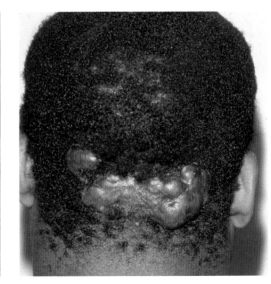

Fig. 3.47 Acne keloid nuchalis

Acute erythematous rash on the face

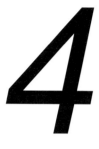

Normal surface

Crust or exudate on surface

Face
Acute erythematous rash
Surface normal/smooth
Widespread patches, papules, plaques, swelling

WIDESPREAD RASH – NO EXUDATE

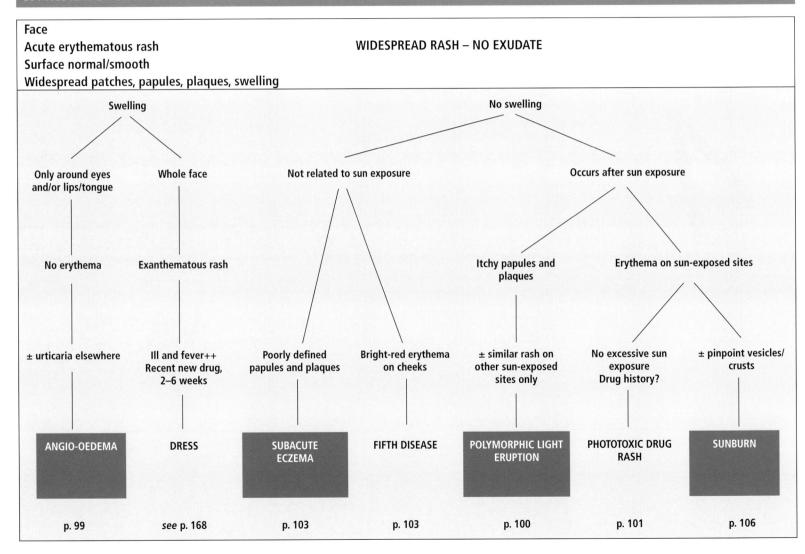

Swelling

No swelling

Only around eyes and/or lips/tongue

Whole face

Not related to sun exposure

Occurs after sun exposure

No erythema

Exanthematous rash

Itchy papules and plaques

Erythema on sun-exposed sites

± urticaria elsewhere

Ill and fever++
Recent new drug, 2–6 weeks

Poorly defined papules and plaques

Bright-red erythema on cheeks

± similar rash on other sun-exposed sites only

No excessive sun exposure
Drug history?

± pinpoint vesicles/ crusts

ANGIO-OEDEMA

DRESS

SUBACUTE ECZEMA

FIFTH DISEASE

POLYMORPHIC LIGHT ERUPTION

PHOTOTOXIC DRUG RASH

SUNBURN

p. 99

see p. 168

p. 103

p. 103

p. 100

p. 101

p. 106

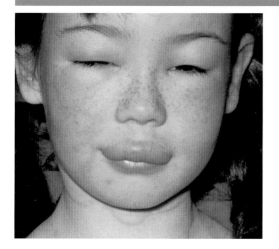

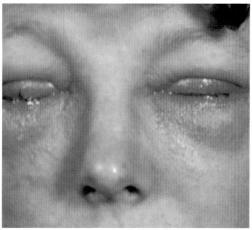

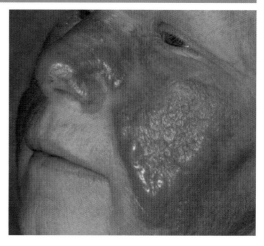

Fig. 4.01 Angio-oedema and urticaria: note oedema around eyes and lips without redness, scaling or exudate

Fig. 4.02 Acute eczema: swelling of eyelids with exudate and crusting

Fig. 4.03 Erysipelas: swelling of eyelids and cheeks with large blisters

ANGIO-OEDEMA

Angio-oedema is oedema in the dermis due to increased vascular permeability. There should be no associated redness. On the face the swelling involves the eyelids and lips. Less commonly the tongue and larynx can be involved, leading to difficulty in swallowing and breathing. The onset is often dramatic. The patient may feel unwell and the eyelid swelling may cause complete closure of the eyes. It should start going down quite quickly but can last up to 48 hours. If there is associated urticaria (*see* p. 171) the diagnosis is easy. When it occurs alone it needs to be distinguished from an acute eczema or erysipelas. The fact that the swelling is not red and there are no blisters or scaling should make the diagnosis easy.

Angio-oedema without weals is often idiopathic, but you should exclude a drug cause or possible C1 esterase deficiency (hereditary angio-oedema), especially if there is a family history or previous episodes of laryngeal oedema or abdominal pain.

TREATMENT: ANGIO-OEDEMA

Use a long-acting non-sedative antihistamine such as cetirizine or loratidine at a high dose, 10–20 mg every 12 hours (maximum of four times the standard hay fever dose) until it settles. In a life-threatening situation in the context of anaphylaxis (not hereditary angio-oedema) with swelling of the larynx or tongue, inject 0.5 mL of 1:1000 adrenaline solution intramuscularly (prescribable to appropriate at-risk patients, with appropriate training, in the form of an EpiPen) with strict directions to attend A&E for follow-up, as its benefits are short term and further treatment may well be required.

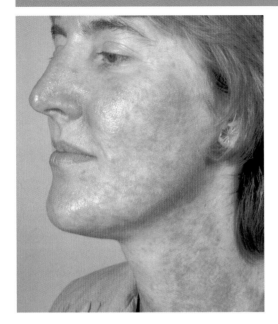

Fig. 4.04 Polymorphic light eruption. Itchy papules and vesicles on face and neck sparing the area under the chin

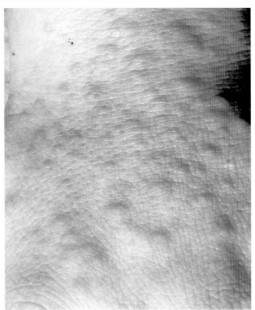

Fig. 4.05 Polymorphic light eruption. Itchy papules on dorsum of hand

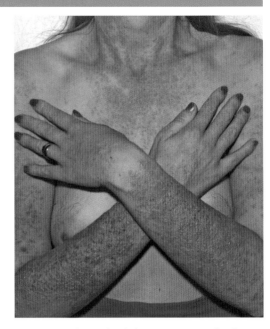

Fig. 4.06 Polymorphic light eruption. Distribution over sun exposed sites

POLYMORPHIC LIGHT ERUPTION

This is a common rash due to ultraviolet light. It occurs in early adult life and affects twice as many females as males. The rash consists of itchy red papules, vesicles or plaques. The size of the papules varies in different patients, from pinpoint up to 5 mm. The plaques may be urticarial (i.e. non-scaly dermal oedema) or eczematous (scaly and poorly defined). Vesicles are less common. It occurs only on sun-exposed parts, especially the backs of the hands, forearms, 'V' of neck and below the ears, as well as the face, but not all sun-exposed sites need to be involved, and quite often the face may be clear.

Most patients are aware of the connection with the sun. The rash typically occurs several hours after sun exposure and, if there is no further exposure, lasts for 2–5 days. It usually occurs in spring and early summer and tends to improve as the summer progresses, due to some form of tolerance. In some patients it only occurs when they are away from home (on holiday) in more intense sunlight.

TREATMENT: POLYMORPHIC LIGHT ERUPTION

- Keep out of strong sunlight, wear protective clothing and use a high-factor sunblock with both medium wave ultraviolet light (UVB) and long-wave ultraviolet light (UVA) protection.
- Refer to dermatology department for TL01, UVB or PUVA desensitisation therapy. This can be given in early summer to prevent the rash developing, or as a treatment to induce tolerance. It is given twice a week for 6 weeks. Following treatment, regular sun exposure is necessary to maintain tolerance.
- Systemic steroids (prednisolone 20 mg/day) may suppress the eruption for the duration of a short 2-week holiday.
- Hydroxychloroquine 400 mg daily may provide partial protection.

PHOTOTOXIC RASHES

A phototoxic rash looks like sunburn but occurs in a patient who has not been exposed to excessive sunlight. It is caused by sunlight plus:

- chemicals applied to the skin, e.g. psoralens in sun creams, photodynamic therapy photosensitizers – aminolevulinic acid
- accidental contamination of the skin by wood tars in creosote
- drugs taken by mouth, e.g.
  — antiarrhythmics: amiodarone (30%–50% of patients on this drug), quinidine
  — antibiotics: tetracyclines (doxycycline and demeclocycline), nalidixic acid, quinolones (e.g. ciprofloxacin)
  — diuretics: thiazides and furosemide
  — hypoglycaemics, sulphonylureas
  — NSAIDs (e.g. naproxen)
  — phenothiazines: chlorpromazine
  — psoralens
  — sulphonamides.

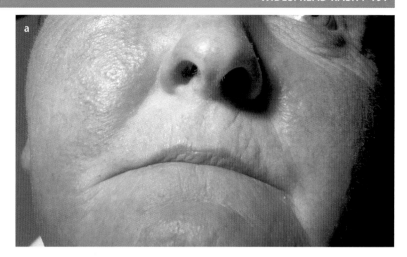

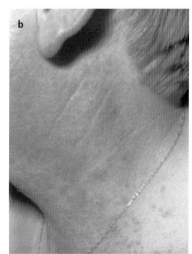

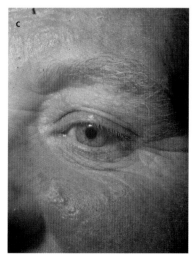

Fig. 4.07 Phototoxic rash showing sparing of shaded sites: a. under nose (top), b. behind ear (above left) and c. upper eye lid (above right).

The diagnosis is suggested by the distribution of the rash with shaded sites (upper eyelids, behind ears, under chin, *see* Fig. 4.07) spared. It can be confused with a contact allergic dermatitis but there should not be any scaling. The history of drug ingestion or creams applied to the face should enable the cause to be identified.

TREATMENT: PHOTOTOXIC RASHES

Stop the drug responsible. If this is not possible, use an opaque total sunblock containing titanium dioxide or zinc oxide to screen out all UVA (almost all drug sensitivity rashes are due to UVA). Note that UVA penetrates glass, so protection is needed even indoors or inside a car.

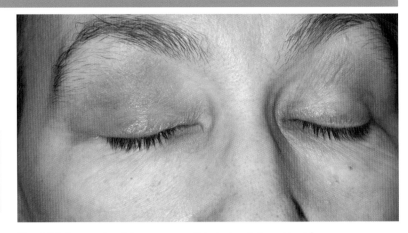

Fig. 4.09 Eczema involving upper eyelids: to be distinguished from photosensitive rashes, which spare this site

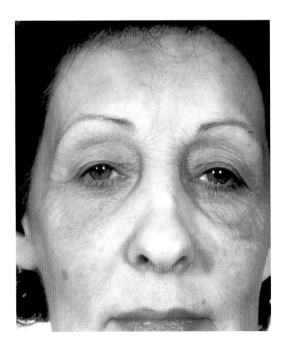

Fig. 4.08 (left) Eczema: ill-defined papules and plaques without exudate or scaling

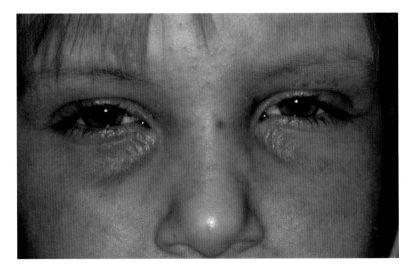

Fig. 4.10 Atopic eczema involving both eyelids as well as cheeks

SUBACUTE ECZEMA

Subacute eczema occurs without obvious vesicles and exudate. There will be erythematous patches and plaques where the border of the rash is ill defined, merging imperceptibly into normal skin. It can be due to an allergic contact dermatitis (to cosmetics, perfumes, medicaments), or to a new occurrence of an unclassified endogenous eczema or an exacerbation of existing eczema (atopic or seborrhoeic).

FIFTH DISEASE (ERYTHEMA INFECTIOSUM)

This is a viral infection due to parvovirus B19. It is characterised by the appearance of red papules on the cheeks that coalesce within hours to form symmetrical, red, oedematous plaques, sparing the nasolabial fold and eyelids, the so-called 'slapped cheek' appearance. Other symptoms are mild (sore throat, pruritis, fever) or even absent. The rash on the face fades after 4 days, but within 48 hours of the onset of the facial erythema, a lace-like pattern of erythema appears on the proximal limbs, extending to the trunk and extremities. This fades within 6–14 days. No treatment is needed, as it gets better on its own.

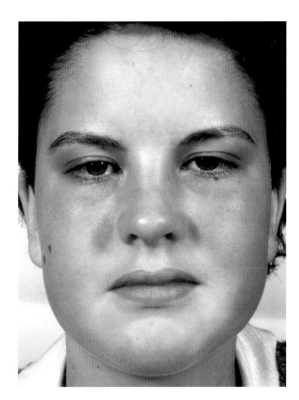

Fig. 4.11 Fifth disease (erythema infectiosum): typical 'slapped cheek' appearance

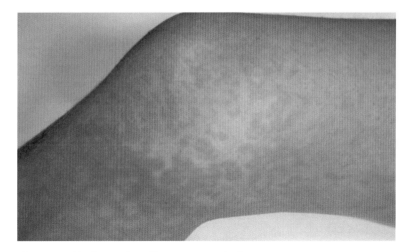

Fig. 4.12 Fifth disease: lace-like pattern on the leg

Face
Acute erythematous rash
Crust or exudate on surface
Papules, plaques, blisters, erosions

CRUST, EXUDATE or BLISTERS

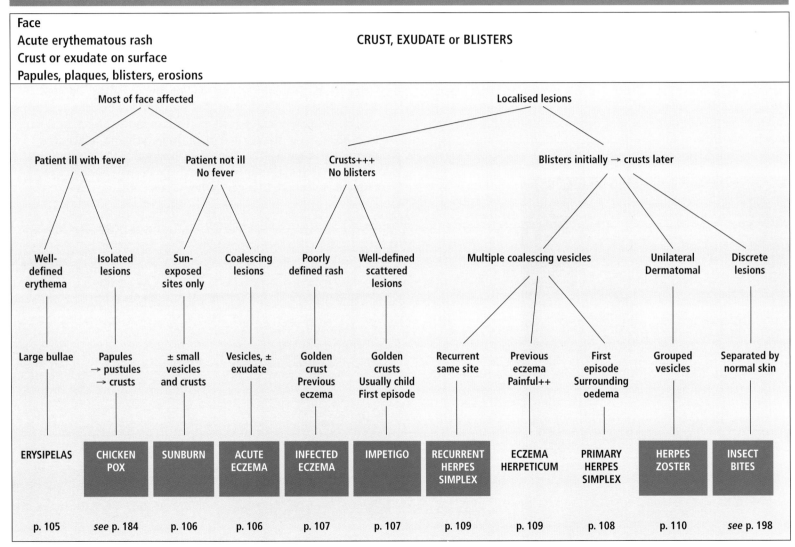

| Most of face affected | | | | Localised lesions | | | | | | | |

| Patient ill with fever | | Patient not ill No fever | | Crusts+++ No blisters | | Blisters initially → crusts later | | | | | |

| Well-defined erythema | Isolated lesions | Sun-exposed sites only | Coalescing lesions | Poorly defined rash | Well-defined scattered lesions | Multiple coalescing vesicles | | | Unilateral Dermatomal | Discrete lesions |

| Large bullae | Papules → pustules → crusts | ± small vesicles and crusts | Vesicles, ± exudate | Golden crust Previous eczema | Golden crusts Usually child First episode | Recurrent same site | Previous eczema Painful++ | First episode Surrounding oedema | Grouped vesicles | Separated by normal skin |

| ERYSIPELAS | CHICKEN POX | SUNBURN | ACUTE ECZEMA | INFECTED ECZEMA | IMPETIGO | RECURRENT HERPES SIMPLEX | ECZEMA HERPETICUM | PRIMARY HERPES SIMPLEX | HERPES ZOSTER | INSECT BITES |

| p. 105 | see p. 184 | p. 106 | p. 106 | p. 107 | p. 107 | p. 109 | p. 109 | p. 108 | p. 110 | see p. 198 |

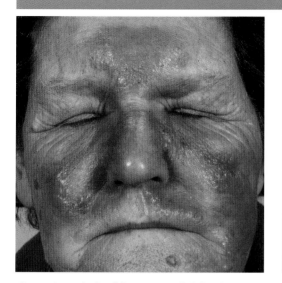

Fig. 4.13 Erysipelas: blisters on well-defined erythema (*see* also Fig. 4.03)

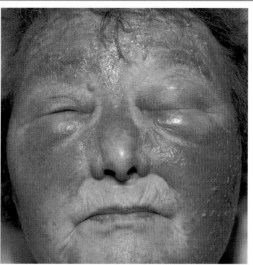

Fig. 4.14 Acute contact dermatitis due to lanolin in moisturising cream: exudate and crusting

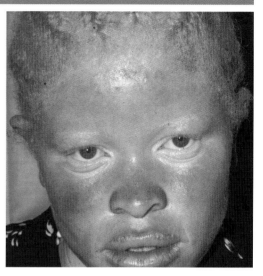

Fig. 4.15 Acute sunburn in an African albino: painful redness and blistering on sun-exposed sites

ERYSIPELAS

This is an acute, rapidly spreading rash usually caused by a group A β-haemolytic streptococcus. The patient is unwell with fever, rigors and general malaise. The rash itself is bright red, well demarcated and may or may not contain large blisters in the centre. There is no associated lymphangitis or lymphadenopathy. It is not usually possible to culture the organism, and measurement of the ASO titre is not helpful. Diagnosis is made on the characteristic clinical picture.

TREATMENT: ERYSIPELAS

Ideally treat with intravenous benzyl penicillin 1200 mg 6 hourly. Alternatively, oral flucloxacillin 1 g every 6 hours will cover *Staph* as well as *Streptococci*. If the patient is allergic to penicillin, use oral clindamycin 300 mg or clarithromycin 500 mg 6 hourly. The patient should be dramatically better within 24 hours.

TREATMENT: ACUTE SUNBURN

Topical calamine lotion will produce symptomatic relief. If severe, a single application of a very potent[UK]/group 1[USA] topical steroid (0.05% clobetasol propionate) ointment will reduce redness and bring instant relief.

ACUTE SUNBURN

Acute sunburn presents as painful erythema with or without blisters, between a few hours to 2 days after sun exposure. Usually the cause will be obvious, as the patient will have been exposed to strong sunlight, although a delay in symptoms can lead to misdiagnosis. Any exposed areas will be burnt.

ACUTE ECZEMA

Acute eczema on the face presents as tiny vesicles, weeping and crusting, and is usually due to a contact allergic dermatitis or atopic eczema. The onset of the rash is sudden with a well-defined erythema followed by vesicles, profuse exudate and crusting. If the eyelids are involved there may be marked oedema and the patient may not be able to open the eyes (*see* Fig. 4.14). The rash is usually symmetrical and uncomfortable and itchy rather than painful as in herpes zoster. Angio-oedema causes swelling only, with no weeping, and there is no associated fever as in erysipelas.

Acute allergic contact dermatitis of the face can be due to medicaments applied to the face or airborne allergens such as sawdust, cement dust, epoxyresins or phosphorus sesquisulphide from the smoke of 'strike anywhere' matches. Common applied allergens include lanolin (in ointment bases), formaldehyde and parabens (preservatives in creams), topical antihistamines or antibiotics, cosmetics and fragrances within perfumes. The exact pattern of the rash depends on the allergen responsible. Airborne allergens cause a symmetrical eczema especially affecting the upper eyelids and cheeks, while allergens in medicaments and cosmetics only involve areas where these have been applied. Linear streaking can be due to nail varnish. A rash around the hair margins and ears can be due to hair dyes or perming solutions (*see* p. 90).

A **photoallergic dermatitis** is identical in appearance to an allergic contact dermatitis but it needs a combination of UVA and a drug to cause it. The commonest drugs are:

- chlorpromazine
- promethazine
- sulphonamides
- alimemazine.

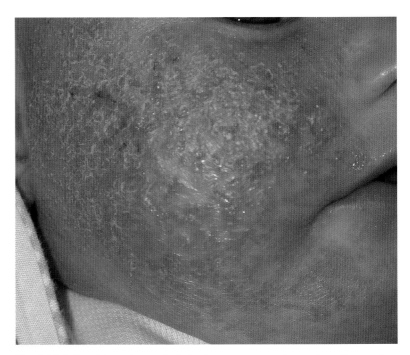

Fig. 4.16 Baby with acute onset of atopic eczema: weeping and crusting on the cheeks

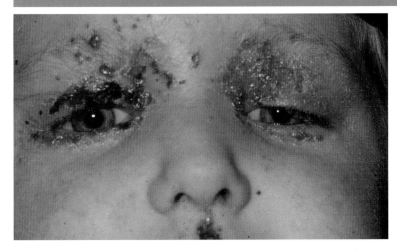

Fig. 4.17 Impetiginised eczema: exudate and golden crusts in a child with atopic eczema

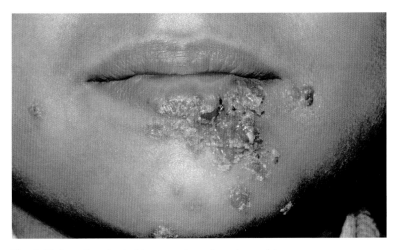

Fig. 4.18 Impetigo: typical honey-coloured crusts on chin

TREATMENT: ALLERGIC CONTACT DERMATITIS

Remove the patient from all possible allergens. Dry up any exudate with wet dressings of potassium permanganate (1:10 000) or aluminium acetate (*see* p. 30) twice a day. Dry the skin and then apply 1% hydrocortisone or 0.05% clobetasone ointment bid. Always use a steroid ointment rather than a cream, which may contain potential allergens. Once the rash is better, refer the patient to a dermatologist for patch testing (*see* p. 21).

IMPETIGINISED ECZEMA

Any itchy rash may become secondarily infected with *Staphylococcus aureus* once scratching has broken the skin. Weeping occurs and a golden-yellow crust forms on the surface. The diagnosis is made by a history of a preceding rash (usually atopic eczema or scabies). Individual lesions may be difficult to distinguish from impetigo.

TREATMENT: IMPETIGINISED ECZEMA

It is best to give a systemic antibiotic, either flucloxacillin or erythromycin four times a day (125 mg dose for children, 250 mg for adults). At the same time, treat the atopic eczema (*see* p. 236) or scabies (*see* p. 248) or the infection will reoccur.

IMPETIGO

This is a very superficial infection of the epidermis (*see* Fig. 7.31, p. 187) due to *S. aureus*, a group Λ β-haemlytic streptococcus or a mixture of both. Children are mainly affected, since the organisms gain entrance through broken skin (cuts and grazes). It is very contagious. Typically it starts as vesicles, which rapidly break down to form honey-coloured crusts; less commonly there may be just a glazed erythema. On the trunk occasionally flaccid cloudy bullae (Fig. 7.32, p. 187) are seen, which burst and form the typical golden crusts.

TREATMENT: IMPETIGO

Because the infection is very superficial, topical antibiotics are more effective than systemic (if present without underlying chronic eczema). If thick crust is present, remove it by applying arachis oil (or olive/sunflower oil) for 15–20 minutes. This will soften it so that it can be wiped off. Once the crust has been removed, apply 2% mupirocin (Bactroban), 2% fusidic acid (Fucidin) or 0.3% neomycin ointment four times a day for 3 days. Apply the antibiotic ointment to the anterior nares at the same time.

In parts of the world where impetigo is commonly due to a group A β-haemolytic streptococcus, the child will need to be treated with oral penicillin V four times a day for 7 days to prevent acute glomerulonephritis from occurring.

PRIMARY HERPES SIMPLEX

Infection with the *Herpesvirus hominis* type 1 most commonly affects the buccal mucosa (*see* p. 143) and occurs in the first 5 years of life. It is usually asymptomatic but may cause an acute gingivostomatitis. A primary infection on the skin causes painful blistering on an oedematous background (*see* Fig. 4.21 and Fig. 13.04, p. 406).

TREATMENT: RECURRENT HERPES SIMPLEX

Most patients need no treatment. Topical aciclovir or penciclovir cream applied every 2 hours for 2 days, beginning as soon as the prodromal symptoms occur, will shorten the attack but will not prevent further episodes. If recurrent episodes occur frequently or result in erythema multiforme, these can be suppressed by giving oral aciclovir 400 mg bid or famciclovir 250 mg daily for at least 6 months.

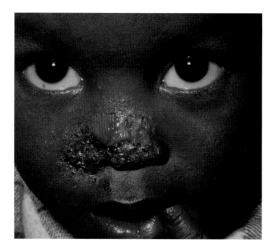

Fig. 4.19 Impetigo: golden-coloured crusts and erosions on nose

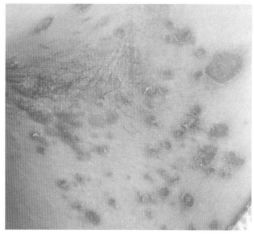

Fig. 4.20 Impetigo: glazed erythema and erosions

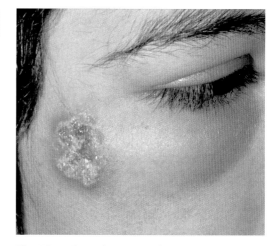

Fig. 4.21 Primary herpes simplex: grouped vesicles associated with marked surrounding oedema

RECURRENT HERPES SIMPLEX

If the primary infection of herpes simplex was in the mouth, recurrent episodes affect the lips or the skin around the lips. Primary infections elsewhere on the skin produce recurrences at the same site (e.g. finger, buttock). Most patients know that a recurrence is beginning because of the prodromal sensation of itching, burning or tingling. A few hours later, small grouped vesicles appear (*see* Fig. 1.29, p. 9), burst, crust and then heal in 7–10 days. These episodes can be precipitated by fever (hence the name 'cold sores'), sunlight, menstruation and stress, and can continue throughout life. Herpes simplex is differentiated from impetigo by the history of recurrent episodes, prodromal pain and initial vesicles containing clear fluid, and in adults it is the more likely diagnosis. If in doubt, a Tzanck smear from the base of a blister will show multinucleate giant cells in herpes simplex.

ECZEMA HERPETICUM

Atopic eczema may become secondarily infected by herpes simplex. The characteristic feature is small umbilicated vesicles that are painful rather than itchy, often with sudden onset and deterioration of previous eczema. The patient will be ill and more miserable than might be expected from normal eczema. Swabs from the vesicles will confirm the presence of the herpes simplex virus. Pemphigus, pemphigoid and Darier's disease may all become similarly infected with herpes simplex virus. Treat the same as herpes zoster (*see* p. 180).

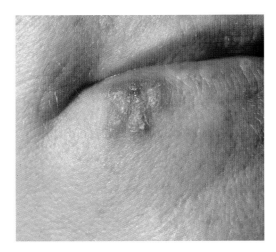

Fig. 4.22 Herpes simplex, recurrent lesions with localised crusts on the lower lip

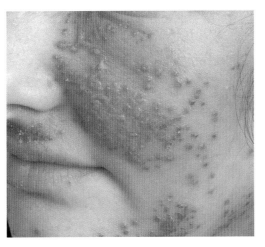

Fig. 4.23 Eczema herpeticum: painful umbilicated vesicles on cheek

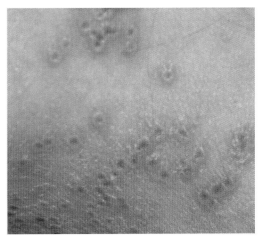

Fig. 4.24 Close up of umbilicated vesicles

HERPES ZOSTER

Herpes zoster on the face is the result of involvement of the trigeminal nerve. It presents as groups of small vesicles on a red background, followed by weeping and crusting. The rash is unilateral. Healing takes 3–4 weeks. With ophthalmic zoster the rash extends from the upper eyelid to the vertex of the skull, but if vesicles occur on the side of the nose (nasocillary branch), the eye is likely to be involved. These patients should be referred to an ophthalmologist. *See* also p. 179.

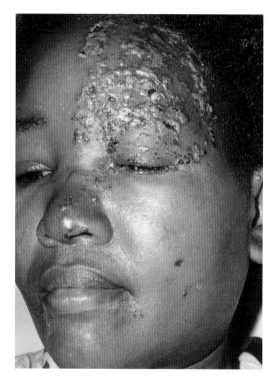

Fig. 4.25 Ophthalmic zoster: vesicles on the side of the nose mean the eye will be involved

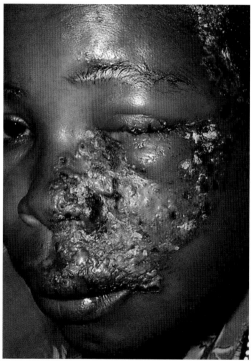

Fig. 4.26 Maxillary zoster affecting the maxillary branch: the eye is not affected

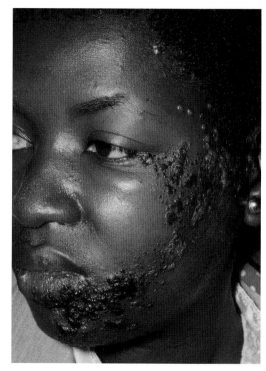

Fig. 4.27 Mandibular zoster: involvement of the mandibular branch of the fifth cranial nerve affects the chin and half of the tongue (*see* Fig. 6.04, p. 143)

Chronic erythematous rash on the face

5

Face

Chronic erythematous lesions MACULES

Surface normal

Macules

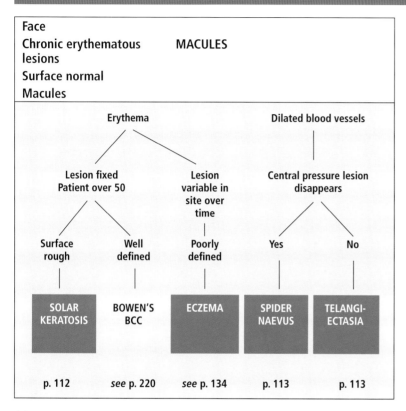

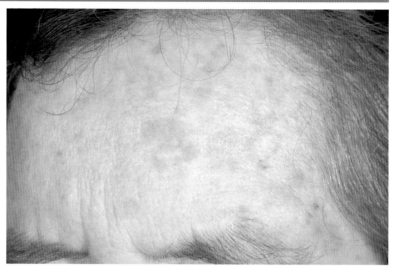

Fig. 5.01 Multiple solar keratoses on forehead: often misdiagnosed as eczema

SOLAR KERATOSIS

Solar keratoses may present as an area of fixed erythema on the face of a middle-aged or elderly fair-skinned individual who has had a lot of sun exposure in the past. They are often misdiagnosed (as eczema), but the key to the diagnosis is to feel the surface, which is rough. The individual lesions remain fixed over a period of time.

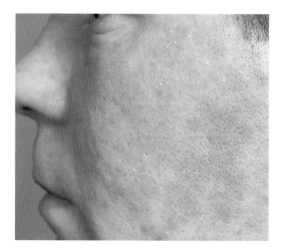

Fig. 5.02 Eczema on the face: the erythema may be variable in extent and time

SPIDER NAEVUS (SPIDER ANGIOMA)

A red papule with a central arteriole and peripheral radiating arms is a common normal finding especially in children. Pressure (use the end of a paper clip) on the central vessel results in obliteration of the lesion. Large numbers occur in pregnancy and in association with chronic liver disease.

TREATMENT: SPIDER NAEVUS

The central feeding vessel can be cauterised with a 'cold point' or fine looped wire cautery or a Hyfrecator. This takes about 1 second so local anaesthetic is not necessary, unless the lesion is very large. The pulse dye laser is also effective – a single shot is all that is necessary, and if available it may be preferable in children.

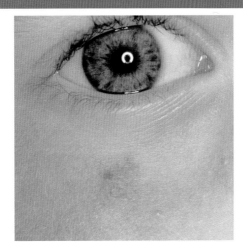

Fig. 5.03 Spider naevus

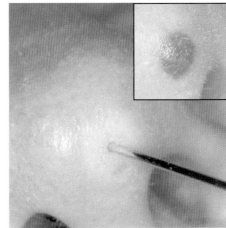

Fig. 5.04 Spider naevus: central arteriole compressed (insert before compression)

TELANGIECTASIA

Small areas of visibly dilated blood vessels where there is no central vessel feeding are called telangiectasia. They are very common on the face due to weathering and may be associated with rosacea, scleroderma and the use of potent topical steroids.

TREATMENT: TELANGIECTASIA

Any vascular laser such as the pulsed dye or KTP laser will remove visible telangiectasia on the face (*see* p. 66). The KTP laser does not cause bruising, so patients can continue to work. Several treatments may be needed at 6-weekly intervals. The patient should not have a suntan otherwise post-inflammatory hyperpigmentation can occur.

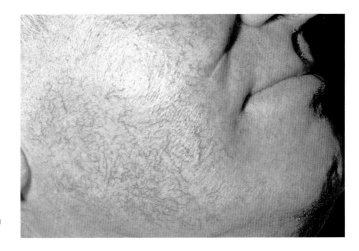

Fig. 5.05 Telangiectasia on the cheek

Face
Chronic erythematous rash
Surface normal
(Single/few lesions, *see* p. 262)

MULTIPLE PAPULES AND PUSTULES

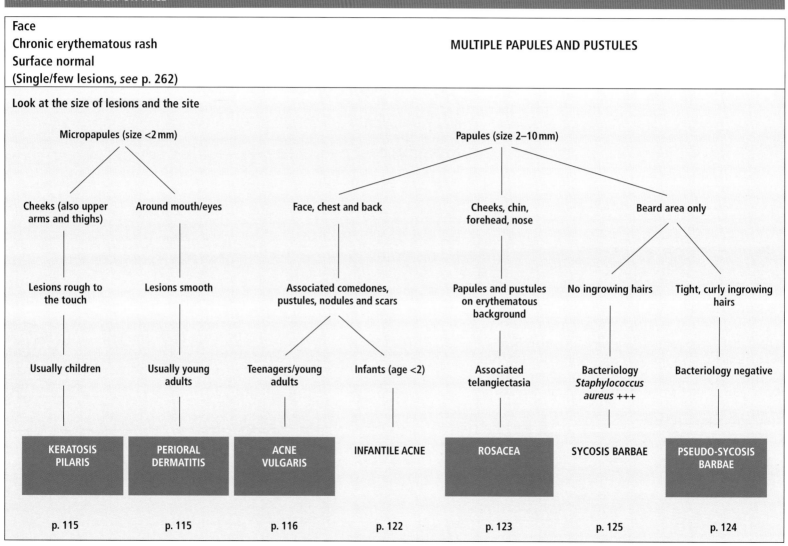

Look at the size of lesions and the site

Micropapules (size <2 mm)

Papules (size 2–10 mm)

Cheeks (also upper arms and thighs)

Around mouth/eyes

Face, chest and back

Cheeks, chin, forehead, nose

Beard area only

Lesions rough to the touch

Lesions smooth

Associated comedones, pustules, nodules and scars

Papules and pustules on erythematous background

No ingrowing hairs

Tight, curly ingrowing hairs

Usually children

Usually young adults

Teenagers/young adults

Infants (age <2)

Associated telangiectasia

Bacteriology *Staphylococcus aureus* +++

Bacteriology negative

KERATOSIS PILARIS

PERIORAL DERMATITIS

ACNE VULGARIS

INFANTILE ACNE

ROSACEA

SYCOSIS BARBAE

PSEUDO-SYCOSIS BARBAE

p. 115

p. 115

p. 116

p. 122

p. 123

p. 125

p. 124

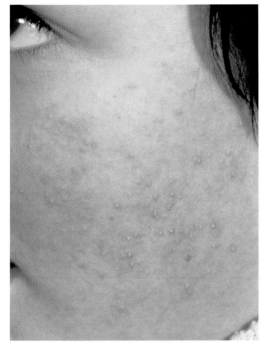

Fig. 5.06 Keratosis pilaris: redness associated with pinhead follicular plugs

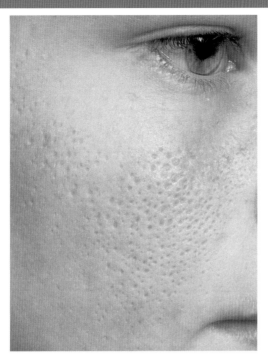

Fig. 5.07 Atrophoderma vermiculata

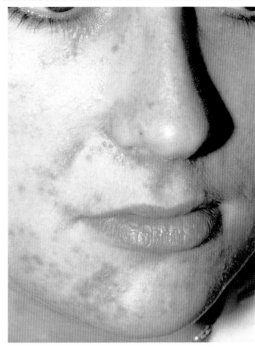

Fig. 5.08 Perioral dermatitis

KERATOSIS PILARIS

Keratosis pilaris may affect the cheeks and eyebrows in children. Redness associated with pinhead follicular plugs is seen, and as the plugs are shed, atrophy can occur (**atrophoderma vermiculata**). On the (outer) eyebrows this is associated with loss of hair follicles. In some cases the forehead may be involved. These changes are usually accompanied by typical keratosis pilaris on the upper arms and thighs (*see* Fig. 9.144, p. 324).

PERIORAL DERMATITIS

Perioral dermatitis is a condition of young adults who have been applying moderately potent or potent topical corticosteroids to the face. Minute red papules and pustules appear around the mouth, typically sparing the skin immediately adjacent to the lips. Occasionally it occurs around the eyes (periocular dermatitis). In some cases there is no history of topical steroid use.

TREATMENT: PERIORAL DERMATITIS

Stop any topical steroid use. This may lead to worsening of the rash initially; warn the patient about this and tell him or her on no account to use the topical steroid again. Oxytetracycline 250 mg bid (on an empty stomach) or lymecycline 408 mg daily taken for 6 weeks usually speeds up its resolution.

ACNE VULGARIS

Acne is a disease of the pilosebaceous unit. The hallmark of the disease is the comedo, a single blocked follicle. Everyone gets some acne. In girls it may appear before menstruation commences, sometimes as early as 9 years of age. In both sexes the peak incidence is 13–16 years, although it may continue into the 20s, 30s and occasionally later. Acne occurs on the face, chest and back, depending on the distribution of the sebaceous follicles in that individual.

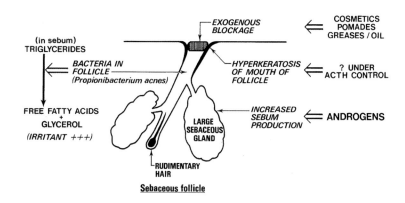

Fig. 5.09 Aetiology of acne

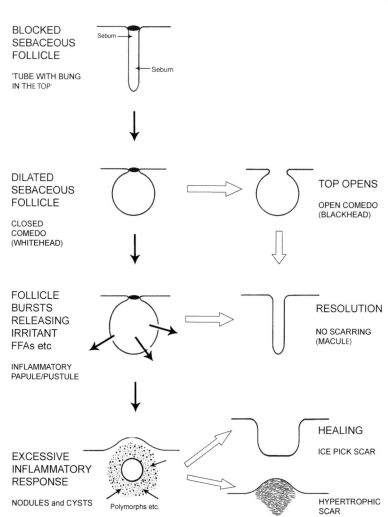

Fig. 5.10 Diagram to show the evolution of acne lesions

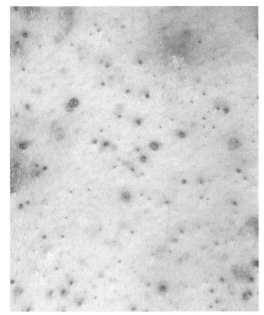

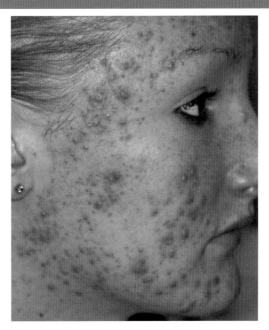

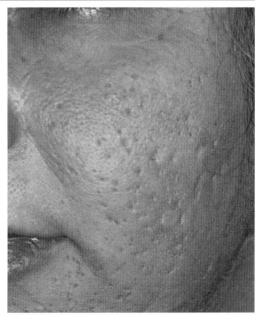

Fig. 5.11 Open and closed comedones with some inflammatory lesions

Fig. 5.12 Typical acne with papules, pustules and few comedones

Fig. 5.13 Ice pick scarring following acne that has resolved

The factors involved in the aetiology are shown in Fig. 5.09. The evolution of acne lesions from a blocked sebaceous follicle is shown in Fig. 5.10. Genetic factors are important in determining the severity, duration and clinical pattern. Recent evidence suggests that diet can influence acne, with high glycaemic loads and excess dairy consumption aggravating severity. The black colour of open comedones is due to melanin, not dirt.

The diagnosis of acne is usually easy, but comedones should be present before it is made. Comedones, papules, pustules, nodules, cysts and scars on the face or trunk of a young person are unique to acne, but occasionally folliculitis or even a papular form of eczema can mimic acne. Multiple epidermoid cysts may be confused with severe nodulocystic acne. Rosacea looks similar on the face but affects an older population. There are no comedones, and the papules and pustules remain the same size and occur over a general erythematous background (*see* Fig. 5.23). In perioral dermatitis there are no comedones, and tiny papules and pustules occur around the mouth (*see* Fig. 5.08).

SUMMARY OF TREATMENT OF ACNE VULGARIS

| | COMEDONAL ACNE | INFLAMMATORY ACNE | | |
		Mild	Moderate	Severe
Lesions	Comedones only	Comedones, papules and pustules	Papules and pustules	Nodules and cysts
First Choice	Topical retinoid e.g. adapalene, isotretinoin, tretinoin (not available in UK)	Topical retinoid plus oral tetracycline e.g. oxytetracycline, lymecycline, doxycycline	Any oral tetracycline for 6 months e.g. oxytetracycline, lymecycline, doxycycline	Oral isotretinoin (urgent referral to dermatologist)
Alternatives	Azelaic acid Benzoyl peroxide	Benzoyl peroxide plus topical antibiotic	Oral isotretinoin if acne persistent over 6 months	High-dose oral antibiotic plus topical retinoid/benzoyl peroxide
Female alternative	As above	As above	Oral anti-androgen plus topical retinoid	Oral isotretinoin plus oral contraceptive
Maintenance	Topical retinoid or benzoyl peroxide			

TREATMENT: ACNE VULGARIS

1. Topical therapy

Topical therapies are slow to work and will not induce complete eradication. They are designed to prevent acne, so should be used daily at night-time regardless of how the skin looks, as opposed to applying to spots that are already present in the hope of clearing them quicker.

Squeezing with the fingers should be avoided, since this can convert a comedo into an inflammatory papule. Female patients can use make-up to cover their spots during the daytime, but they must wash it off at night so that the follicles do not become blocked.

COMEDONES

Keratolytic agents remove the surface keratin and unplug the follicular openings. Retinoids are the most effective, for example:
- adapalene 0.1% cream or gel (Differin)
- isotretinoin 0.05% gel (Isotrex[UK])

Instruction for the use of keratolytic agents
Before going to bed the patient should wash the skin with soap and water (medicated washes are not any better) and then apply the weakest strength of retinoid cream or benzoyl peroxide. Build up slowly by applying to a small area initially or by short contact and rinsing off after a few minutes' application. Emphasise the need to induce tolerance to side effects and that there is a slow onset in benefit. Online advice and application videos are available from various pharmaceutical companies.

If the skin becomes too sore, stop the treatment for a few days and then restart on alternate nights. In the morning, if the skin becomes dry apply a non-greasy moisturiser. Increase the strength of the keratolytic if side effects are tolerated.

Ultraviolet light has a similar effect and a suntan tends to hide acne spots.

INFLAMMATORY LESIONS
If **inflammatory lesions** are present as well as the comedones, use:
- benzoyl peroxide (2.5%, 5%, 10%) as a cream, lotion or gel
- benzoyl peroxide combined (5%) with

 — 1% clindamycin (Duac[UK])
 — 0.5% potassium hydroxyquinoline sulphate (Quinoderm)
 note that benzoyl peroxide can bleach bed linen and clothing
- 0.1% adapalene cream or gel (Differin)
- 15%–20% azelaic acid cream (Azelex[USA], Finacea[UK], Skinoren[UK]).

Topical antibiotics
- Erythromycin (Stiemycin[UK], Zineryt[UK])
- Clindamycin (Dalacin T[UK], Zindaclin[UK])

These work nearly as well as systemic antibiotics but have the disadvantage of causing resistant bacteria. Using a combination such as Duac (clindamycin and benzoyl peroxide) can reduce this. They are useful in pregnancy, as there is negligible systemic absorption. There is no evidence that combining topical and systemic antibiotics is beneficial.

2. Systemic antibiotics

A single daily dose of lymecycline 408 mg or doxycycline 100 mg is preferred by teenagers over oxytetracycline 500 mg bid because the latter has to be taken 30 minutes before or 2 hours after food. The cost benefit of oxytetracycline is likely to be outweighed by probable lack of compliance. Maintenance treatment must be continued until the acne gets better spontaneously, however long that is.

Do not use tetracyclines in those under the age of 12, in females who are pregnant or breastfeeding (it causes staining of teeth in the foetus and in children) or if renal function is impaired. Side effects are few – diarrhoea and vaginal candidiasis. At this dose they do not interfere with the absorption of the contraceptive pill, although extra precautions are needed for the first month of treatment as the gut flora changes.

Erythromycin 500 mg bid or trimethoprim 200–300 mg bid are useful alternatives. Treatment with antibiotics should be given for at least 6 months.

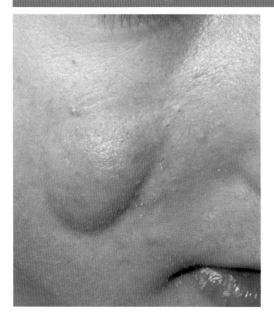

Fig. 5.14 Acne cyst: this can be injected with 10 mg/mL triamcinolone, which will reduce the size

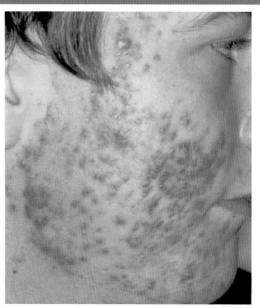

Fig. 5.15 Severe acne before treatment with isotretinoin

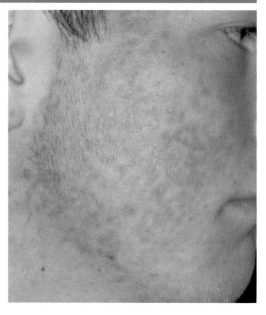

Fig. 5.16 Same patient as Fig. 5.15 after 4 months' treatment with isotretinoin

3. Anti-androgens

Anti-androgens are useful in female patients if antibiotics have not worked and they are already on a contraceptive pill. They should be avoided in patients with a family history of thromboembolic disease or personal history of hemiplegic migraine. Co-cyprindiol (Dianette) contains 2 mg of cyproterone acetate plus 35 µg of oestrogen. It will act as a contraceptive pill as well as an anti-acne agent. The maximum effect does not occur for 2–3 months and treatment needs to be continued long term.

4. Isotretinoin

INDICATIONS FOR ORAL ISOTRETINOIN
- Severe acne that will lead to permanent scarring
- Acne that has not responded to 6 months or more of oral antibiotics or anti-androgens
- Patients who are depressed by the state of their skin (even though isotretinoin has been associated with depressive episodes, if the acne is the cause of the depression, then its use is likely to be beneficial; close psychiatric follow-up is advised)

(cont)

- Persistent low-grade acne in patients over the age of 30
- Patients with acne excoriée

Isotretinoin is given as a single daily dose (0.5–1 mg/kg body weight/day) with food for 4–6 months (120 mg/kg total course dose). Early use can prevent scarring. A single course of treatment gives long-term remission (permanent in over 70% of individuals). Recurrence is more likely with lower doses or incomplete courses. For the side effects of isotretinoin, *see* p. 50. Female patients (of childbearing age) should be on established contraception during the course and for 1 month after stopping. Pregnancy testing before (and during) treatment is recommended.

Isolated acne cysts can be injected with 10 mg/mL triamcinolone.

DRUG- AND CHEMICAL-INDUCED ACNE

A rash that looks like acne occurring in the wrong site or in the wrong age group may be due to drugs, chemicals or systemic hormonal imbalance. Anabolic steroids (which can be purchased on the internet for bodybuilding), corticosteroids (including pituitary tumour and adrenal causes) or isoniazid may worsen or precipitate acne. Chlorinated aromatic hydrocarbons used in insecticides, fungicides and wood preservatives cause severe acne, which may continue after exposure has ceased. Insoluble cutting oils, coal tars, corticosteroids and cosmetics may induce acne when applied topically to the skin (*see* Fig. 5.19).

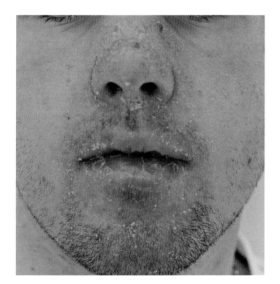

Fig. 5.17 Dry lips and skin during isotretinoin treatment

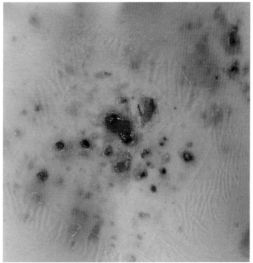

Fig. 5.18 Pyogenic granuloma-like lesions on chest during treatment with isotretinoin

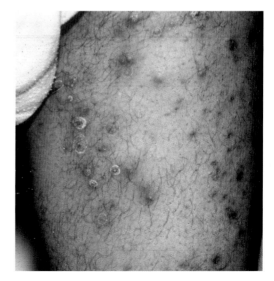

Fig. 5.19 Oil acne on thigh

INFANTILE ACNE

Acne is occasionally seen in boys in the first 2 years of life. It is confined to the face, with comedones, papules, pustules and nodules. It gets better spontaneously and is presumably due to maternal androgens. It is not seen in girls.

TREATMENT: INFANTILE ACNE

A trial of topical antibiotics is worthwhile but systemic antibiotics for 4–6 months are usually needed. All forms of tetracycline are contraindicated because they stain developing teeth. Co-trimoxazole paediatric suspension 240 mg bid or erythromycin 125 mg bid can be used, although the latter needs replacing weekly. If there are only comedones present a keratolytic agent can be used.

STEROID ROSACEA

Application of potent topical fluorinated steroids to the face can result in a rosacea-like rash. Telangiectasia is the most obvious feature, although small papules and pustules may also be present.

TREATMENT: STEROID ROSACEA

The topical steroids must be stopped or the rash will not get better. Usually when the steroids are stopped the rash gets very much worse. You will need to warn the patient about this and it is a good idea to see him or her 3 days later for reassurance or he or she may be tempted to restart the topical steroid.

The resolution of the rash can be speeded up by taking oxytetracycline 250 mg bid or lymecycline 408 mg daily for 6 weeks. If the patient wants to use a topical preparation for dry skin or itching, prescribe a moisturiser that can be used as often as he or she likes.

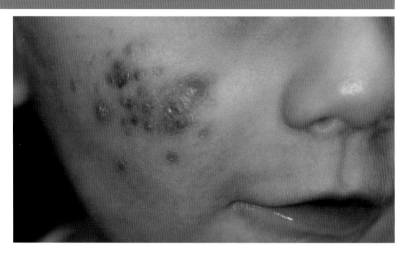

Fig. 5.20 Infantile acne

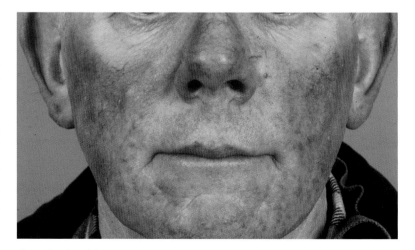

Fig. 5.21 Steroid rosacea

ROSACEA

Rosacea is a rash that looks like acne but on a red background. Red patches (erythema and telangiectasia) occur on the cheeks, chin, forehead and tip of nose. On top of this there are papules and pustules, but no comedones. If the patient is undressed, papules and pustules may be seen on the upper trunk as well. Rosacea affects women more commonly than men, and the main incidence is over the age of 40 (although it can occur at any age). Complications, such as sore, red eyes (blepharitis, conjunctivitis and keratitis), chronic lymphoedema of the face (*see* Fig. 5.24) and rhinophyma (*see* Fig. 5.25) occur more commonly in men.

Rosacea needs to be distinguished from acne, seborrhoeic eczema and perioral dermatitis. Acne occurs at a younger age and there should be comedones present as well as papules and pustules. Seborrhoeic eczema may be confused with rosacea. Seborrhoeic eczema is scaly, there are no pustules and the nasolabial folds rather than cheeks are affected; scaling will also be present in the scalp and possibly elsewhere (*see* p. 135). Perioral dermatitis (*see* p. 115) occurs around the mouth in young adults. Systemic lupus erythematous (*see* p. 131) causes redness of the face but there are no papules or pustules and the patient is usually unwell.

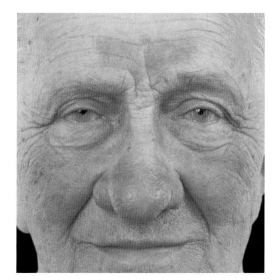

Fig. 5.22 Erythematous rosacea showing distribution: flushing and redness are the main features

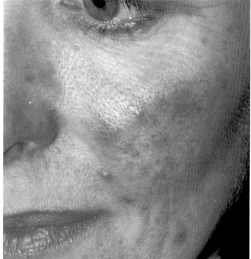

Fig. 5.23 Papulopustular rosacea on cheek: papules and pustules on background erythema

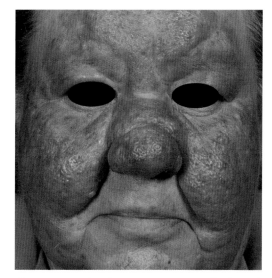

Fig. 5.24 Lymphoedematous rosacea on cheeks and nose with overgrowth of sebaceous tissue

TREATMENT: ROSACEA

The papular form of rosacea responds well to broad-spectrum antibiotics, but how they work is not understood. Oxytetracycline or lymecycline for 2 months are the best options. One course clears up a third of patients; another third respond to a second course; while a third may need more long-term therapy. There is no harm in giving a tetracycline indefinitely if necessary.

Other options include erythromycin 250 mg bid, or metronidazole 200 mg tid. If you do not want to use a systemic antibiotic, 0.75% metronidazole cream (Rosex^UK) or gel applied twice a day is effective in some instances. Minocycline should not be used, as long-term use can lead to blue-grey pigmentation on the face (see Fig. 1.74, p. 15).

Telangiectasia alone does not respond to oral antibiotics but can be treated with a vascular laser (see p. 65). Redness is more difficult to treat but intense pulsed light therapy (see p. 68) can be very effective. It is not available on the National Health Service.

If flushing is a problem, the patient should reduce the things that induce it, such as hot drinks, spicy foods, and so forth. Clonidine 25–50 mg bid may be helpful.

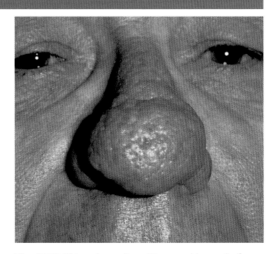

Fig. 5.25 Rhinophyma in a 68-year-old man before shaving off the excess tissue

RHINOPHYMA

Enlargement of the skin of the nose due to hyperplasia of the sebaceous glands can occur in individuals with rosacea. Contrary to popular belief it is not associated with excessive alcohol intake.

TREATMENT: RHINOPHYMA

First treat any active rosacea. The excess sebaceous tissue can then be shaved off under a local or general anaesthetic using a suitable electrocautery machine or a carbon dioxide laser. Provided the shave is no deeper than the base of the sebaceous glands, complete healing without scarring occurs in 4 weeks.

PSEUDO-SYCOSIS BARBAE

Pseudo-sycosis barbae is a condition caused by ingrowing hairs in the beard area. It occurs in men with tight, curly hair. The inflammatory papules and pustules are due to a foreign body reaction to the ingrowing hair.

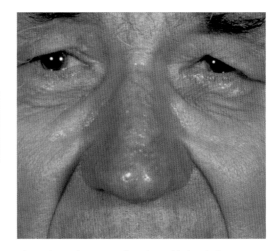

Fig. 5.26 After 4 weeks when skin healed

TREATMENT: PSEUDO-SYCOSIS BARBAE

This is not an infection, so antibiotics are not needed. If the patient will grow a beard or put up with a short stubble by shaving less closely, the hairs will uncurl as they get longer and the problem will be solved. The only other alternative is to persuade a partner to uncurl the ingrowing hairs with a needle each day, which is both time-consuming and tedious.

SYCOSIS BARBAE

This is folliculitis of the beard area caused by infection with *S. aureus*. Shaving results in spread and inoculation of the bacteria over the beard area. The organism is often cultured from the nose as well as the infected follicles. It occurs only in men who shave, and it presents with follicular papules and pustules in the beard area.

TREATMENT: SYCOSIS BARBAE

Take swabs for bacteriology culture from a pustule and from the anterior nares before starting treatment. Start with flucloxacillin 500 mg qid orally for 7 days. If staphylococci are grown from the nose, apply topical mupirocin (Bactroban) qid for 2 weeks. Recurrent infection may require long-term antibiotics for 6 months or more with erythromycin 500 mg bid or co-trimoxazole 480–960 mg bid.

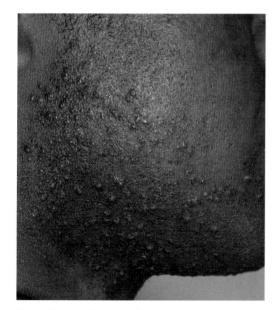

Fig. 5.27 Pseudo-sycosis barbae

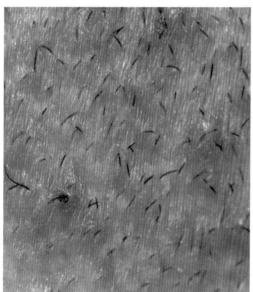

Fig. 5.28 Pseudo-sycosis barbae: close-up of ingrowing hairs

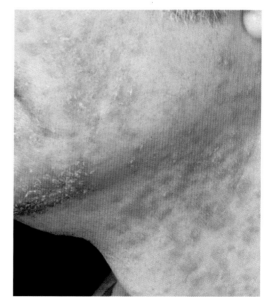

Fig. 5.29 Sycosis barbae

Face
Chronic erythematous rash
Normal surface
Well-defined patches, plaques, nodules

PATCHES, PLAQUES AND NODULES
WELL-DEFINED BORDER

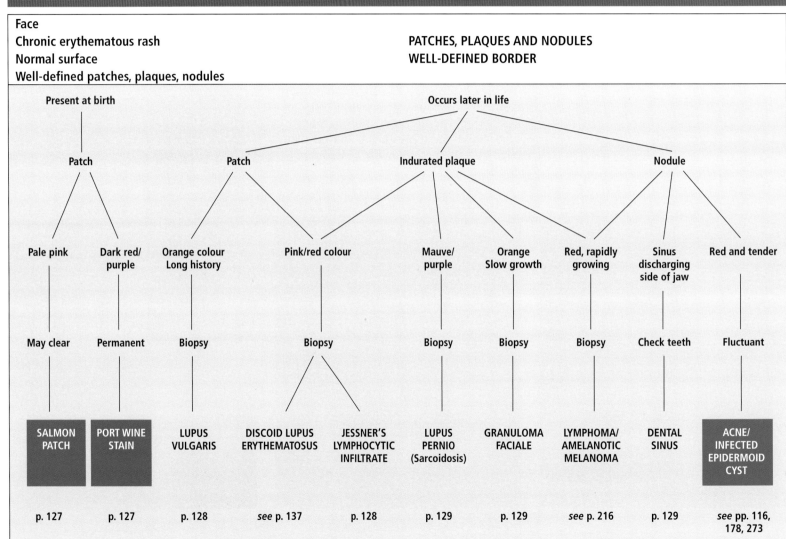

SALMON PATCH (NAEVUS FLAMMEUS)

This is a pale pink patch that has been present since birth and is situated on the nape of the neck, forehead or eyelid. Pressure over the area will cause blanching, showing that it is due to dilated blood vessels. Those on the face usually disappear during the first year of life; those on the nape of the neck do not, usually persisting throughout life. Often the occipital patch is not noticed unless there has been hair loss at this site. No treatment is needed because it is usually covered by hair.

PORT WINE STAIN (CAPILLARY MALFORMATION)

A permanent, more obvious and cosmetically disfiguring birthmark, being darker in colour than a salmon patch. It is present at birth and is usually unilateral. It increases in size only in proportion with growth. Port wine stains are very variable in size and colour. They tend to darken with age and may develop papules within them. If involving trigeminal (V^1) area, the port wine stain may rarely be associated with ocular and intracranial angiomas, sometimes resulting in blindness, focal epilepsy, hemiplegia or mental retardation (Sturge–Weber syndrome). Palpable segmental capillary malformations have increased association with internal abnormalities and should be referred for imaging and specialist investigation.

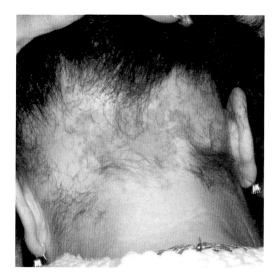

Fig. 5.30 Naevus flammeus on occiput

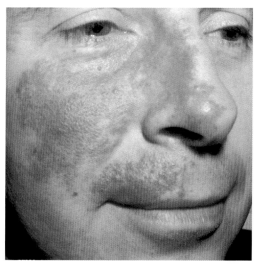

Fig. 5.31 Port wine stain, before laser treatment

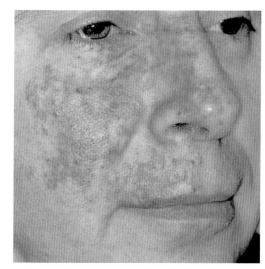

Fig. 5.32 Port wine stain after 15 treatments with the pulsed dye laser: improved but not cleared

TREATMENT: PORT WINE STAIN

> The pulsed dye laser is the treatment of choice, although results are variable. Only 10% of patients get complete clearance. The majority respond but do not totally clear (*see* Figs 5.31 and 5.32). Recurrence can occur later. Treatment is painful, so children will need a general anaesthetic. If laser treatment is not successful or possible, then cosmetic camouflage can be used to hide the mark.

TREATMENT: LUPUS VULGARIS

> Triple therapy as for pulmonary tuberculosis: isoniazid 300 mg/day single dose, rifampicin 600 mg/day single dose and pyrazinamide 20 mg/kg body weight three to four times day or ethambutol 15 mg/kg weight as single dose. After 2 months two drugs can be used for the next 4 months, usually isoniazid and rifampicin. This treatment is usually instigated via respiratory teams with monitoring schemes in place.

LUPUS VULGARIS

Lupus vulgaris is a chronic tuberculous infection of the skin. A slowly enlarging orange-pink plaque is typical. Nowadays it is exceedingly rare but it is a diagnosis that still needs to be considered. Confirm the diagnosis by biopsy.

JESSNER'S LYMPHOCYTIC INFILTRATE

Fixed, red, indurated plaque(s) with a smooth, non-scaly surface are scattered over the face or trunk. Individual lesions are round, oval or serpiginous in outline. The diagnosis can be confirmed by taking a skin biopsy, which shows a dense perivascular lymphocytic infiltrate in the dermis. A biopsy will distinguish this condition from discoid lupus erythematosus and a lymphoma. It tends to be unresponsive to treatment but antimalarials (*see* discoid lupus erythematosus, p. 137) can be tried.

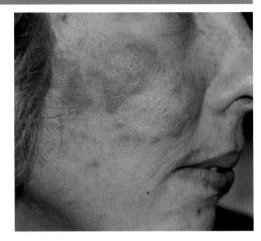

Fig. 5.34 Jessner's lymphocytic infiltrate

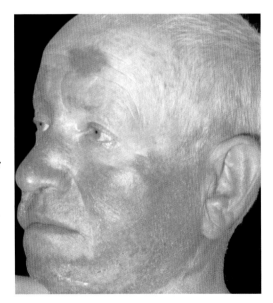

Fig. 5.33 Lupus vulgaris: this orange patch had been present for 40 years and was assumed to be a birthmark

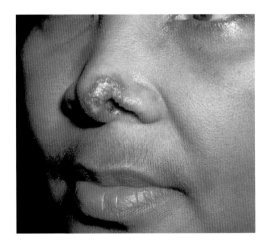

Fig. 5.35 Lupus pernio in black skin

SARCOIDOSIS – LUPUS PERNIO

Around a quarter of patients with sarcoid have skin involvement. Sarcoid of the skin can present with macules, papules, patches and plaques. They can be red, orange or purple in colour. On the face the commonest appearance is of a mauve/purple plaque (lupus pernio) on the nose or cheek. Sarcoid seems to be commoner in black skin. Diagnosis is made by skin biopsy, and if positive, look for evidence of sarcoid elsewhere.

TREATMENT: SARCOIDOSIS

Refer the patient to a dermatologist and respiratory physician to confirm the diagnosis and to look for sarcoid elsewhere. For multi-system disease the patient will need systemic steroids; this will also improve the skin lesions. Steroid-sparing regimens include methotrexate (10–25 mg/week), azathioprine (100–150 mg/day), hydroxychloroquine (200 mg bid) or acitretin (25 mg/day). If there is only lupus pernio, inject triamcinalone (5 mg/mL) intradermally every 4–6 weeks. Err on the side of caution because steroid-induced atrophy of the skin may be unsightly and permanent.

GRANULOMA FACIALE

Granuloma faciale is characterised by a chronic nodule or indurated plaque with an orange colour and prominent follicular openings. Histologically both a granuloma and a vasculitis are present.

DENTAL SINUS

This is due to a tooth abscess that discharges through to the skin on the cheek, chin or under the jaw. The diagnosis can be confirmed by looking in the mouth, where a rotten tooth is usually seen. The offending tooth needs to be removed.

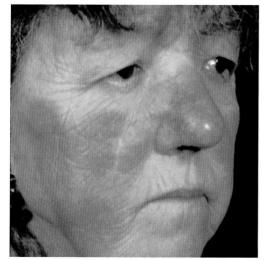

Fig. 5.36 Lupus pernio

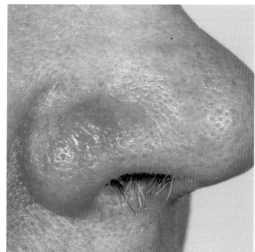

Fig. 5.37 Granuloma faciale

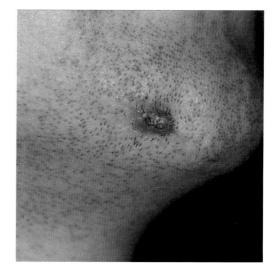

Fig. 5.38 Dental sinus from rotten pre-molar tooth

Face
Chronic erythematous rash
Normal/smooth surface
Poorly defined patches/plaques

PATCHES AND PLAQUES
POORLY DEFINED BORDER

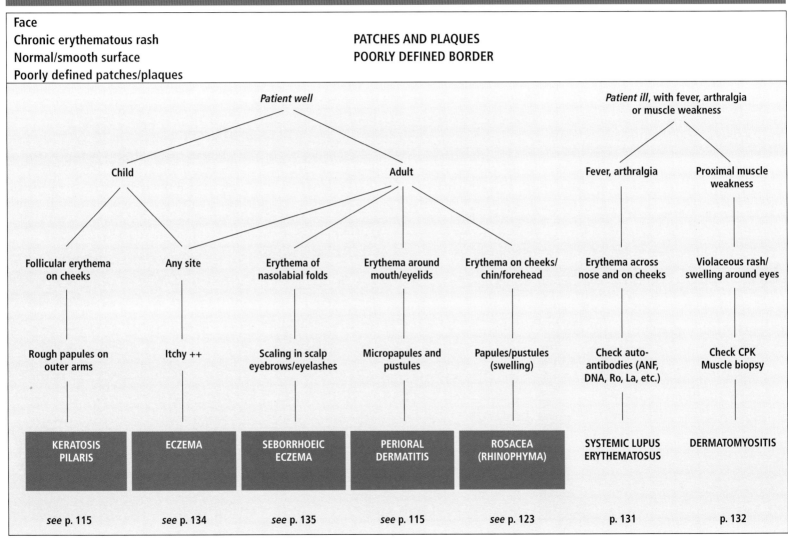

Patient well

Child

Adult

Patient ill, with fever, arthralgia
or muscle weakness

Fever, arthralgia

Proximal muscle
weakness

Follicular erythema
on cheeks

Any site

Erythema of
nasolabial folds

Erythema around
mouth/eyelids

Erythema on cheeks/
chin/forehead

Erythema across
nose and on cheeks

Violaceous rash/
swelling around eyes

Rough papules on
outer arms

Itchy ++

Scaling in scalp
eyebrows/eyelashes

Micropapules and
pustules

Papules/pustules
(swelling)

Check auto-
antibodies (ANF,
DNA, Ro, La, etc.)

Check CPK
Muscle biopsy

| KERATOSIS PILARIS | ECZEMA | SEBORRHOEIC ECZEMA | PERIORAL DERMATITIS | ROSACEA (RHINOPHYMA) | SYSTEMIC LUPUS ERYTHEMATOSUS | DERMATOMYOSITIS |

see p. 115   *see* p. 134   *see* p. 135   *see* p. 115   *see* p. 123   p. 131   p. 132

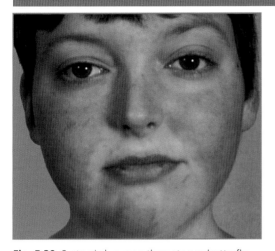

Fig. 5.39 Systemic lupus erythematosus: butterfly erythema on face

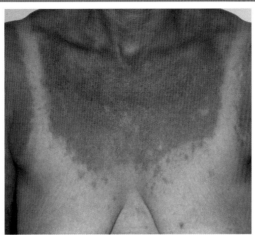

Fig. 5.40 Systemic lupus erythematosus showing photo-accentuated distribution

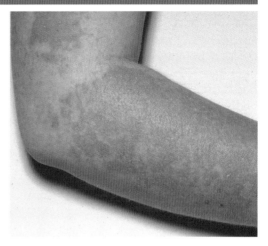

Fig. 5.41 Subacute cutaneous LE on forearm

SYSTEMIC LUPUS ERYTHEMATOSUS

An erythema on the face associated with fever and arthralgia in a female patient is suggestive of systemic lupus erythematosus (SLE). The rash characteristically occurs in a 'butterfly' distribution (cheeks and bridge of nose), but does not always do so. There is also nail-fold telangiectasia with ragged cuticles. Although the site may be similar to rosacea, there are no papules or pustules. The patient may have renal involvement, psychiatric or neurological symptoms, pericarditis, pleurisy or abdominal pain. Chilblains and Raynaud's phenomenon are likely. A positive anti-nuclear factor will confirm the diagnosis. Drugs such as procainamide, hydralazine, minocycline and the anti-TNF monoclonal biologic therapies can cause an illness identical to SLE. **Subacute cutaneous lupus erythematosus** looks like SLE or consists of non-scaly plaques on the face. There may be positive auto-antibodies, but systemic symptoms are absent.

TREATMENT: SYSTEMIC LUPUS ERYTHEMATOSUS

Referral to a specialist (rheumatologist, physician or dermatologist) with an interest in this condition is necessary. Treatment depends on which organs are involved. Severe disease involving the kidneys, pleura, pericardium, central nervous system or blood requires high doses of systemic steroids, starting with prednisolone 1.0 mg/kg/day. Steroid-sparing agents such as azathioprine, methotrexate or mycophenolate mofetil are used long term as well as newer biologics such as anti-TNFs and anti-IL6 (*see* p. 56).

The skin should be protected from the sun by using a high-factor sunscreen (SPF 30 or above).

If the joints are the main problem, non-steroidal anti-inflammatory drugs will be the treatment of choice. If it is only the skin and joints involved, hydroxychloroquine 200 mg bid or mepacrine 100 mg bid can be used.

DERMATOMYOSITIS

Weakness and tenderness of proximal muscles associated with a mauve or pink rash on the face, 'V' of the neck, upper eyelids or in lines along the backs of the fingers and over the metacarpal bones (*see* Fig. 5.43) is typical. There may be considerable oedema on the face and arms (*see* Fig. 5.42) and dilatation of the nail-fold capillaries (*see* Fig. 5.44). The diagnosis can be confirmed by measuring muscle enzymes (creatine phosphokinase), muscle biopsy or electromyography. In patients over the age of 40 there may be an associated internal malignancy.

TREATMENT: DERMATOMYOSITIS

Refer urgently to a dermatologist for diagnosis and treatment. A search for an internal malignancy is essential (especially carcinoma of the lung, stomach, ovary or breast); if found and treated successfully, the dermatomyositis will disappear. If the cancer is not curable it may be very difficult to control the dermatomyositis.

Initial treatment is with prednisolone 1.0 mg/kg/day. This is gradually reduced as the disease comes under control. Steroid-sparing agents such as azathioprine, methotrexate or mycophenolate mofetil may also be needed. Patients not responding to these may require high dose intravenous immunoglobulin as well.

Muscle enzyme levels can be used to monitor disease activity. In the acute phase rest is important; later, passive muscle exercises and physiotherapy will be needed.

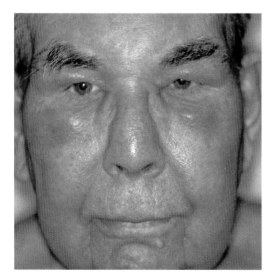

Fig. 5.42 Dermatomyositis: oedema of upper and lower eyelids

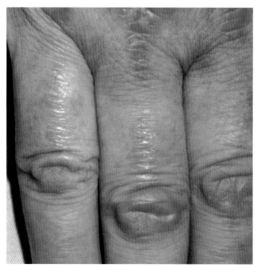

Fig. 5.43 Linear erythema along back of the fingers

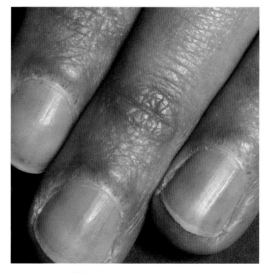

Fig. 5.44 Nail-fold telangiectasia seen in systemic lupus erythematosus and dermatomyositis

Face
Chronic erythematous rash   SCALY SURFACE
Scaly surface
Papules and plaques

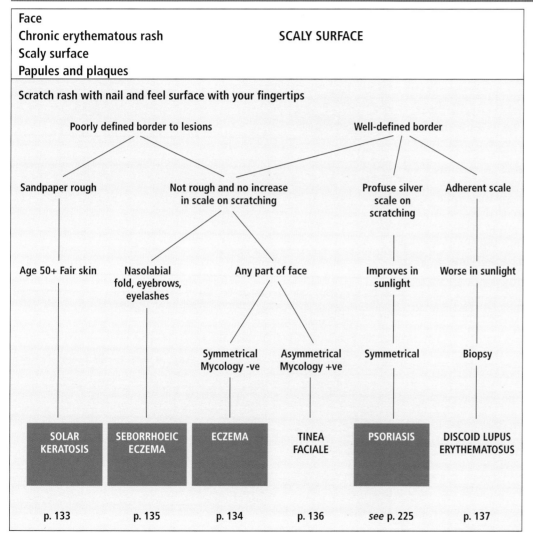

Scratch rash with nail and feel surface with your fingertips

Poorly defined border to lesions   Well-defined border

Sandpaper rough   Not rough and no increase   Profuse silver   Adherent scale
                         in scale on scratching   scale on
                                                            scratching

Age 50+ Fair skin   Nasolabial   Any part of face   Improves in   Worse in sunlight
                     fold, eyebrows,   sunlight
                     eyelashes

                                  Symmetrical   Asymmetrical   Symmetrical   Biopsy
                                  Mycology -ve   Mycology +ve

| SOLAR KERATOSIS | SEBORRHOEIC ECZEMA | ECZEMA | TINEA FACIALE | PSORIASIS | DISCOID LUPUS ERYTHEMATOSUS |

        p. 133   p. 135   p. 134   p. 136   see p. 225   p. 137

SOLAR KERATOSES

Widespread solar keratoses may be confused with eczema on the face but will feel rough to the touch. The patient will probably be over 50, have fair skin (burn rather than tan on sun exposure) and blue eyes. Often there will be a history of working out of doors or living abroad (20+ years ago). Solar elastosis (*see* p. 287) will be present – this is a yellowish discolouration of the skin with increased skin markings and follicular openings on the face, neck and back of the neck. These 'wrinkles' are not due to ageing per se but to long term sun damage.

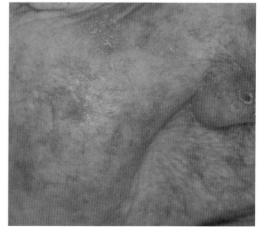

Fig. 5.45 Solar keratoses on face of elderly patient with sun-damaged type I fair skin

ECZEMA ON THE FACE

The most likely cause of poorly defined, red, scaly plaques on the face is chronic eczema. The distribution and age of the patient determine the type of eczema.

Atopic eczema. Eczema on the face in infants and children is likely to be due to atopic eczema. In infants it often starts on the cheeks and scalp before affecting the rest of the body, especially the anticubital and popliteal fossae (*see* p. 236). Atopic eczema persisting into adult life is often lichenified (*see* Fig. 5.48).

Allergic contact dermatitis may be due to cosmetics, nail varnish (from the fingernails touching the face), creams applied to the face and from airborne allergens such as cement dust or sawdust. Plastic and metal frames from glasses can result in a patch of eczema on the sides of the nose and behind the ears. All unexplained instances of facial eczema should be referred to a dermatologist for patch testing.

Seborrhoeic eczema on the face involves the nasolabial folds and hairy areas such as eyebrows, eyelids, scalp and beard.

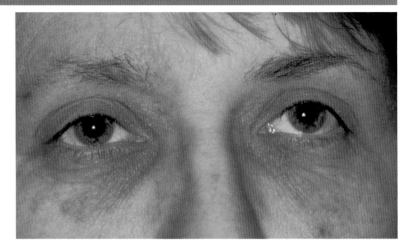

Fig. 5.46 Eczema around the eyes: a common pattern

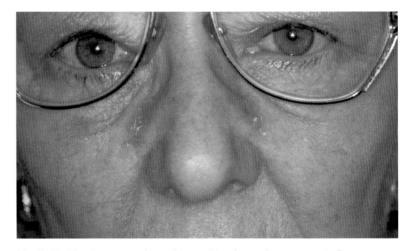

Fig. 5.47 Allergic contact dermatitis on side of nose from spectacle frames

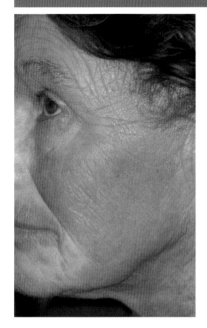

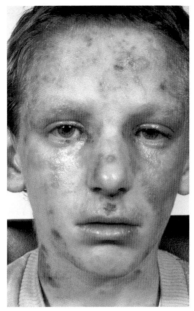

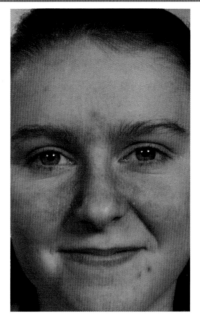

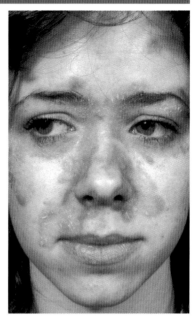

Fig. 5.48 Lichenified atopic eczema

Fig. 5.49 Atopic eczema on face of a 9-year-old boy

Fig. 5.50 Seborrhoeic eczema

Fig. 5.51 Psoriasis of the face

TREATMENT: ECZEMA ON THE FACE

On the face use only a weak[UK]/group 7[USA] topical steroid such as 1% hydrocortisone. Use an ointment if the skin is particularly dry or an allergic contact dermatitis is suspected (creams can contain preservatives that are potential sensitisers). Instead of soap use a wash product such as Dermol lotion, and moisturise with a leave-on emollient such as Cetroben, Dermol or Diprobase creams.

Tacrolimus 0.1% ointment and pimecrolimus cream are alternatives in atopic eczema (*see* p. 34), and can be used prophylactically twice a week.

SEBORRHOEIC ECZEMA

In adults this common type of eczema is due to an overgrowth of the yeast *Pityrosporum ovale*. It is diagnosed by its distribution on the skin (*see* Fig. 5.53) – scalp, eyebrows, eyelashes, nasolabial folds, external ear, centre of chest and centre of back (*see* also p. 201, 205). On the face you will see greasy scaling spreading out from the nasolabial folds onto the cheeks. The hairy areas are usually involved – eyebrows, eyelashes, hairy scalp and beard. Scaling can also be seen around the external auditory meatus and behind the ear (*see* Fig. 6.46, p. 163).

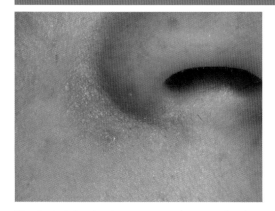

Fig. 5.52 Seborrhoeic eczema: erythema and scale in the nasolabial fold

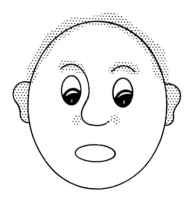

Fig. 5.53 Distribution of seborrhoeic eczema on the face

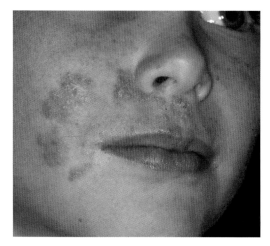

Fig. 5.54 Tinea around mouth caught from a puppy: always think of this diagnosis with an asymmetrical rash

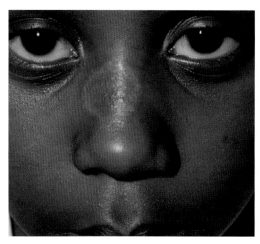

Fig. 5.55 Tinea on nose of black child

TREATMENT: SEBORRHOEIC ECZEMA

Only treat seborrhoeic eczema when it is present. Start with 2% ketoconazole (Nizoral) cream twice a day until it is clear. This will reduce the pityrosporum yeasts.

If it does not work use 1% hydrocortisone cream twice a day or 2% miconazole plus 1% hydrocortisone cream (Daktacort). Treat the scalp with ketoconazole shampoo (see p. 89).

TINEA ON THE FACE

Ringworm is uncommon on the face. It should be suspected if a red scaly rash is unilateral or very much more on one side than the other. It will have a well-demarcated edge, with relatively normal skin in the centre. It is often itchy and slowly gets bigger. The border needs to be scraped and the scale sent off for mycology (see p. 20).

TREATMENT: TINEA ON THE FACE

Apply either terbinafine (Lamasil) cream once daily for 7–10 days or an imidazole cream twice a day for 2 weeks. All the imidazoles work equally well. Systemic antifungals are not needed.

DISCOID LUPUS ERYTHEMATOSUS

Discoid lupus erythematosus is a benign form of lupus erythematosus where the skin is involved usually without any systemic involvement (although 5% of patients have autoantibodies). Females are more commonly affected than males and it usually starts between the ages of 25 and 40 years. Well-defined, red, scaly plaques occur on the face and scalp. The scale is quite different from that occurring in psoriasis or eczema. Scratching with the fingernail does not produce silver scaling as in psoriasis and the scale is rougher and more adherent than that of eczema. Follicular plugging, atrophy and a change in pigment (both hypo- and hyperpigmentation) may also be present. It is exacerbated by sunlight, so it often starts or worsens in the summer. The diagnosis should only be considered when more common causes of scaling on the face are excluded. On occasions indurated non-scaly plaques are seen and the diagnosis will need to be confirmed by skin biopsy.

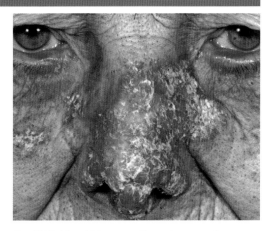

Fig. 5.56 Discoid lupus erythematosus: scaly plaques on face

TREATMENT: DISCOID LUPUS ERYTHEMATOSUS

Discoid lupus erythematosus is the only condition where a very potent[UK]/group 1[USA] topical steroid can be used on the face. 0.05% clobetasol propionate (Dermovate[UK], Temovate[USA]) ointment should be applied carefully to the plaques twice daily until they disappear. Only use while there are active lesions present (the plaques are red and scaly). It will not help atrophy or pigment change.

Discoid lupus erythematosus is also made worse by sunlight, so use a sunscreen (SPF 30+) in the summer. Topical 0.1% tacrolimus (Protopic) and pimecrolimus (Elidel) can be useful steroid-sparing agents in preventing flares but are rarely effective for acute flares.

If topical steroids do not help or if there are extensive lesions, use an antimalarial by mouth instead. Try hydroxychloroquine 200 mg bid or mepacrine 100 mg bid for at least 3 months.

Hydroxychloroquine can affect the retina, so check the visual acuity and fields yearly. It may also stain the nails a greyish-blue colour. Mepacrine makes the patient's skin and urine yellow and can also cause vomiting or diarrhoea. The patient should be warned about these side effects.

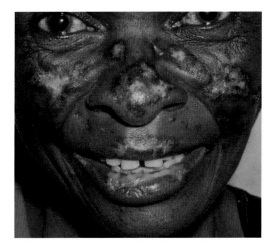

Fig. 5.57 Discoid lupus erythematosus in black skin with hypo- and hyperpigmentation

CRUST, EXUDATE OR EXCORIATED SURFACE

Face
Chronic erythematous rash
Crust, excoriated or eroded surface
Papules, plaques, erosions, ulcers

SURFACE CRUST, EROSION, EXCORIATION

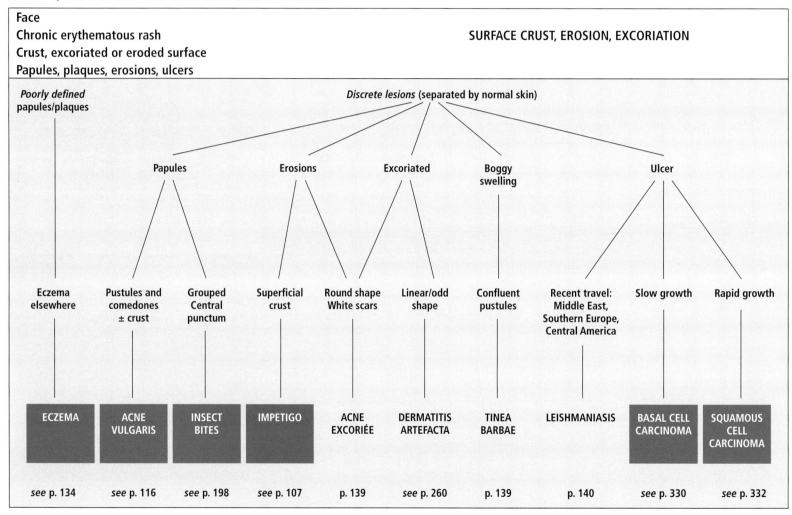

ECZEMA	ACNE VULGARIS	INSECT BITES	IMPETIGO	ACNE EXCORIÉE	DERMATITIS ARTEFACTA	TINEA BARBAE	LEISHMANIASIS	BASAL CELL CARCINOMA	SQUAMOUS CELL CARCINOMA
see p. 134	see p. 116	see p. 198	see p. 107	p. 139	see p. 260	p. 139	p. 140	see p. 330	see p. 332

ACNE EXCORIÉE

This variety of acne occurs predominantly in women over the age of 30. The acne is usually mild but most of the lesions are excoriated. Round or oval, white scars are the most obvious finding confirming that the condition is largely self-induced.

TREATMENT: ACNE EXCORIÉE

It usually responds well to low-dose isotretinoin (20 mg/day) on a long-term basis (*see* pp. 49 and 121). Adequate contraception is essential if this is going to be used.

TINEA BARBAE

Tine barbae is an uncommon infection due to animal ringworm (usually *Trichophyton verrucosum* from calves). It usually occurs in farm workers. A confluent boggy swelling is studded with multiple pustules. The hairs come out easily and can be examined for fungi. Secondary infection with staphylococci can produce a misleading positive bacterial culture.

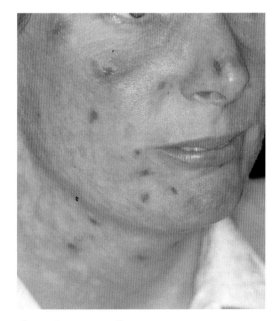

Fig. 5.58 Acne excoriée

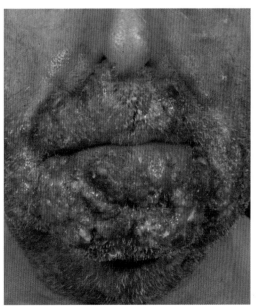

Fig. 5.59 Tinea barbae: kerion in beard area

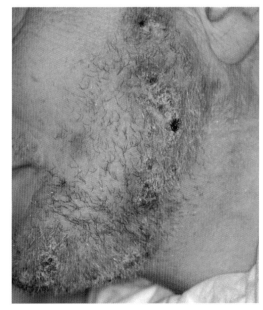

Fig. 5.60 Tinea barbae: crusting in beard area

TREATMENT: TINEA BARBAE

> Oral griseofulvin 500 mg daily with food for 4–6 weeks works better for animal ringworm than terbinafine.

LEISHMANIASIS

Leishmaniasis results from the bite of an infected sandfly. It is a common disease around the southern Mediterranean, in the Middle East, North Africa, India, Pakistan and Central and South America. A few weeks after the sandfly bite, a boil-like nodule appears at the site of the bite. It gradually flattens off to form a plaque, which may or may not ulcerate. One or more lesions appear on exposed sites – face, arms and legs. They are painless and heal spontaneously after about 1 year to leave a cribriform scar. Some patients with leishmaniasis develop a chronic form of the disease in which new granulomatous papules or plaques occur around the edge of the scar (lupoid leishmaniasis, *see* Fig. 5.62). This condition may continue for many years.

In Central and South America, a much more destructive picture is seen (New World leishmaniasis) with ulcerated nodules, and later systemic spread to mucous membranes (mucocutaneous leishmaniasis). Refer to a specialist for diagnosis and treatment.

TREATMENT: LEISHMANIASIS

> - Leave alone to heal spontaneously
> - Weekly intralesional injection with sodium stibogluconate (Pentostam) or N-methylglucamine antimonate (Glucantime) until healed
> - Intraveneous (through a peripherally inserted central catheter line) of sodium stibogluconate at a daily dose of 20 mg/kg body weight for 20 days; this is particularly recommended for New World leishmaniasis

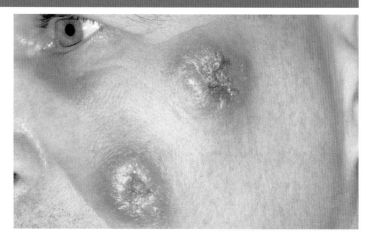

Fig. 5.61 Cutaneous leishmaniasis: ulcerated nodules on cheek

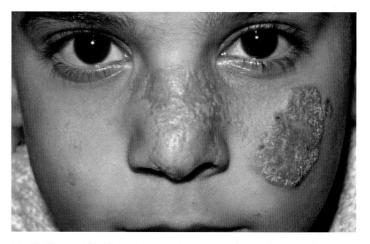

Fig. 5.62 Lupoid leishmaniasis on cheek, note the previous scarring on the nose

Mouth, tongue, lips and ears

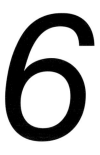

MOUTH

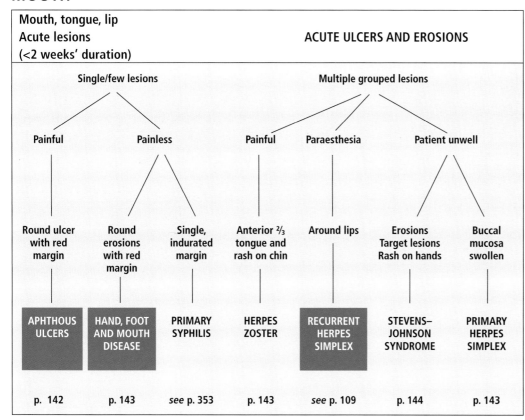

Mouth, tongue, lip
Acute lesions
(<2 weeks' duration)

ACUTE ULCERS AND EROSIONS

Single/few lesions

Painful — Round ulcer with red margin — **APHTHOUS ULCERS** — p. 142

Painless — Round erosions with red margin — **HAND, FOOT AND MOUTH DISEASE** — p. 143

Single, indurated margin — **PRIMARY SYPHILIS** — *see* p. 353

Multiple grouped lesions

Painful — Anterior ⅔ tongue and rash on chin — **HERPES ZOSTER** — p. 143

Paraesthesia — Around lips — **RECURRENT HERPES SIMPLEX** — *see* p. 109

Patient unwell — Erosions Target lesions Rash on hands — **STEVENS–JOHNSON SYNDROME** — p. 144

Buccal mucosa swollen — **PRIMARY HERPES SIMPLEX** — p. 143

TREATMENT: APHTHOUS ULCERS

This is a self-limiting condition that often needs no treatment. Most patients will use things like Bonjela (choline salicylate and cetalkonium chloride) for symptomatic relief. For more troublesome ulcers consider one of the following:

- 2% sodium cromoglicate nasal spray (Rynacrom) sprayed directly onto the ulcers three times a day – about 50% of patients find this extremely helpful; it is not known how it works
- Tetracycline mouthwash, 250 mg/5 mL, held in the mouth and swished around for about 5 minutes four to five times a day; do not use in children under 12, since it stains teeth
- 0.1% triamcinolone acetonide (Adcortyl) in Orabase applied to the ulcers three times a day
- Beclometasone dipropionate inhaler, 50 g/puff, can be sprayed on the ulcers several times a day until they heal
- 10% hydrocortisone in equal parts of glycerine and water as a mouthwash three times a day; the patient must spit it out after use rather than swallow it, to make sure that not too much steroid is absorbed
- 2.5% hydrocortisone sodium succinate (Corlan) pellet, held against the ulcer(s) until the pellet dissolves, twice daily.

APHTHOUS ULCERS

Aphthous ulcers are the commonest cause of recurrent mouth ulcers. The single or multiple small, round ulcers with a red margin last 7–10 days before healing spontaneously. They begin in the teens and may continue throughout life. Aphthous ulcers may be rarely associated with Crohn's disease, ulcerative colitis or coeliac disease.

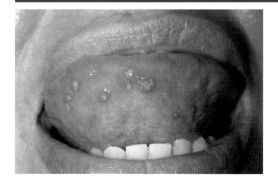

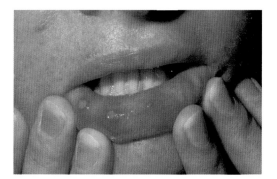

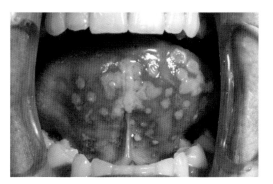

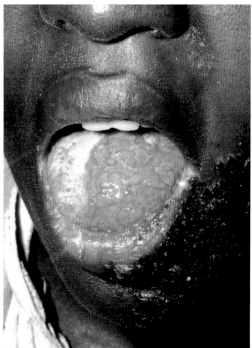

HAND, FOOT AND MOUTH DISEASE

This mild infection is due to Coxsackie virus A16. Round erosions with a red margin are seen in the mouth. They look like small aphthous ulcers but are associated with small, grey blisters with a red halo on the fingers and toes (*see* Fig. 13.03, p. 405). The condition gets better spontaneously in a few days.

PRIMARY HERPES SIMPLEX

Most primary infections with the herpes simplex virus occur in early childhood and are asymptomatic, with only a few vesicles/erosions on the hard palate or buccal mucosa. Occasionally it may cause an acute gingivostomatitis associated with fever and general malaise.

HERPES ZOSTER

Herpes zoster involving the mandibular branch of the fifth cranial nerve is uncommon, but it presents with unilateral vesicles and ulceration on the anterior two-thirds of the tongue, as well as the characteristic vesicles on the same side of the chin.

Fig. 6.01 (top left) Aphthous ulcers on the tongue

Fig. 6.02 (middle left) Hand, foot and mouth disease: blisters and erosions on lower lip

Fig. 6.03 (bottom left) Primary herpes simplex, blisters and erosions on tongue

Fig. 6.04 (above) Herpes zoster affecting the mandibular branch of the fifith cranial nerve: blisters and ulceration on anterior two-thirds of tongue and a rash on the side of the chin

STEVENS–JOHNSON SYNDROME

Erythema multiforme involving the mouth presents with multiple irregular erosions on the buccal mucosa. Extensive involvement of the mouth, lips, conjunctiva and genitalia is called Stevens–Johnson syndrome. The causes of this are the same as for erythema multiforme (*see* p. 174) but usually drugs (often co-trimoxazole) rather than infections are the cause. Toxic epidermal necrolysis (*see* p. 192), Stevens–Johnson syndrome and erythema multiforme are a clinical continuum of decreasing severity.

TREATMENT: STEVENS–JOHNSON SYNDROME

Many of these patients will need to be admitted to hospital because they are unable to eat or drink. Frequent mouth washes with glycerine and thymol (made up by dissolving a glycerine and thymol tablet in a tumbler of water) should be swished around the mouth for several minutes every hour, or applied on a cotton wool swab by a nurse if the patient cannot manage a mouthwash by him- or herself. This will keep the buccal mucosa relatively comfortable. If this is not done, the lips can stick together, which initially will make eating and drinking even more difficult, and will at some stage necessitate surgical separation. Benzydamine hydrochloride (Difflam) or chlorhexidine gluconate (Corsodyl) are alternative mouthwashes.

For the eyes, frequent bathing with normal saline and insertion of hypromellose eye drops (artificial tears) will be needed to keep them comfortable. If there are extensive skin lesions as well as extensive mucosal involvement, the patient may need nursing in a burns unit where there are facilities to prevent ulceration of the skin.

There is no evidence that systemic steroids are helpful.

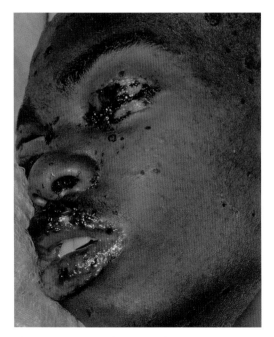

Fig. 6.06 Stevens–Johnson syndrome

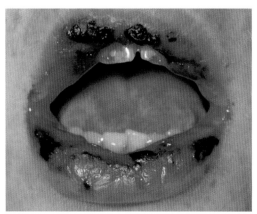

Fig. 6.05 Stevens–Johnson syndrome

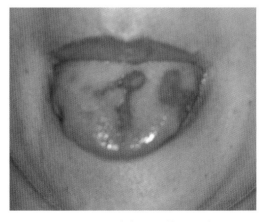

Fig. 6.07 Erythema multiforme affecting the tongue

Mouth
Ulcers and erosions
Chronic lesions (>2 weeks' duration)

CHRONIC MOUTH ULCERS

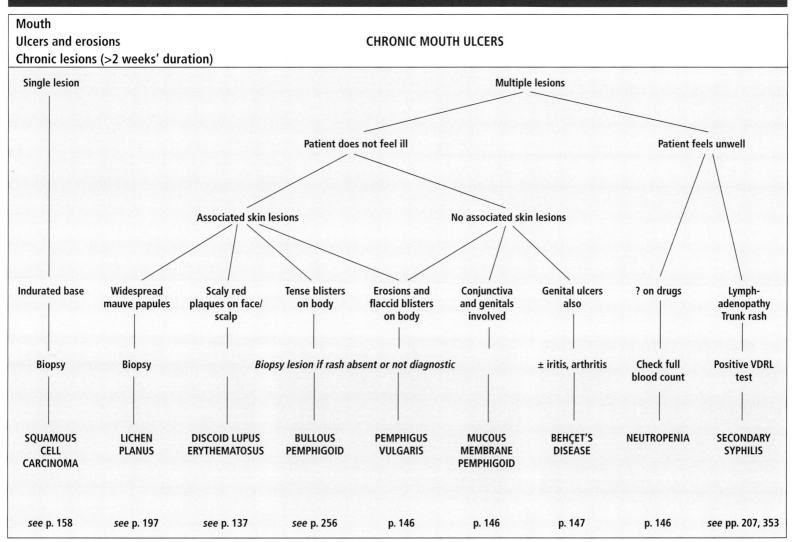

SQUAMOUS CELL CARCINOMA	LICHEN PLANUS	DISCOID LUPUS ERYTHEMATOSUS	BULLOUS PEMPHIGOID	PEMPHIGUS VULGARIS	MUCOUS MEMBRANE PEMPHIGOID	BEHÇET'S DISEASE	NEUTROPENIA	SECONDARY SYPHILIS

see p. 158   see p. 197   see p. 137   see p. 256   p. 146   p. 146   p. 147   p. 146   see pp. 207, 353

PEMPHIGUS VULGARIS

Blisters and erosions in the mouth are usually the first sign of pemphigus vulgaris; the rash often comes later (*see* p. 257).

MUCOUS MEMBRANE PEMPHIGOID

This is a rare autoimmune disease in which there are antibodies against the epidermal basement membrane. Mucous membranes (mouth, eyes and genitalia) are predominantly involved with blisters, erosions and scarring. Blisters can also occur on the skin adjacent to orifices. The diagnosis is usually made by looking in the eyes. Scarring and adhesions between the palpebral conjuctivae are characteristic, and can lead to blindness if not treated. **Bullous pemphigoid** less commonly involves the mucous membranes. The diagnosis is made from the characteristic skin rash (*see* p. 256).

TREATMENT: MUCOUS MEMBRANE PEMPHIGOID

Unlike bullous pemphigoid, mucous membrane pemphigoid does not respond well to systemic steroids. There is no single treatment that always works and it is a question of finding the right drug for any individual patient. Start with dapsone 50 mg tid, as this is the safest choice. It can cause haemolytic anaemia and/or methaemoglobinaemia, so check the full blood count after 1 week and every 2–3 months. To prevent this, also give the patient cimetidine 400 mg tid. If this fails to work cyclophosphamide 50 mg bid is more effective but you will need to check the full blood count regularly (monthly). A third alternative is azathioprine 50 mg tid. If there is scarring of the conjunctivae, it may sometimes be necessary to inject steroids intralesionally to inactivate the disease. All patients with this rare disorder should be under the care of a dermatologist or ophthalmologist.

BLOOD DYSCRASIA

Agranulocytosis and neutropenia can cause mouth ulcers. They may be the first manifestation of leukaemia, or they may be a side effect of cytotoxic drugs such as methotrexate.

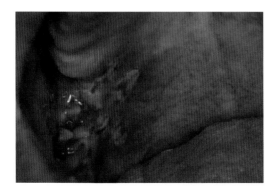

Fig. 6.08 Pemphigus: erosions on palate

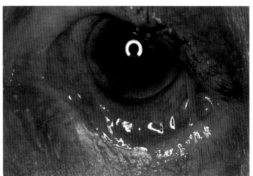

Fig. 6.09 Mucous membrane pemphigoid with conjunctival adhesions in corner of the eye

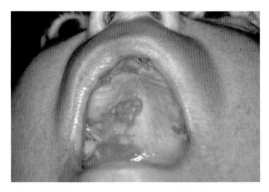

Fig. 6.10 Mucous membrane pemphigoid: ulcers on hard palate

BEHÇET'S SYNDROME

Behçet's syndrome is a rare condition mainly affecting young men. You should think of it in any patient with recurrent oral and genital ulceration. The ulcers tend to be larger, deeper and last longer than aphthous ulcers. There will also be one or more of the following: iritis, arthritis, thrombophlebitis, sterile pustules on the skin, erythema nodosum and meningoencephalitis. Such patients should be referred to hospital for treatment.

TREATMENT: BEHÇET'S SYNDROME

Since the cause is unknown, treatment is empirical and often unsatisfactory. The drugs used are:
- colchicine 500 μg bid
- azathioprine 2 mg/kg body weight/day (average = 50 mg tid)
- thalidomide 100 mg nocte given 'on a named patient basis'.

For the mouth ulcers it is worth the patient trying:
- **10% hydrocortisone** in equal parts of glycerine and water, used as a mouthwash after each meal – the patient should be warned that it has a very bitter taste; it should be spat out so that the steroid is not absorbed
- **Steroid inhaler**: beclometasone dipropionate, 50 g/puff, is usually used for asthma, but instead of inhaling it, the patient sprays it on the ulcers several times a day until the ulcers heal.

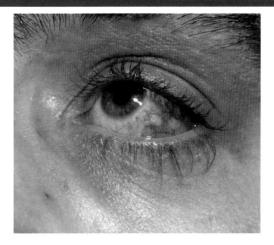

Fig. 6.11 Behçet's syndrome: eye conjunctivitis

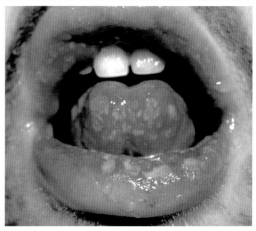

Fig. 6.12 Behçet's syndrome: erosions on tongue and lips

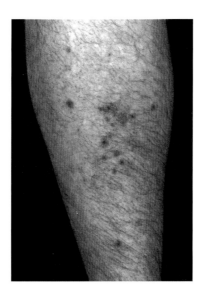

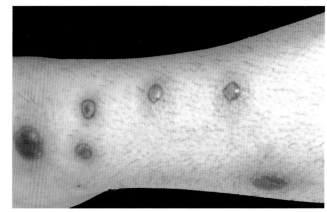

Fig. 6.13 (left) Behçet's syndrome: pustules on lower leg

Fig. 6.14 (above) Behçet's syndrome: vasculitic pustules on lower leg

Mouth lesions
Macules, patches, papules and plaques   WHITE/YELLOW/BROWN

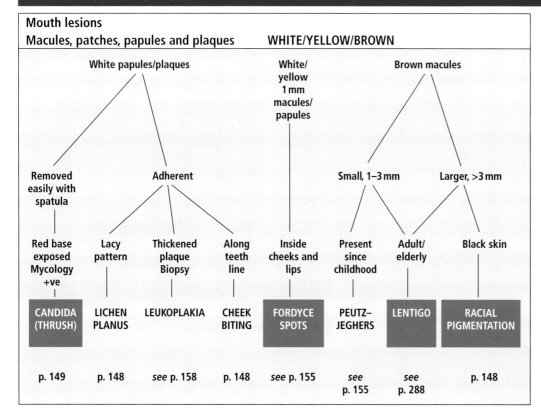

PIGMENTATION IN THE MOUTH

Melanin pigmentation in the mouth and on the tongue is a normal finding in patients with black skin. If present from childhood, multiple small, brown macules may be due to Peutz–Jeghers syndrome (*see* p. 155). In later life pigmented macules are likely to be lentigines (*see* p. 288).

TREATMENT: ORAL LICHEN PLANUS

Most oral lichen planus is asymptomatic and needs no treatment. Treatment of erosive lichen planus is unsatisfactory. The following can be tried:

- ordinary mouthwashes as used for aphthous ulcers (*see* p. 142); if these fail to work, some kind of systemic therapy is necessary
- prednisone 15–30 mg/day may occasionally be needed for the most severe forms of ulceration; the dose is reduced to a maintenance dose of 5–10 mg/day as soon as the ulceration is healed – you want to get the patient off steroids as soon as possible, because otherwise he or she will end up taking them for years
- rarely one of the oral retinoids may be needed as an alternative to systemic steroids (acitretin, 0.5–1 mg/kg body weight/day, *see* p. 49).

LICHEN PLANUS

Lichen planus in the mouth is usually asymptomatic. The diagnosis is made from the typical skin rash (*see* p. 197). In the mouth there is a white lacy pattern on the buccal mucosa. Rarely there may be erosions and ulceration and the patient will have a sore mouth and find eating painful. The edge of the ulcer is usually white. At the start there may have been the characteristic rash of lichen planus, but ulceration can go on for years, and can continue long after the rash is gone. It needs to be distinguished from **cheek biting**, where a fold of mucous membrane is seen heaped up along the teeth line.

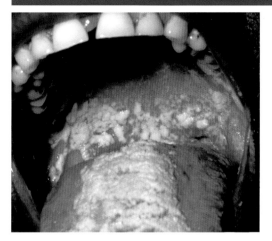

Fig. 6.15 Candida of the tongue and hard palate (may extend down the oesophagus)

ORAL CANDIDIASIS

Thrush occurs in the very young, the very old and patients who are immunosuppressed or who are taking antibiotics or cytotoxic drugs. Small, white papules scrape off easily with a spatula to leave a red surface. If these are mixed with potassium hydroxide, the spores and hyphae are easily seen on direct microscopy (*see* Fig. 10.15, p. 342) or can be cultured on Sabouraud's medium.

TREATMENT: ORAL CANDIDIASIS

- In infancy, miconazole gel applied directly to the plaques by an adult's finger four times daily
- In adults, nystatin oral suspension (1 mL) swirled around the mouth several times before swallowing, four times a day; continue for 48 hours after clinical cure
- Alternatives are nystatin pastilles or amphotericin B lozenges sucked until they dissolve, four times a day
- Oral itraconazole (100 mg/day for 2 weeks) or fluconazole (50 mg/day for 7–14 days); if the patient is on antibiotics, treatment will need to be continued until they are finished; if the patient has cancer or is immunosuppressed, treatment may need to be prolonged

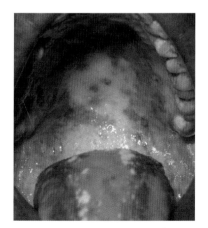

Fig. 6.16 Racial pigmentation involving the palate and tongue

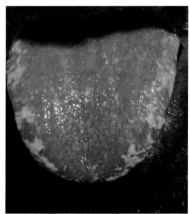

Fig. 6.17 Oral candida of the tongue: easily scraped off with a spatula

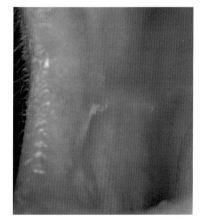

Fig. 6.18 Bite line along buccal mucosa

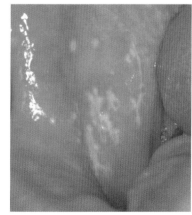

Fig. 6.19 Lichen planus of buccal mucosa: white lacy pattern

ABNORMALITIES OF THE TONGUE

ORAL HAIRY LEUKOPLAKIA

A white plaque consisting of multiple papules (looking like hairs) is found along the side of the tongue. It is due to the Epstein–Barr virus and is found in patients with HIV infection. It is usually asymptomatic.

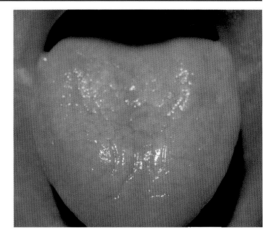

Fig. 6.21 Smooth tongue due to pernicious anaemia

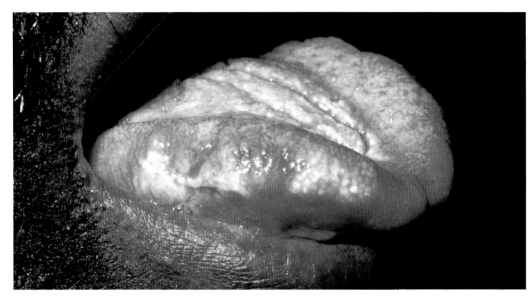

Fig. 6.20 Oral hairy leukoplakia in patient with HIV

LARGE TONGUE (MACROGLOSSIA)

The tongue may be large from birth or from early childhood in individuals with Down's syndrome or with a lymphangioma, haemangioma or neurofibroma of the tongue. Intermittent enlargement of the tongue (lasting <24 hours) is due to angio-oedema (*see* p. 99) and is usually associated with urticaria. After middle age, enlargement of the tongue should make you think of systemic amyloid.

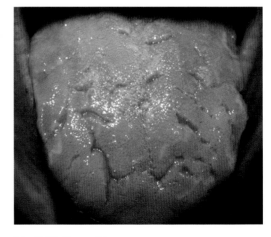

Fig. 6.22 Fissured tongue

SMOOTH TONGUE

A smooth tongue may be associated with iron deficiency, malabsorption or pernicious anaemia. A **dry tongue** is associated with Sjögren's syndrome.

FISSURED TONGUE

Deep grooves in the tongue may be a congenital abnormality or seen together with facial nerve palsy and swelling of the lips in **Melkersson–Rosenthal syndrome** (*see* p. 155).

GEOGRAPHIC TONGUE

Geographic tongue is a very common benign condition where smooth red patches appear on the dorsum of the tongue, giving a map-like appearance. These move about from day to day. The condition is generally asymptomatic although its appearance can cause alarm.

Any soreness can be treated with glycerine and thymol mouthwash. Tell the patient to avoid acidic foods such as citrus fruits or vinegar.

FURRED AND BLACK HAIRY TONGUE

These common conditions are due to hypertrophy of the filiform papillae and are completely harmless. They are asymptomatic and not indicative of any internal disease.

Apply 0.05% isotretinoin (Isotrex) gel and brush it off with a soft toothbrush 5 minutes later. This is repeated daily until it clears (about 2 weeks).

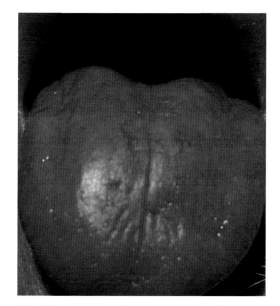

Fig. 6.23 Dry tongue due to Sjögren's syndrome

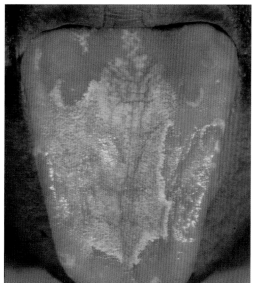

Fig. 6.24 Geographic tongue

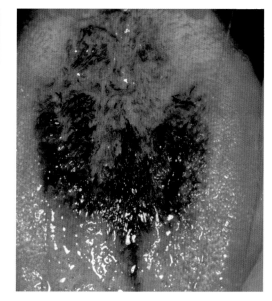

Fig. 6.25 Black hairy tongue

LIPS

Lips
Lesions
Normal surface

LIPS: NORMAL SURFACE

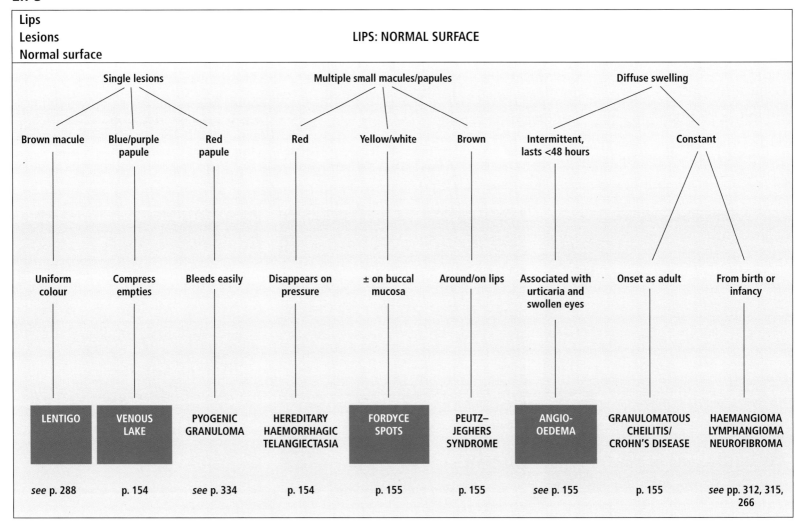

Single lesions

Brown macule — Uniform colour — **LENTIGO** — *see* p. 288

Blue/purple papule — Compress empties — **VENOUS LAKE** — p. 154

Red papule — Bleeds easily — **PYOGENIC GRANULOMA** — *see* p. 334

Multiple small macules/papules

Red — Disappears on pressure — **HEREDITARY HAEMORRHAGIC TELANGIECTASIA** — p. 154

Yellow/white — ± on buccal mucosa — **FORDYCE SPOTS** — p. 155

Brown — Around/on lips — **PEUTZ–JEGHERS SYNDROME** — p. 155

Diffuse swelling

Intermittent, lasts <48 hours — Associated with urticaria and swollen eyes — **ANGIO-OEDEMA** — *see* p. 155

Constant

Onset as adult — **GRANULOMATOUS CHEILITIS/ CROHN'S DISEASE** — p. 155

From birth or infancy — **HAEMANGIOMA LYMPHANGIOMA NEUROFIBROMA** — *see* pp. 312, 315, 266

Lips

Scale, fissures, hyperkeratotic, crust, warty, surface
Chronic papules, plaques, ulcers

(Acute ulcers and erosions, *see* p. 142)

LIPS: ABNORMAL SURFACE

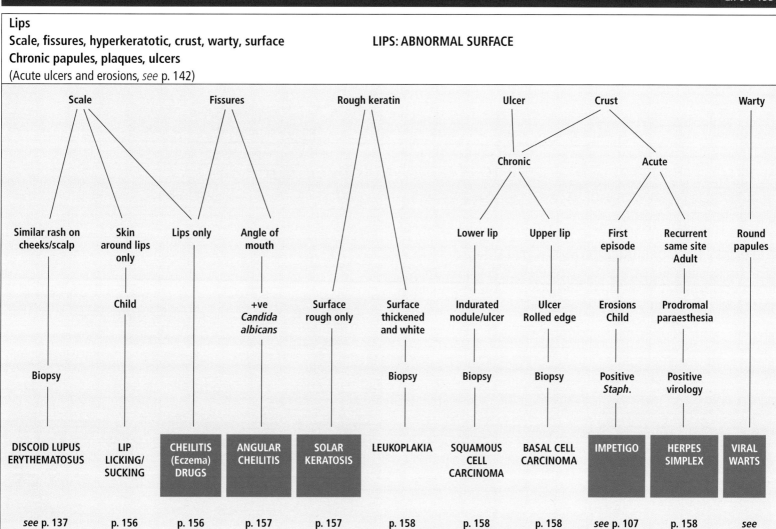

Scale			Fissures		Rough keratin		Ulcer	Crust		Warty
								Chronic	Acute	
Similar rash on cheeks/scalp	Skin around lips only	Lips only	Angle of mouth				Lower lip	Upper lip	First episode / Recurrent same site Adult	Round papules
	Child		+ve *Candida albicans*	Surface rough only	Surface thickened and white		Indurated nodule/ulcer	Ulcer Rolled edge	Erosions Child / Prodromal paraesthesia	
Biopsy					Biopsy		Biopsy	Biopsy	Positive *Staph.* / Positive virology	
DISCOID LUPUS ERYTHEMATOSUS	LIP LICKING/ SUCKING	CHEILITIS (Eczema) DRUGS	ANGULAR CHEILITIS	SOLAR KERATOSIS	LEUKOPLAKIA		SQUAMOUS CELL CARCINOMA	BASAL CELL CARCINOMA	IMPETIGO / HERPES SIMPLEX	VIRAL WARTS
see p. 137	p. 156	p. 156	p. 157	p. 157	p. 158		p. 158	p. 158	*see* p. 107 / p. 158	*see* p. 318

VENOUS LAKE

A solitary soft, purple papule on the upper or lower lip is common in the middle-aged or elderly.

TREATMENT: VENOUS LAKE

Most patients do not seem to mind having these lesions on their lips. If they want them removed there are various ways of doing it.

- Surgical excision under a local anaesthetic: the lip will heal well if the excision line is sited perpendicularly across the lip.
- The pulsed dye laser can be used without any anaesthetic and gives excellent cosmetic results. This is the treatment of choice if there is one in use near where the patient lives.

HEREDITARY HAEMORRHAGIC TELANGIECTASIA

Small red macules and papules occur on the lips, tongue and fingers associated with nosebleeds and gastro-intestinal bleeding. It is inherited as an autosomal dominant trait.

TREATMENT: HEREDITARY HAEMORRHAGIC TELANGIECTASIA

The skin lesions do not need any treatment, although the pulsed dye laser is very effective at removing them. Nosebleeds may need cauterising if they will not stop with ordinary pressure. Anaemia due to recurrent bleeding from the nose or gastro-intestinal tract will need treating with oral iron. The familial nature of the disorder should be explained to the patient and his or her family.

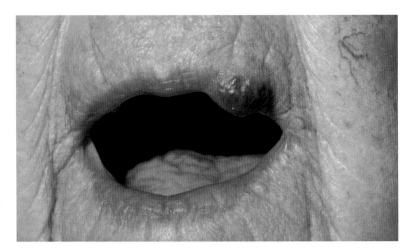

Fig. 6.26 Venous lake

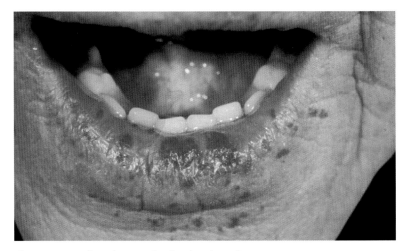

Fig. 6.27 Hereditary haemorrhagic telangiectasia

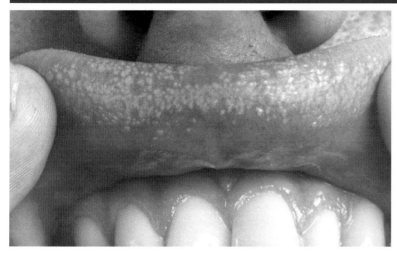

Fig. 6.28 Fordyce spots on inside of the upper lip

FORDYCE SPOTS

These are small, discrete, white or yellow papules on the lips or buccal mucosa due to sebaceous gland hyperplasia. They are very common and completely harmless.

PEUTZ–JEGHERS SYNDROME

A rare genetically determined condition, transmitted as an autosomal dominant trait. Brown macules on the lips, the skin around the mouth and on the fingers and toes occur in early childhood. They may be associated with small bowel polyps that can cause intussusception.

ANGIO-OEDEMA

Intermittent swelling of the lips lasting less than 24 hours before starting to go down is usually associated with urticaria and swelling around the eyes (*see* p. 99).

GRANULOMATOUS CHEILITIS

In granulomatous cheilitis the whole lip (upper or lower) (*see* Fig. 6.31) is swollen. Initially this may fluctuate quite a lot, but eventually the swelling becomes permanent. The cause is unknown, although it can sometimes be due to an allergic contact dermatitis to toothpaste. If the buccal mucosa is also thickened consider **Crohn's disease**. Ask about abdominal symptoms and look inside the mouth for the characteristic cobblestone appearance of the buccal mucosa. If necessary, do a barium follow-through and a biopsy. If there is an associated facial nerve palsy and/or a fissured tongue (*see* p. 151) consider **Melkersson–Rosenthal syndrome**. Injection of triamcinolone 5 mg/mL into the swollen lip is often helpful.

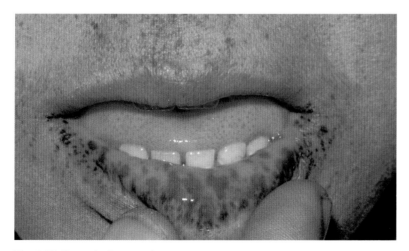

Fig. 6.29 Peutz–Jeghers syndrome

ECZEMA ON THE LIPS (CHEILITIS)

Allergic contact eczema can occur on the lips from lipstick, lip salves, toothpaste or mouthwashes. The diagnosis is confirmed by patch testing (*see* p. 21). Atopic eczema may affect the lips as well as the rest of the skin of the face (*see* p. 236). Many children suck or lick their lips, causing a red scaly rash around the mouth that only extends as far as the tongue can reach (*see* Fig. 6.33).

Oral retinoids cause dryness and scaling of the lips and the skin around the mouth (*see* Fig. 5.17, p. 121).

TREATMENT: LIP ECZEMA

It is important to use white soft paraffin[UK]/petrolatum[USA] as a regular moisturiser. A weak[UK]/group 7[USA] topical steroid such as 1% hydrocortisone ointment will be effective if applied twice a day.

Lip licking/sucking in children can usually be stopped once the parents realise what is happening. Applying a thick paste (e.g. Lassar's paste) will discourage the habit.

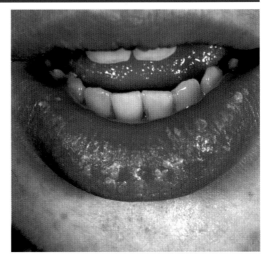

Fig. 6.30 Cheilitis: eczema on the lower lip

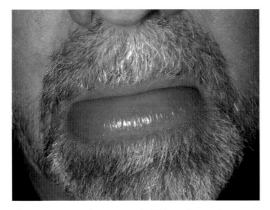

Fig. 6.31 Granulomatous cheilitis on lower lip

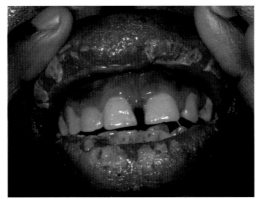

Fig. 6.32 Cheilitis (contact allergic dermatitis) to toothpaste

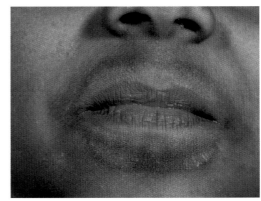

Fig. 6.33 Lip licking

ANGULAR CHEILITIS

Cheilitis means inflammation of the lips, and in angular cheilitis only the corners of the lips are involved. It occurs in individuals who wear dentures, and it is usually due to infection with *Candida albicans* from under the top denture. Poorly fitting dentures may also lead to overlap of the lower by the upper lip resulting in angular cheilitis.

TREATMENT: ANGULAR CHEILITIS

First scrape the underside of the denture and examine for the spores and hyphae of *C. albicans* or send for culture. Tell the patient to clean his or her dentures after every meal with a hard toothbrush and soap. Specific anti-candida treatment is not usually necessary.

ACTINIC CHEILITIS & SOLAR KERATOSES

Chronic sun exposure to the lower lip in older fair skinned (Type I) individuals leads to atrophy, loss of the normal creases and vermilion border. Histologically epithelial dysplasia is seen which may progress to in-situ or invasive SCC.

Rough keratin on the lower lip in older patients who have had a lot of sun exposure on the lip are solar keratoses. This change is not seen on the upper lip. If there is any induration under the keratosis, then a biopsy is necessary to exclude a squamous cell carcinoma

TREATMENT ACTINIC CHEILITIS & SOLAR KERATOSES

Cryotherapy is the treatment of choice for solar keratoses. Extensive involvement of the lower lip can be treated with 5-fluorouracil cream, imiquimod or photodynamic therapy, or the whole lower lip can be excised, and by pulling forward the buccal mucous membrane can be sutured back onto the vermilion border.

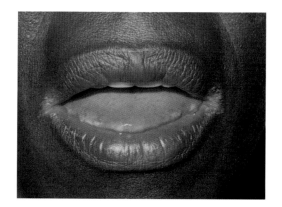

Fig. 6.34 Angular cheilitis

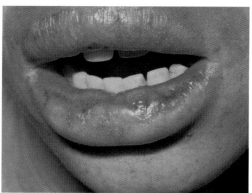

Fig. 6.35 Actinic cheilitis in African albino

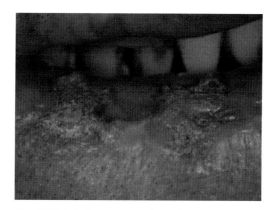

Fig. 6.36 Solar keratoses on lower lip

LEUKOPLAKIA

This is a persistent white, hyperkeratotic plaque in the mouth or on the tongue or lips due to epithelial dysplasia or carcinoma in situ.

TREATMENT: LEUKOPLAKIA

Since leukoplakia is usually caused by smoking, the first thing for the patient to do is to stop smoking. This may result in the lesion(s) disappearing. If it does not, consider one of the following.

- If the area involved is small, excise it.
- If it is too large for excision, it can be frozen with liquid nitrogen (two freeze–thaw cycles, *see* p. 58).
- Widespread involvement can be treated by removing the lip epidermis with the carbon dioxide laser and allowing the epidermis to regenerate.

Such patients are probably best cared for by an oral surgeon.

SQUAMOUS AND BASAL CELL CARCINOMAS

Squamous cell carcinomas occur on the lower lip as ulcers or indurated nodules and will need urgent referral for removal. Squamous cell carcinomas on mucous membranes are more likely to spread than those on exposed skin (*see* p. 332).

An ulcer or nodule on the upper lip, often involving the vermilion border, is more likely to be a basal cell carcinoma (*see* p. 330).

RECURRENT HERPES SIMPLEX

Recurrent herpes simplex is usually preceded by prodromal itching, burning or tingling on the lips. Small grouped vesicles appear, burst, crust and then heal in 7–10 days (*see* also p. 109).

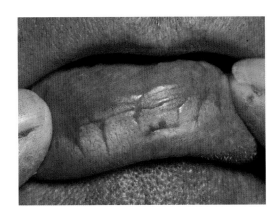

Fig. 6.37 Leukoplakia on lower lip

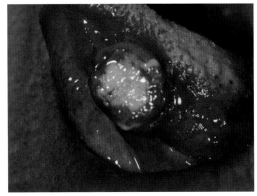

Fig. 6.38 Squamous cell carcinoma on underside of the tongue

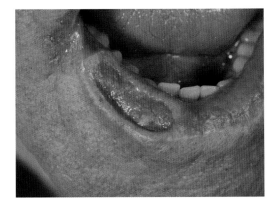

Fig. 6.39 Squamous cell carcinoma on lower lip

EARS

Ears

Patches and plaques   RASH ON EARS

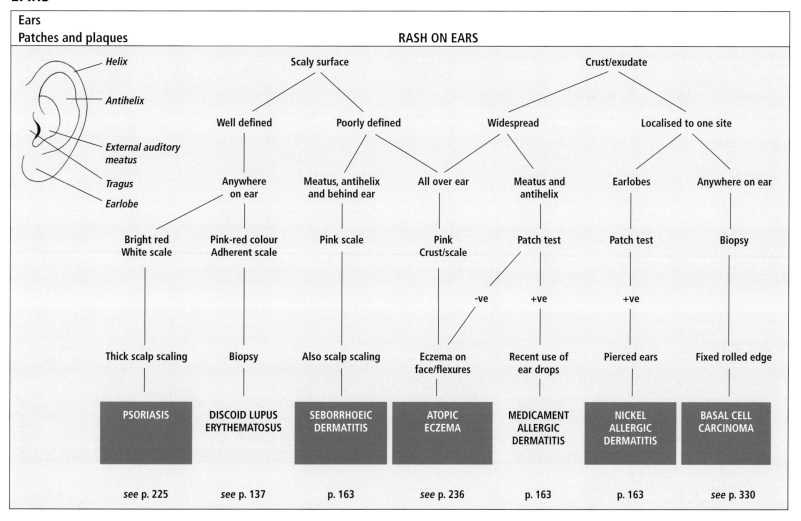

PSORIASIS	**DISCOID LUPUS ERYTHEMATOSUS**	

Helix
Antihelix
External auditory meatus
Tragus
Earlobe

Scaly surface
Crust/exudate

Well defined
Poorly defined
Widespread
Localised to one site

Anywhere on ear
Meatus, antihelix and behind ear
All over ear
Meatus and antihelix
Earlobes
Anywhere on ear

Bright red White scale
Pink-red colour Adherent scale
Pink scale
Pink Crust/scale
Patch test
Patch test
Biopsy

-ve   +ve   +ve

Thick scalp scaling
Biopsy
Also scalp scaling
Eczema on face/flexures
Recent use of ear drops
Pierced ears
Fixed rolled edge

PSORIASIS | **DISCOID LUPUS ERYTHEMATOSUS** | **SEBORRHOEIC DERMATITIS** | **ATOPIC ECZEMA** | **MEDICAMENT ALLERGIC DERMATITIS** | **NICKEL ALLERGIC DERMATITIS** | **BASAL CELL CARCINOMA**

see p. 225   see p. 137   p. 163   see p. 236   p. 163   p. 163   see p. 330

Ears
Papules and nodules

LESIONS ON EARS

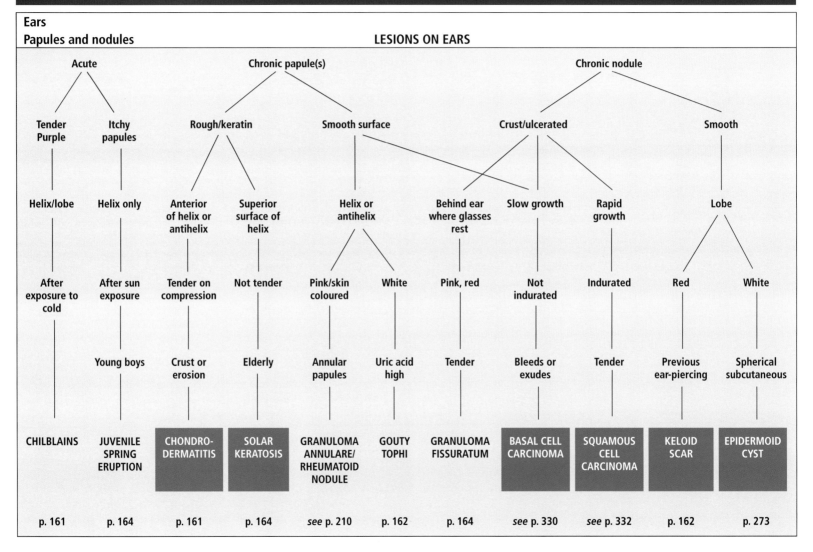

p. 161   p. 164   p. 161   p. 164   see p. 210   p. 162   p. 164   see p. 330   see p. 332   p. 162   p. 273

CHILBLAINS

Tender, itchy, mauve papules and nodules on the earlobes and helix occur in cold weather and last up to 2 weeks. Similar lesions can occur on other exposed sites, e.g. fingers, toes and nose. They occur in individuals who get very cold and warm up too quickly. The lesions are due to an abnormal reaction to cold where constriction of arterioles is followed by exudation of fluid into the tissues on rewarming.

TREATMENT: CHILBLAINS

Prevention is better than cure, i.e. do not allow the skin to get too cold. Those at risk, particularly individuals who work out of doors and the elderly who live in unheated accommodation, should wear warm gloves, boots and hats in the winter. When they come in from the cold they should warm up slowly.

Nifedipine retard 20 mg tid can reduce the pain, soreness and irritation of chilblains. For patients who get severe recurrent chilblains, it is worth considering continuing the drug for several weeks if the weather is particularly cold.

CHONDRODERMATITIS

Chondrodermatitis nodularis helicis chronica is a painful skin-coloured or pink papule on the helix or antihelix. There may be a central area of scaling or crusting. A history of pain in bed at night when the patient lies on that side differentiates it from solar keratoses and skin tumours, which, if painful, hurt all the time.

TREATMENT: CHONDRODERMATITIS

Excision biopsy of the painful papule together with the underlying cartilage is usually curative. Removing the cartilage is more important than removing the skin. It is usually necessary to take the adjoining cartilage away to prevent a new pressure point occurring and the problem returning.

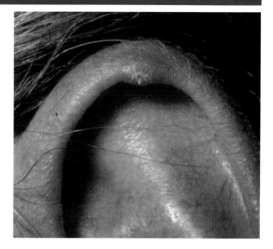

Fig. 6.41 Chondrodermatitis at pressure point at top of helix

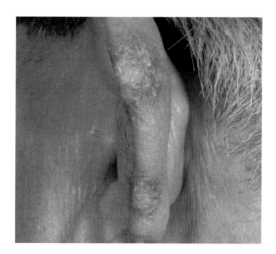

Fig. 6.40 Chilblains on the helix

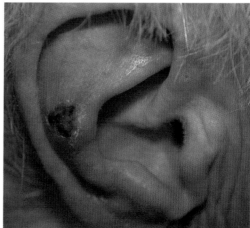

Fig. 6.42 Chondrodermatitis on the antihelix

GOUTY TOPHI

These are hard white or cream-coloured papules or plaques due to deposition of sodium urate crystals in the dermis. Classically they occur on the helix or antihelix of the ear, but occasionally they are found on the dorsum of the hands and feet (*see* Fig. 13.12, p. 411). Patients with tophi are likely to suffer from gout.

TREATMENT: GOUTY TOPHI

Allopurinol competitively inhibits the enzyme xanthine oxidase, which oxidises xanthine to uric acid. It causes a rapid fall in serum uric acid. Start with 100 mg daily as a single oral dose, and gradually increase to 300–400 mg a day, which will need to be continued indefinitely. By gradually increasing the dose you will hope to avoid precipitating acute attacks of gout at the beginning of treatment. With this treatment the tophi gradually become smaller and disappear.

KELOID SCAR

A round pink or purple papule or nodule may develop on the earlobe following ear-piercing. It may gradually increase in size and become unsightly. It is differentiated from an inclusion epidermoid cyst (due to epidermis being implanted into the dermis at the time of ear-piercing) by its colour, an epidermoid cyst being white or skin coloured.

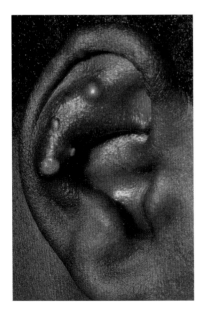

Fig. 6.43 Gouty tophi on antihelix

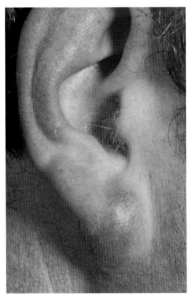

Fig. 6.44 Epidermoid cyst on earlobe

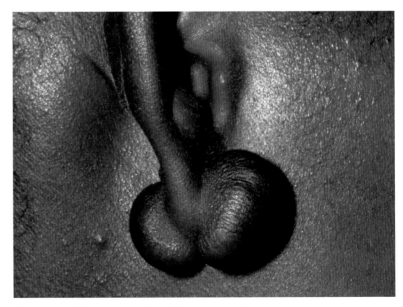

Fig. 6.45 Keloid scar on earlobe following ear-piercing

ECZEMA ON THE EAR

Allergic contact dermatitis on the ears presents with an acute eczema (vesicles, exudate and crusting, *see* Fig. 6.47). On the earlobes this is usually due to nickel in cheap earrings. In the external auditory meatus and on the rest of the ear it is usually due to antibiotic or antihistamine ear drops, creams or ointments.

Chronic eczema on the ear usually occurs in association with eczema elsewhere. **Otitis externa**, i.e. eczema of the external auditory canal and meatus, is usually due to seborrhoeic eczema (*see* Fig. 6.46), and there will be other evidence of this, e.g. scaling in the scalp (*see* p. 88). **Psoriasis** is red rather than pink and there

will be typical plaques elsewhere, with or without thick scaly plaques in the scalp (*see* p. 88). **Discoid lupus erythematosus** (*see* p. 137) usually involves the antihelix but not the external auditory canal. A biopsy will be needed to confirm this diagnosis.

Because of the narrow ear canal, eczema here can cause problems:
- scale tends to accumulate, blocking the ear and causing pain
- secondary infection (with *Staphylococcus aureus*, Gram-negative organisms, *C. albicans* and *Aspergillus*) is common, especially in wet conditions (e.g. after swimming)
- the itching encourages the patient to poke things down the ear canal.

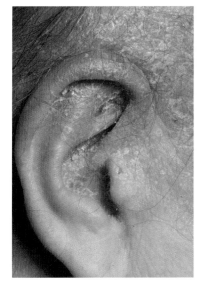 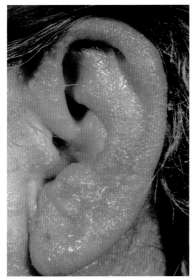 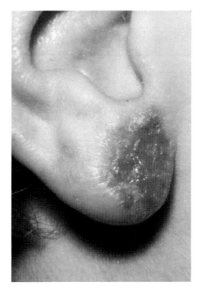 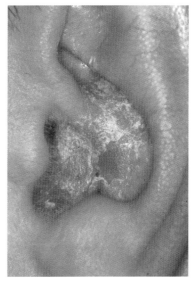

Fig. 6.46 Seborrhoeic eczema with associated scaling in scalp

Fig. 6.47 Acute contact allergic dermatitis from neomycin ear drops

Fig. 6.48 Contact allergic dermatitis to nickel from earrings

Fig. 6.49 Psoriasis in external auditory meatus

TREATMENT: OTITIS EXTERNA

If the eczema is dry and scaly, the treatment is the same as for seborrhoeic eczema elsewhere, i.e. 1% hydrocortisone cream or 2% ketoconazole cream used twice a day until it is better.

If there is a lot of scale and/or pain, the patient should see an ear, nose and throat surgeon. A perforated eardrum and a co-existant otitis media must be excluded. Aural toilet, with removal of the excess scale can be done in the ear, nose and throat clinic, which will help the pain.

If there is an acute weeping eczema, do not be tempted to use one of the topical steroid/antibiotic/antifunga ear drops or sprays. You will only make things worse by exposing the patient to the risk of developing a further acute allergic contact dermatitis on top of what he or she already has. Take a swab for bacteriology and mycology culture. If there is a bacterial infection present, use a systemic antibiotic depending on the sensitivities (probably flucloxacillin or erythromycin 250 mg qid for 7 days). If there is a fungal infection, ketoconazole will be required rather than a topical steroid. First dry up the exudate with an astringent such as 13% aluminium acetate ear drops. When it is dry, use 1% hydrocortisone ointment twice a day until it is better. Send the patient for patch testing when the rash has settled to exclude an allergic contact dermatitis.

An ichthammol wick inserted into the ear canal is useful in patients with recurrent otitis externa.

GRANULOMA FISSURATUM

Granuloma fissuratum occurs from the pressure of spectacles and occurs at the side of the bridge of the nose or behind the ear (*see* Fig. 6.50). It looks like a basal cell carcinoma and is distinguished by skin biopsy. Changing from heavy- to light-framed glasses usually resolves the problem.

EAR CONDITIONS INDUCED BY SUN EXPOSURE

The ears, especially in males, are exposed to the sun. In young boys and men with short hair, itchy papules can occur on the helix (*see* Fig. 6.51) 2–12 hours after sun exposure in spring, and can last about 2 weeks. It is a form of polymorphic light eruption (*see* p. 100) called **juvenile spring eruption**.

Chronic sun exposure, especially in skin types I and II, leads to **solar keratoses** developing on the superior aspect of the helix, usually in men. These are rough papules that can be felt better than seen (*see* p. 326). **Squamous cell carcinoma** and **keratoacanthomas** (*see* pp. 328), also due to chronic sun exposure, present as rapidly growing nodules on the helix with an ulcerating or keratotic surface. **Basal cell carcinomas** (*see* p. 330) tend to grow slowly, and can occur anywhere on the ear. They usually present with bleeding or exudate that the patient notices on the pillow.

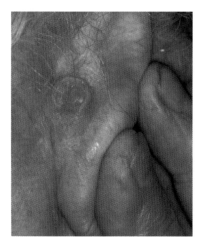

Fig. 6.50 Granuloma fissuratum: a tender nodule behind the ear where glasses rest

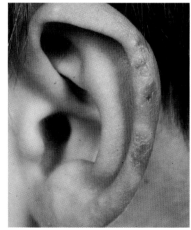

Fig. 6.51 Juvenile spring eruption: itchy papules on sun-exposed site

Acute erythematous rash on the trunk and limbs

Trunk and limbs
Acute progressive erythematous rash
Surface normal
Macules and papules

ACUTE MACULO-PAPULAR RASH

(Erythematous maculopapular rashes consist of small, red macules and papules that coalesce to become confluent)

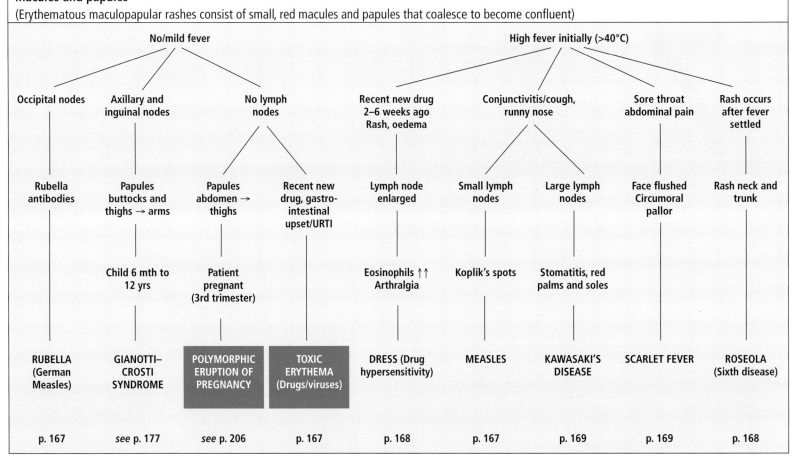

| No/mild fever | | | High fever initially (>40°C) | | | | |

| Occipital nodes | Axillary and inguinal nodes | No lymph nodes | Recent new drug 2–6 weeks ago Rash, oedema | Conjunctivitis/cough, runny nose | | Sore throat abdominal pain | Rash occurs after fever settled |

| Rubella antibodies | Papules buttocks and thighs → arms | Papules abdomen → thighs | Recent new drug, gastro-intestinal upset/URTI | Lymph node enlarged | Small lymph nodes | Large lymph nodes | Face flushed Circumoral pallor | Rash neck and trunk |

| | Child 6 mth to 12 yrs | Patient pregnant (3rd trimester) | | Eosinophils ↑↑ Arthralgia | Koplik's spots | Stomatitis, red palms and soles | | |

| RUBELLA (German Measles) | GIANOTTI–CROSTI SYNDROME | POLYMORPHIC ERUPTION OF PREGNANCY | TOXIC ERYTHEMA (Drugs/viruses) | DRESS (Drug hypersensitivity) | MEASLES | KAWASAKI'S DISEASE | SCARLET FEVER | ROSEOLA (Sixth disease) |

| p. 167 | *see* p. 177 | *see* p. 206 | p. 167 | p. 168 | p. 167 | p. 169 | p. 169 | p. 168 |

TOXIC ERYTHEMA

This is a rash in which pink/red macules and papules appear and then coalesce to become a widespread erythema. The rash may look like measles (morbilliform), rubella (rubelliform) or roseola (roseoliform). There are no prodromal symptoms. It is usually due to an enterovirus (ECHO or Coxsackie) or a drug (*see* p. 176).

MEASLES

Measles is caused by a paramyxovirus. After an incubation period of about 10 days, the child becomes miserable with a high fever, runny nose, conjunctivitis, photophobia, brassy cough, and inflamed tonsils. Koplik's spots on the buccal mucosa are diagnostic at this stage (look like grains of salt on a red base). On day 4 of the illness a red macular rash appears behind the ears and spreads onto the face, trunk and limbs. The macules may become papules, which join together to become confluent. It lasts up to 10 days, leaving brown staining and some scaling.

RUBELLA (GERMAN MEASLES)

Rubella is a common viral illness of children due to a rubivirus. It is spread by inhalation of infected droplets. After an incubation period of 14–21 days, a macular rash begins on the face and neck. It spreads down the body over 24–48 hours and then clears from the face downwards over the next 2–3 days. It is often associated with enlarged occipital and posterior cervical lymph nodes, and sometimes arthritis. The child is infectious from 5 days before to 3 days after the rash appears.

If the diagnosis is suspected rubella antibody titres should be measured immediately and after 10 days so that the diagnosis can be confirmed. Many other viral infections look like rubella but do not carry the same risk to pregnant mothers (foetal cataracts, nerve deafness and cardiac abnormalities) if infection occurs in the first trimester.

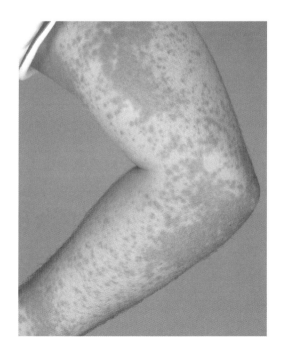

Fig. 7.01 Toxic erythema on arm

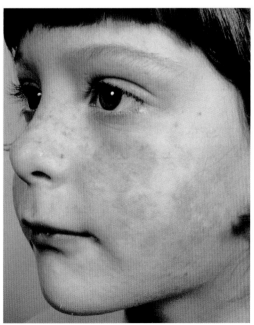

Fig. 7.02 Rubella

ROSEOLA INFANTUM (SIXTH DISEASE)

This is the commonest rash of this kind in children under the age of 2, and is due to the human herpes virus-6. The rash is preceded by a high fever but the child remains well. After 3–5 days the fever goes and the rash, which looks like rubella, appears on the trunk. It lasts only 1–2 days and then disappears.

TREATMENT: MEASLES AND OTHER VIRAL EXANTHEMS

Treatment is symptomatic since they get better spontaneously. Bed rest is necessary if the child is sick, and the pyrexia can be treated with cool sponging and paracetamol elixir.

Measles and rubella can be prevented by immunisation, but with reduced uptake of vaccines, these diseases are becoming more common.

DRESS

DRESS (drug reaction with eosinophilia and systemic symptoms) starts 2–6 weeks after first taking a drug, initially as a morbilliform rash, which later becomes more oedematous. Vesicles and bullae may occur, and there is often oedema of the face. Lymph nodes are enlarged and systemic symptoms include severe arthralgia. The diagnosis is made by the combination of a severe drug rash, a high eosinophil count and abnormalities in liver function tests and renal function.

Drugs implicated include:

- anticonvulsants (phenobarbitone, carbamazepine, phenytoin)
- sulphonamides
- minocycline
- allopurinol
- dapsone
- gold salts
- HIV drugs.

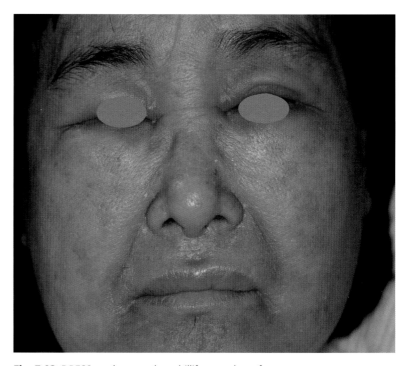

Fig. 7.03 DRESS: oedema and morbilliform rash on face

TREATMENT: DRESS

It is essential that the offending drug is identified and stopped immediately. Systemic corticosteroids are usually effective (prednisolone 40 mg daily). They should be continued till the systemic symptoms have resolved, and then slowly tapered off to prevent relapse.

KAWASAKI'S DISEASE (MUCOCUTANEOUS LYMPH NODE SYNDROME)

This disease may be confused with measles, but it must be recognised because of the potentially serious association with myocarditis. It occurs in young children under the age of 5 (50% under 2 years age). The onset is acute with fever, red eyes, dry lips and prominent papillae on the tongue. The most characteristic signs are the large glands in the neck, the rash on the trunk and limbs, and the red palms and soles that later peel.

TREATMENT: KAWASAKI'S DISEASE

If given immediately, a high dose of intravenous γ-globulin (2 g/kg body weight) as a single infusion over 10 hours will reduce the overall morbidity.

SCARLET FEVER

Scarlet fever is due to an infection with a group A β-haemolytic streptococcus that produces an erythrogenic toxin. The condition seems to be less common than it used to be. After an incubation period of 2–5 days there is a sudden fever with anorexia and sore throat. The tonsils are swollen with a white exudate and there is painful lymphadenopathy in the neck. The tongue is furred initially, but later it becomes red with prominent papillae (strawberry tongue). The rash appears on the second day as a widespread punctate erythema, which rapidly becomes confluent. The face is flushed except for circumoral pallor. After about a week the rash fades followed by skin peeling. *Streptococcus pyogenes* can be grown from the throat and the antistreptolysin O titre is raised.

TREATMENT: SCARLET FEVER

Give oral phenoxymethylpenicillin (Penicillin V) 62.5–125 mg every 6 hours for 10 days depending on the child's age. Gargling with paracetamol suspension (120 mg/5 mL) every 4 hours and then swallowing it may help the sore throat.

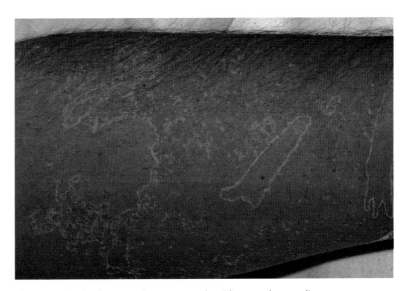

Fig. 7.04 Scarlet fever: erythematous rash with secondary peeling on arm

Trunk and limbs
Acute erythematous rash
Surface normal
Widespread multiple papules, patches, plaques

ACUTE ERYTHEMATOUS RASHES

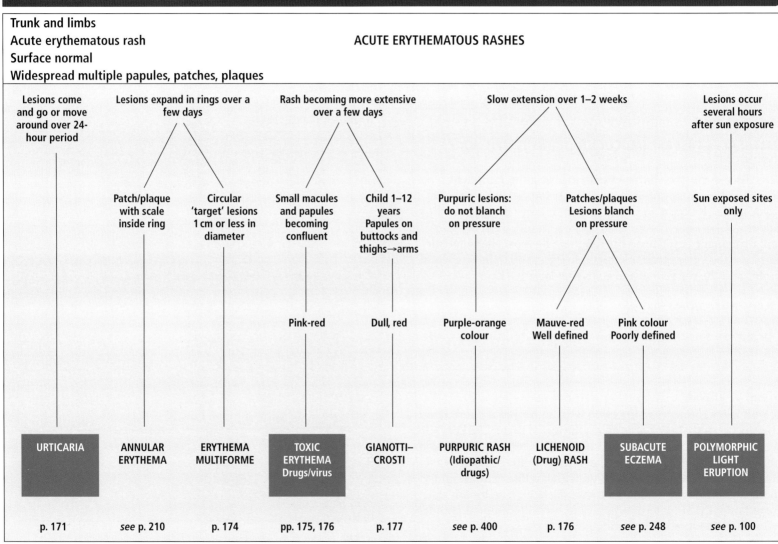

Lesions come and go or move around over 24-hour period	Lesions expand in rings over a few days		Rash becoming more extensive over a few days		Slow extension over 1–2 weeks			Lesions occur several hours after sun exposure
	Patch/plaque with scale inside ring	Circular 'target' lesions 1 cm or less in diameter	Small macules and papules becoming confluent	Child 1–12 years Papules on buttocks and thighs→arms	Purpuric lesions: do not blanch on pressure	Patches/plaques Lesions blanch on pressure		Sun exposed sites only
			Pink-red	Dull, red	Purple-orange colour	Mauve-red Well defined	Pink colour Poorly defined	
URTICARIA	**ANNULAR ERYTHEMA**	**ERYTHEMA MULTIFORME**	**TOXIC ERYTHEMA** Drugs/virus	**GIANOTTI– CROSTI**	**PURPURIC RASH** (Idiopathic/ drugs)	**LICHENOID** (Drug) RASH	**SUBACUTE ECZEMA**	**POLYMORPHIC LIGHT ERUPTION**
p. 171	see p. 210	p. 174	pp. 175, 176	p. 177	see p. 400	p. 176	see p. 248	see p. 100

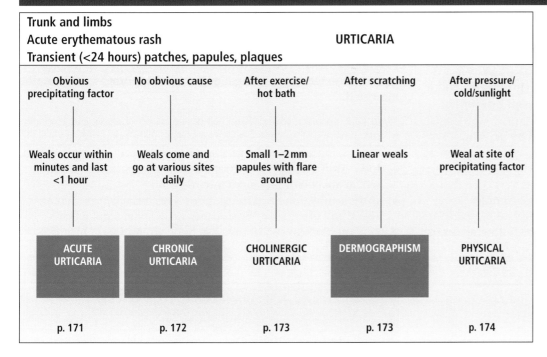

Trunk and limbs Acute erythematous rash Transient (<24 hours) patches, papules, plaques		URTICARIA		
Obvious precipitating factor	No obvious cause	After exercise/ hot bath	After scratching	After pressure/ cold/sunlight
Weals occur within minutes and last <1 hour	Weals come and go at various sites daily	Small 1–2 mm papules with flare around	Linear weals	Weal at site of precipitating factor
ACUTE URTICARIA	**CHRONIC URTICARIA**	CHOLINERGIC URTICARIA	**DERMOGRAPHISM**	PHYSICAL URTICARIA
p. 171	p. 172	p. 173	p. 173	p. 174

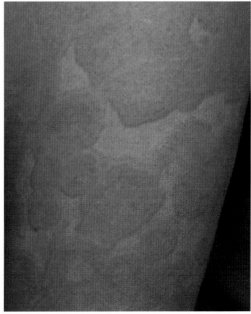

Fig. 7.05 Acute urticaria: large weals

ACUTE URTICARIA

Acute urticaria is defined as urticaria that has been present for less than 6 weeks. Individual lesions last for less than 24 hours ('here today and gone tomorrow'). A central itchy white papule or plaque due to dermal oedema (weal) is surrounded by an erythematous flare. The lesions are variable in size and shape, and may be associated with swelling of the soft tissues of the eyelids, lips and tongue (angio-oedema, *see* p. 99). To identify how long the weals last, draw around one, and ask to see the patient the following day. Lesions that last for longer than 24 hours should be classified as **urticarial dermatoses** and require a biopsy for diagnosis. The weal is the result of degranulation of mast cells releasing histamine and other mediators of inflammation; degranulation can be stimulated by allergic (IgE) and non-allergic stimuli.

Acute urticaria may be caused by:

1. **A type 1 allergic response** that occurs within a few minutes of contact with an allergen either on the skin (e.g. nettle rash, latex allergy, *see* p. 405) or ingested (e.g. strawberries or penicillin). The rash disappears spontaneously within an hour. Contact with the same allergen again will result in a further episode.
2. **Direct release of histamine from mast cells by aspirin, codeine or opiates**. IgE is not involved. This is the commonest cause of infrequent acute episodes of urticaria, occurring when a patient takes aspirin for a cold or headache.
3. **Drugs** that cause serum sickness (an immune complex reaction): urticaria, arthralgia, fever and lymphadenopathy are the hallmarks of this. It may be caused by the following drugs:
   - penicillin
   - nitrofurantoin
   - phenothiazines
   - thiazide diuretics
   - thiouracils.

TREATMENT: ACUTE URTICARIA

Use a non-sedative, long-acting antihistamine such as cetirizine or loratadine at high doses (10–20 mg bid), or, if in extremis, intravenous chlorpheniramine 10 mg. If life-threatening swelling of the larynx or tongue occurs, inject 0.5 mL of 1:1000 adrenaline/epinephrine solution intramuscularly via an EpiPen. Do not give systemic steroids except in serum sickness.

CHRONIC URTICARIA

Urticaria is classified as chronic if the weals come and go over a period of more than 6 weeks. Individual lesions always last less than 24 hours, but new lesions appear daily or every few days.

These can occur at any time of the day or night. This is not a type I allergic response.

Possible causes of chronic urticaria can be identified by a good history, so extensive investigation, unless supported by this, is not indicated.

Most cases will be **idiopathic**. No cause can be found, but exclude:

- psychological factors – ongoing stress; very hectic lifestyle
- regular ingestion of drugs such as aspirin, codeine and opiates
- food additives such as tartrazines, benzoates, and so forth, which are chemically similar to aspirin
- chronic infections and infestations – bacterial (sinus, dental, chest, gall bladder), fungal (candidiasis), intestinal worms
- general medical conditions, e.g. hyperthyroidism, chronic active hepatitis, systemic lupus erythematosus.

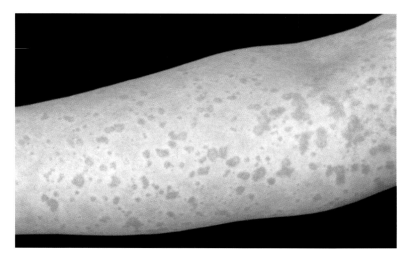

Fig. 7.06 Cholinergic urticaria

Around 40% of patients show a positive autologous skin test (used as a research tool). The patient's own serum is injected intradermally into the forearm and produces a weal. This indicates that IgE is present in the serum, which will degranulate mast cells in the skin.

TREATMENT: CHRONIC URTICARIA

Ask the patient to avoid aspirin (and proprietary cold and flu remedies), codeine, and foods containing azo dyes (tartrazine – orange yellow) and benzoic acid (used as a preservative in peas and bananas).

Long-acting, non-sedative antihistamines need to be given regularly and in sufficient dosage to prevent the urticaria. Try one of the following:
- cetirizine 10–40 g daily (Zirtek^{UK}/Zyrtec^{USA}) or levocetirizine 5–20 mg daily (Xyzal)
- fexofenadine 180 mg daily (Telfast^{UK}/Allegra^{USA})
- loratadine 10 mg or desloratadine 5 mg (Neoclarityn)

If standard (hay fever) doses do not control it, increase up to four time this. Although this is not licensed, it is recommended in UK guidelines. Do not mix antihistamines. Once the patient has been free of the rash for 4 weeks, the antihistamine can be stopped. If it reoccurs then further long-term treatment is needed, and in some cases this can last for months.

If non-sedative antihistamines do not work try:
- a sedative antihistamine such as hydroxyzine (Atarax) 10–50 mg 2 hours before bedtime (the dose depending on effect and degree of sedation produced)
- an H$_2$ blocker such as ranitidine 150 mg bid as well.

Then refer to a dermatologist for consideration of:
- oral ciclosporin (useful in patients with a positive autologous skin test not responding to antihistamines)
- omalizumab (a monoclonal antibody that targets IgE) has been shown to be effective in severe recalcitrant cases.

Do not use systemic steroids in urticaria. They do work but generally the problem reoccurs on stopping and there is a risk of long-term dependence.

CHOLINERGIC URTICARIA
Small red papules (1–3 mm diameter) surrounded by an area of vasoconstriction occur after exercise or hot baths, mainly in young adults. The diagnosis can be confirmed by making the patient exercise vigorously for a few minutes.

DERMOGRAPHISM
Weals occur only after scratching or rubbing the skin. Obviously the more the skin is scratched in response to itch, the worse the lesions can become. Dermographism is not usually associated with urticaria.

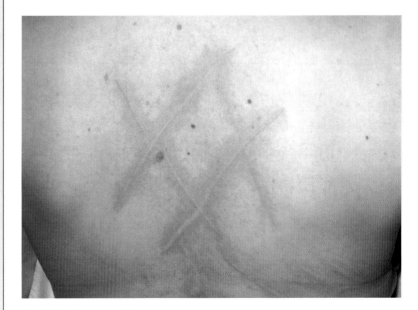

Fig. 7.07 Dermographism

PHYSICAL URTICARIA

Cold, pressure, water and sunlight can all induce an immediate urticarial reaction. **Delayed pressure urticaria** occurs after a delay of 30 minutes to 12 hours and occurs at sites of prolonged pressure. Weals or deeper oedema occur, which are itchy and painful, and persist for several days. It can occur on the feet from tight shoes, on soles after climbing a ladder, around the waist, on palms from gripping, and so forth. Diagnosis requires specific questioning.

TREATMENT: CHOLINERGIC AND PHYSICAL URTICARIA

The options are to take a long-acting antihistamine on a regular basis to prevent the attacks, or take a short-acting one (such as chlorphenamine 4–8 mg) before exercise or the precipitating cause.

Avoidance of exercise or the physical cause should be an obvious priority.

ERYTHEMA MULTIFORME

Multiple small (<1 cm diameter), round blisters made up of rings of different colours ('target' or 'iris' lesions) occur on the palms, dorsum of hands and forearms, knees and dorsum of the feet. It may be very itchy.

The rash occurs 10–14 days after some precipitating cause:
- viral infections, especially herpes simplex– this is the commonest cause of recurrent episodes of erythema multiforme (90%)
- immunisations
- bacterial infections, especially streptococcal sore throats
- mycoplasma pneumoniae infection
- drugs – sulphonamides, phenylbutazone and other non-steroidal anti-inflammatory drugs (NSAIDs).

Occasionally the skin lesions may be widespread and associated with blisters or erosions in the mouth. **Stevens–Johnson syndrome** is erythema multiforme with extensive mucous membrane involvement (*see* p. 144).

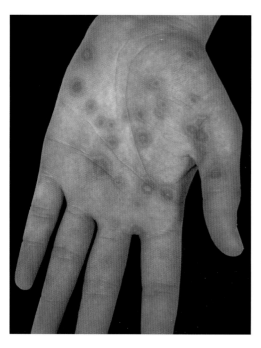

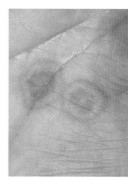

Fig. 7.09 (above) Close-up of 'target lesions'

Fig. 7.08 (left) Erythema multiforme on the palm

TREATMENT: ERYTHEMA MULTIFORME

Erythema multiforme gets better on its own after 2 weeks and does not require treatment. Even in severe episodes the case for systemic steroids is controversial. Treatment is symptomatic. Causes of erythema multiforme should be sought and treated if necessary.

DRUG RASHES

Some drug rashes are life-threatening and it is essential that the offending drug is stopped. Although immediate life-threatening IgE-mediated anaphylactic reactions can occur, delayed (type IV) reactions are more common but tend to be idiosyncratic and unpredictable. Mostly they are asymptomatic and get better whether or not the drug is stopped. Unfortunately there is no simple test to identify the cause of a drug rash, and if patients are taking numerous drugs it is often not possible to be sure of the exact cause or even whether a drug is responsible (a **viral exanthem** may look identical). This leaves the doctor with a problem, not only during the current episode but also in the future, because he or she needs to know whether it is safe to prescribe the drug again.

If you think the patient has a drug rash you need to find out the following.
- A complete list of all drugs the patient is taking (prescribed, over-the-counter or borrowed).
- The exact date each one was started and stopped. It is more likely that a rash is from a recently started drug than one that has been taken for years. A drug rash is unlikely to have developed in less than 4 days if the drug has not been taken before. Most drug rashes take 7–10 days to occur, but they sometimes do not appear for 28 days (especially if concomitant immunomodulating drugs are being taken). Look for the drug that was started 7–14 days before the rash began.
- Has the suspected drug or any chemically related drug been taken before?
- Has there ever been an adverse reaction to a drug before and to which one?

Avoid drug rashes by remembering the following:
- only prescribe drugs that are necessary
- always ask the patient if he or she has had any previous drug allergies
- make sure you know what is in a tablet or injection when you prescribe it; always use proper names
- do not give ampicillin/amoxicillin for sore throats.

List of drug rashes covered elsewhere
Acne, *see* p. 121
Bullous, *see* p. 183
Exanthematous (morbiliform), *see* p. 176
Erythema multiforme, *see* p. 174
Erythema nodosum, *see* p. 378
Erythrodermic, *see* p. 194
Drug reaction with eosinophia, *see* p. 168
Lichenoid, *see* p. 176
Fixed drug eruption, *see* p. 181
Hair loss, *see* p. 84
Hyperpigmentation, *see* p. 298
Hypertrichosis, *see* p. 72
Lupus erythematosus, *see* p. 131
Photoallergic, *see* p. 106
Phototoxic, *see* p. 101
Purpuric/vasculitic, *see* p. 401
Serum sickness, *see* p. 172
Toxic epidermal necrolysis, *see* p. 192
Urticarial drug rashes, *see* p. 172

EXANTHEMATOUS DRUG RASH

This is the most common kind of drug rash. In the United Kingdom, antibiotics, sleeping tablets and tranquillisers are the most frequent causative agents. The rash mimics the common viral exanthems and is made up of symmetrical red or pink macules or papules mainly on the trunk; on the legs it may be purpuric. Almost any drug can cause this kind of reaction but the commonest are:

- ampicillin (amoxicillin)
- benzodiazepines
- carbamazepine
- phenothiazines
- thiazide diuretics
- other penicillins
- captopril
- NSAIDs
- sulphonamides
- thiouracils.

LICHENOID DRUG REACTION

Rarely, a rash that looks like lichen planus (although usually atypical) can be due to a drug. The rash has the typical mauve hue of lichen planus but the lesions are larger and more confluent. Histology shows lichenoid features. Drugs that can cause it include:

- β-blockers
- chlorpropamide
- gold
- methyldopa
- quinine
- chloroquine
- ethambutol
- mepacrine
- penicillamine
- thiazide diuretics.

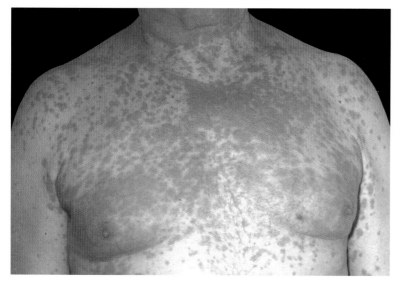

Fig. 7.10 Exanthematous rash due to sulphonamide

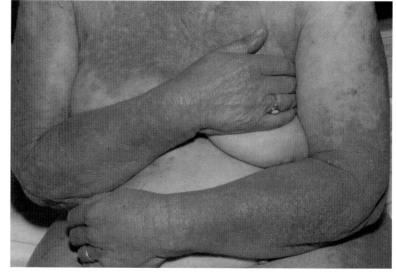

Fig. 7.11 Lichenoid drug rash

GIANOTTI–CROSTI SYNDROME

Gianotti–Crosti syndrome is a papular eruption occurring in children between the ages of 6 months and 12 years and is usually a response to a viral infection especially hepatitis B. A profuse papular rash starts on the buttocks and thighs, and quickly spreads over 3–4 days to the arms and face. The lesions may be a dull-red colour. There is often an associated lymphadenopathy of inguinal and axillary glands. The rash fades after 2–8 weeks. Always check the liver function tests.

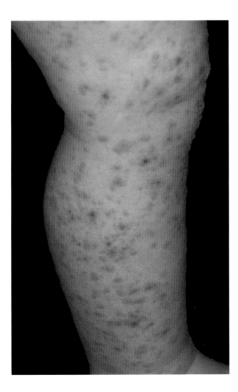

Fig. 7.12 Gianotti–Crosti syndrome on leg of infant

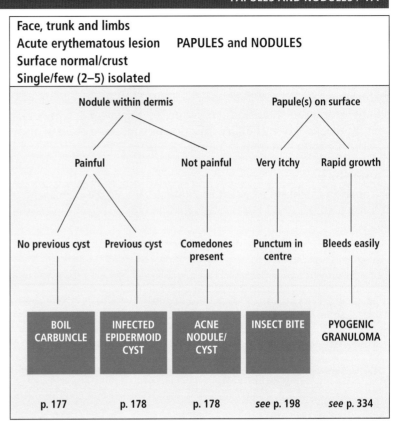

BOIL/FURUNCLE

A boil is an abscess of a single hair follicle (*see* Fig. 7.31) caused by *Staphylococcus aureus*, which may also be isolated from the nose or perineum. Single or multiple tender, red nodules with a central punctum can occur anywhere on the body except the palms or soles. Without treatment the abscess will eventually point on the surface, discharge and heal leaving a scar.

Acne cysts are not due to an infection but to a sudden severe inflammatory reaction in an acne nodule. They usually respond quite rapidly to an injection of intralesional steroid (triamcinolone 10 mg/mL).

Epidermoid cysts have a microscopic opening and through this, staphylococci can enter. Sudden painful enlargement of a previous cyst is indicative of secondary infection or rupture of the cyst and a subsequent foreign body reaction (*see* also p. 273).

CARBUNCLE

An abscess of several adjacent hair follicles is called a **carbuncle**. It looks just like a boil but is larger and has several openings to the surface.

TREATMENT: BOILS, CARBUNCLES AND INFECTED CYSTS

Check the patient's blood to exclude diabetes (fasting blood sugar or HbA1c). If the boil is already pointing, it can be lanced to let the pus out. Otherwise, treat with oral flucloxacillin (or erythromycin) 500 mg qid for 7 days. Take swabs for bacteriology from the boil, the nose, perianal skin and any rash. The infection usually comes from the patient him- or herself, so carriage sites should be treated with topical mupirocin, fucidic acid or neomycin ointment twice daily for 2 weeks. If recurrent boils occur even if carriage sites have been treated, take swabs from other members of the family and treat them if infected. Long-term low-dose antibiotics (flucloxacillin or erythromycin 250 mg bid) may be necessary if the boils reoccur or persist. For cysts, excise after the infection has settled down, not at the time the cyst is red and painful.

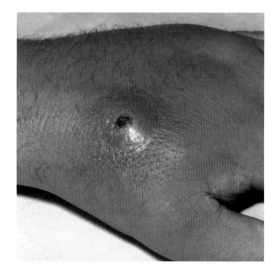

Fig. 7.13 Boil on back of hand

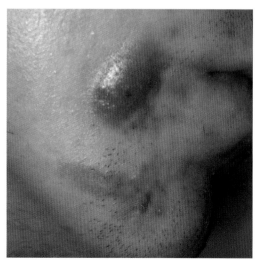

Fig. 7.14 Acne cyst on right cheek

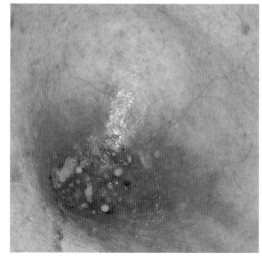

Fig. 7.15 Carbuncle on back with multiple openings

Trunk and limbs
Acute erythematous rash/lesions
Vesicles and bullae

VESICLES AND BULLAE

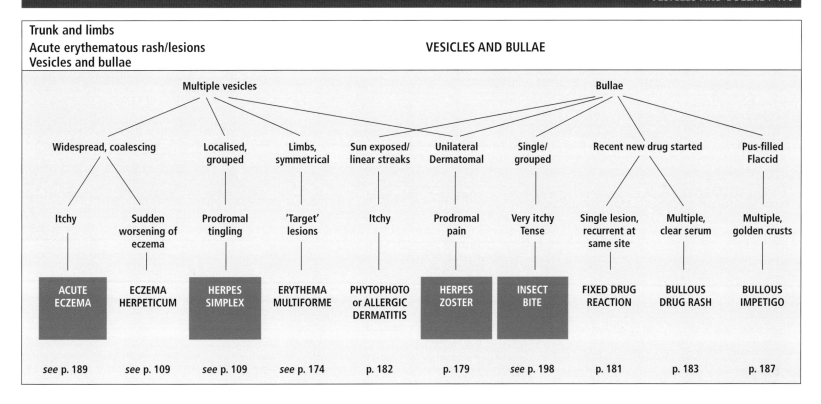

Multiple vesicles						Bullae	

| Widespread, coalescing | | Localised, grouped | Limbs, symmetrical | Sun exposed/ linear streaks | Unilateral Dermatomal | Single/ grouped | Recent new drug started | | Pus-filled Flaccid |

| Itchy | Sudden worsening of eczema | Prodromal tingling | 'Target' lesions | Itchy | Prodromal pain | Very itchy Tense | Single lesion, recurrent at same site | Multiple, clear serum | Multiple, golden crusts |
| **ACUTE ECZEMA** | **ECZEMA HERPETICUM** | **HERPES SIMPLEX** | **ERYTHEMA MULTIFORME** | **PHYTOPHOTO or ALLERGIC DERMATITIS** | **HERPES ZOSTER** | **INSECT BITE** | **FIXED DRUG REACTION** | **BULLOUS DRUG RASH** | **BULLOUS IMPETIGO** |

| *see* p. 189 | *see* p. 109 | *see* p. 109 | *see* p. 174 | p. 182 | p. 179 | *see* p. 198 | p. 181 | p. 183 | p. 187 |

HERPES ZOSTER (SHINGLES)

Herpes zoster occurs in people who have previously had chickenpox. The virus, varicella zoster, lies dormant in the dorsal root ganglion following chickenpox and later travels down the cutaneous nerves to infect the epidermal cells. Destruction of these cells results in the formation of intraepidermal vesicles. For several days before the rash appears there is pain or an abnormal sensation in the skin. Then comes the rash – groups of small vesicles on a red background, followed by weeping and crusting. Healing takes 3–4 weeks. The rash is unilateral and confined to one or two adjacent dermatomes with a sharp cut-off at or near the midline. This feature and the associated pain makes any other diagnosis unlikely. The pain may continue until healing occurs, but in the elderly may go on for months or even years.

TREATMENT: HERPES ZOSTER

If the patient is seen during the *prodromal phase* of pain or paraesthesia, or *within 48 hours of the development of blisters*, treat with a 7-day course of an oral antiviral agent such as:

- aciclovir 800 mg 5 times a day
- famciclovir 250 mg tid
- valaciclovir 1 g tid.

These drugs are competitive inhibitors of guanosine and because they are converted to the triphosphate by viral thymidine kinase, they are effective only in the presence of actively replicating virus. They are all very expensive so should only be given in the early phase of the disease.

Give regular analgesics for the pain, e.g. paracetamol 1 g every 4 hours, two co-dydramol tablets 4-hourly, or dihydrocodeine prolonged-release tablets 60 mg 12-hourly. In the elderly, prophylactic amitriptyline 10–25 mg taken at night, gradually increasing to 75 mg, may help to prevent post-herpetic neuralgia if given as soon as the rash appears.

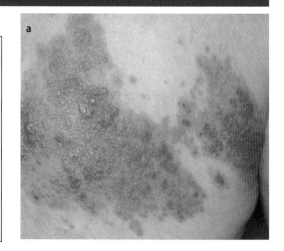

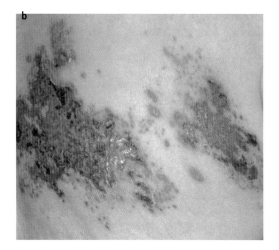

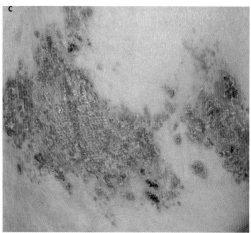

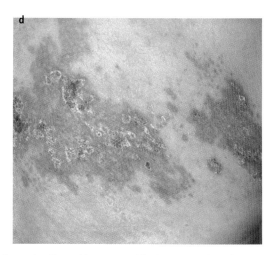

Fig. 7.16 Herpes zoster $T_{1,2}$ at: (a) 7 days – vesicular stage; (b) 14 days – erosions; (c) 21 days – crusting; (d) 28 days – healing with some residual crusts and erythema

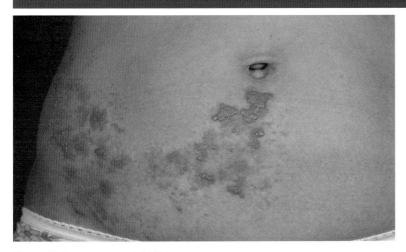

Fig. 7.17 Herpes zoster: right T$_{11,12}$

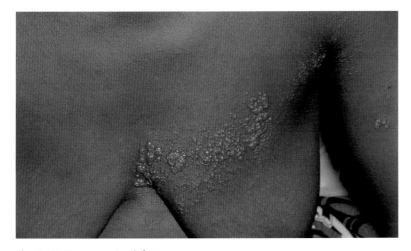

Fig. 7.18 Herpes zoster: left T$_3$

FIXED DRUG ERUPTION

This is a curious reaction, whereby each time a drug is given, a well-demarcated, round or oval, red plaque with/without blistering occurs at the same site, usually within 2 hours, and certainly within 24 hours. The only differential diagnosis is a recurrent herpes simplex infection. Any drug can cause it. In the United Kingdom and the United States the common ones are:

- barbiturates
- benzodiazepines
- sulphonamides
- tetracycline
- phenophthalein (in *over-the-counter* laxatives)
- NSAIDs
- quinine (tablets and in tonic water or bitter lemon drinks).

The redness and swelling disappears after about 10 days to leave a dark-brown patch that remains for several months (*see* p. 297). Stopping the drug will resolve the problem. You can confirm which drug is the cause, as giving it again will produce the same reaction at the same site within 2 hours.

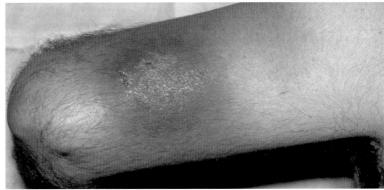

Fig. 7.19 Fixed drug reaction after taking Septrin: erythema and blisters on arm

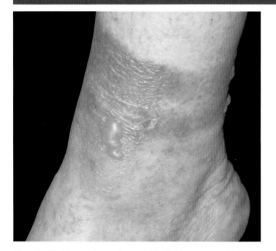

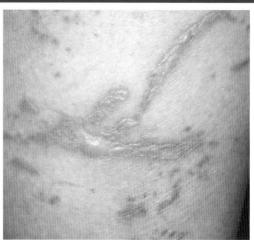

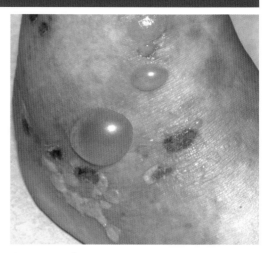

Fig. 7.20 Phytophotodermatitis (strimmer rash): sun-exposed skin below the trouser where plant juices containing psoralens have triggered a phototoxic reaction

Fig. 7.21 Allergic contact dermatitis to *Primula obconica* plant: streaks where plant juices have touched forearm; no sun is necessary for this reaction; poison Ivy will produce a similar reaction

Fig. 7.22 Bullous drug rash on the ankle: this occurs within days of starting the drug (nitrofurantoin)

PHYTOPHOTODERMATITIS

Phytophotodermatitis is due to plant juices containing photoactive chemicals (usually psoralens) being accidentally brushed onto the skin. In the presence of sunlight this causes an irritant or phototoxic dermatitis. Giant hogweed, rue, mustard and St John's wort are common causes. The patient gives a history of having been in the garden clearing weeds, often using a strimmer, or walking in the countryside on a sunny day. The rash is characteristically linear, made up of blisters where the plants have touched the skin, usually on the lower legs or arms.

PLANT CONTACT DERMATITIS

Several plants (*Primula obconica*, *Rhus* – poison ivy) can cause an allergic contact dermatitis. Linear blisters (*see* Fig. 7.21) are seen where the leaves have brushed against the skin, affecting hands, forearms and face). Sometimes the distribution affects the exposed or light-aggravated sites of face, neck, hands and arms with a chronic lichenified dermatitis (chrysanthemums and other compositae). Tulip bulbs and garlic can affect the fingertips (*see* p. 415).

Compositae dermatitis occurs in florists and gardeners, and if suspected it should be patch tested for. Poison ivy, oak or sumac dermatitis is very common in North America and the Far East. The rash generally takes around 24 hours to develop and lasts up to 2 weeks.

TREATMENT: PHYTOPHOTO AND PLANT CONTACT DERMATITIS

Ideally the plant involved should be identified, so that it can be avoided in the future, but this is often not possible. If the rash is due to strimming, the patient should wear trousers tucked inside his or her socks or boots in future. If the rash is very acute with blistering and weeping, dry it with potassium permanganate[UK] or aluminium acetate[USA] soaks (*see* p. 30). Once dry, apply a potent[UK]/group 2–3[USA] topical steroid ointment until better.

BULLOUS DRUG REACTIONS

Bullae at the site of pressure can occur in unconscious patients due to the following drugs:

- barbiturates
- imipramine
- methadone
- meprobamate
- nitrazepam.

Bullous pemphigoid can on occasions be induced by:

- clonidine
- diclofenac
- furosemide
- ibuprofen.

A **pemphigus type** of drug reaction is seen with:

- captopril
- penicillamine
- rifampicin.

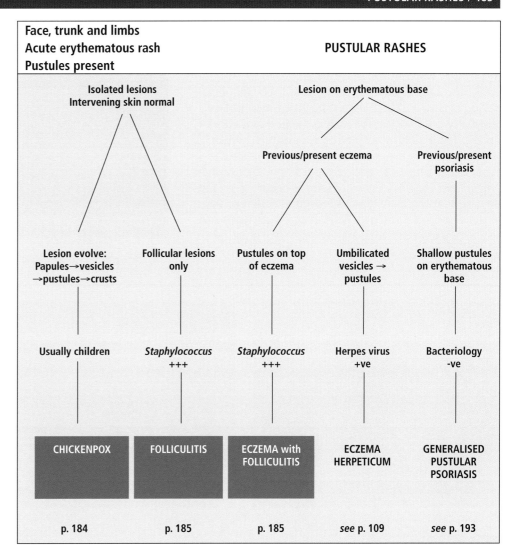

Face, trunk and limbs
Acute erythematous rash
Pustules present

PUSTULAR RASHES

Isolated lesions
Intervening skin normal

Lesion on erythematous base

Previous/present eczema

Previous/present psoriasis

Lesion evolve:
Papules→vesicles
→pustules→crusts

Follicular lesions only

Pustules on top of eczema

Umbilicated vesicles → pustules

Shallow pustules on erythematous base

Usually children

Staphylococcus +++

Staphylococcus +++

Herpes virus +ve

Bacteriology -ve

CHICKENPOX

FOLLICULITIS

ECZEMA with FOLLICULITIS

ECZEMA HERPETICUM

GENERALISED PUSTULAR PSORIASIS

p. 184

p. 185

p. 185

see p. 109

see p. 193

CHICKENPOX (VARICELLA)

Chickenpox (varicella zoster) is a highly infectious illness spread by droplet infection from the upper respiratory tract. In urban communities most children under the age of 10 have been infected. The incubation period is usually 14–15 days. The prodromal illness is usually mild so that the rash is the first evidence of illness. The lesions start off as pink macules, which develop quickly into papules (*see* Fig. 7.23), tense vesicles (*see* Fig. 7.24), pustules (*see* Fig. 7.25) and then crusts (*see* Fig. 7.26). Crops of lesions occur over a few days so that there are always lesions at different stages of development present. The spots are very itchy and secondary infection may lead to pock-like scarring (*see* Fig. 7.27). Typically it occurs on the face and trunk rather than the limbs.

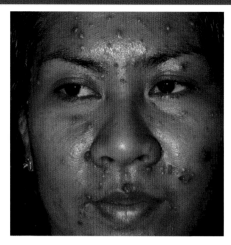

Fig. 7.25 Chickenpox pustules on adult face

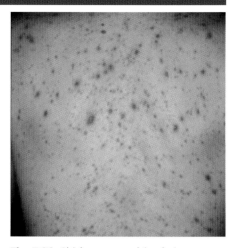

Fig. 7.26 Chickenpox resolving lesions on back of adult

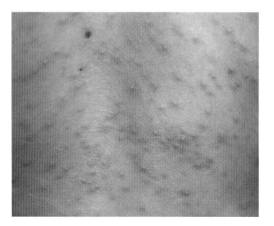

Fig. 7.23 Chickenpox: early lesions showing papules and vesicles

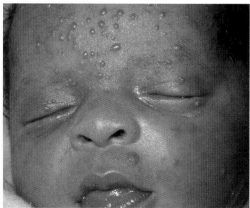

Fig. 7.24 Chickenpox: vesicles on baby's face

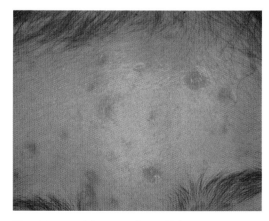

Fig. 7.27 Resolving scars from chickenpox

FOLLICULITIS

Superficial infection of hair follicles is very common. A small bead of pus sits around a protruding hair and there may be slight erythema at the base. One or several follicles may be involved, but there is no tenderness or involvement of the deep part of the follicle. It is usually due to *S. aureus*, which may be carried in the patient's nose or perineum. It can be caused by, or made worse by, the application of greasy ointments to the skin, tar preparations or plasters. The wearing of oily overalls may precipitate folliculitis of the thighs (**oil acne**).

TREATMENT: CHICKENPOX

In most instances chickenpox requires no treatment. In adults and immunocompromised patients, treatment with famciclovir or valaciclovir will reduce the severity of the disease (*see* p. 180 for doses).

TREATMENT: FOLLICULITIS

Take swabs from a pustule and any possible carriage sites (anterior nares, perineum and any other skin rash). Stop applying greasy ointments to the site. If this is the cause then nothing else is necessary. If folliculitis occurs in a patient with atopic eczema, change the patient's steroid ointment to a cream for a few weeks.

Oral flucloxacillin or erythromycin 500 mg qid for a week will clear most cases. Treat any infected carriage sites with topical mupiricin, fucidin or neomycin cream bid for 2 weeks. Persistent folliculitis may require long-term suppressive treatment with low-dose oral antibiotics (250 mg bid for up to 6 months).

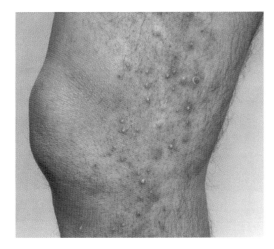

Fig. 7.28 Folliculitis on thigh: *Staphylococcus* aureus grown from pustules

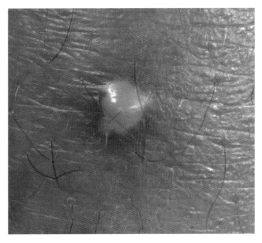

Fig. 7.29 Folliculitis: bead of pus at opening of a hair follicle

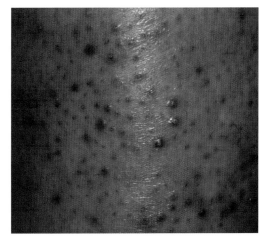

Fig. 7.30 Folliculitis on leg from applying greasy ointments

Trunk and limbs
Acute erythematous lesions
Surface crust/exudate
Erosions and ulcers

CRUST AND EXUDATE

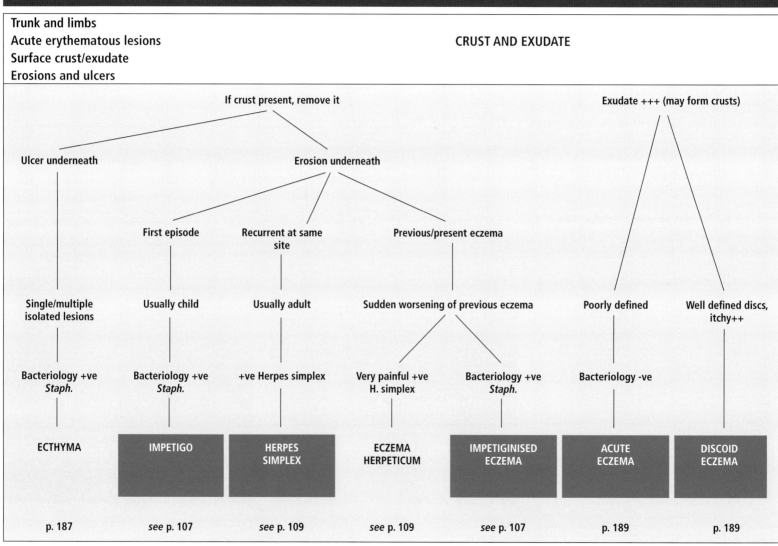

STAPHYLOCOCCAL SKIN INFECTIONS

Pathogenic *S. aureus* can cause a variety of skin infections depending on the depth of inoculation (*see* Fig. 7.31). An infection just under the stratum corneum causes impetigo (*see* Fig. 4.18, p. 107) where the superficial blisters rapidly break to form erosions with golden crusts on the surface. In the newborn you may see intact blisters with pus in them (bullous impetigo, *see* Fig. 7.32). Ecthyma is an infection of the full thickness of the epidermis (*see* below). Folliculitis is a superficial infection of the hair follicle with a pustule at the opening of the follicle (*see* p. 185). Deeper infection results in either a boil, if the whole follicle is involved, or a carbuncle, if multiple adjacent follicles are involved (*see* pp. 177, 178).

A new strain of *S. aureus* producing **Panton–Valentine leukocidin** (**PVL**) has been identified recently. PVL is a cytotoxin that can destroy white blood cells and cause extensive tissue necrosis. PVL-positive *S. aureus* is usually methicillin resistant but is acquired in the community, unlike methicillin-resistant *S. aureus*. It causes recurrent skin abscesses and cellulitis, which do not respond to routine doses of flucloxacillin or erythromycin. Infection with PVL-positive *S. aureus* should be suspected in anyone with recurrent or antibiotic-resistant furunculosis (boils), abscesses or necrotising fasciitis. Swabs should be sent to the laboratory with a request to screen for PVL.

ECTHYMA

Ecthyma can be caused by either *S. aureus* or *Steptococcus pyogenes* and is always secondary to a break in the skin (following an injury, insect bite or scabies). It presents as a round, punched-out ulcer with a thick crust on top. It is usually seen in children but may occur in adults, especially in hot humid climates, and those infected with PVL-positive *S. aureus*. The lesions will heal with scarring.

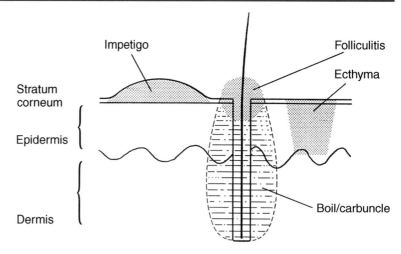

Fig. 7.31 Sites of involvement of staphylococcal infection of the skin

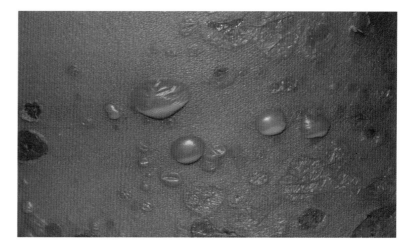

Fig. 7.32 Bullous impetigo: pus-filled bullae on trunk of newborn

TREATMENT: ECTHYMA

Take swabs and give oral flucloxacillin or erythromycin by mouth, 125–500 mg qid for 7–10 days depending on age. Do not treat with topical antibiotics, as the infection is deep and they will not work. The ulcer itself will take at least 4 weeks to heal, but antibiotics do not need to be continued for this long. Extensive tissue necrosis should raise the possibility of PVL-positive *S. aureus*.

TREATMENT: PVL-POSITIVE *S. AUREUS*

Cases not responding to flucloxallin 500 mg qid acquired in the community should be treated with:

- clindamycin 450 mg qid
- rifampicin 300 mg bid plus doxycycline 100 mg bid (not for children <12 years); the doxycycline can be replace by fucidic acid 500 mg tid or trimethoprim 200 mg bid.

Treat carriage sites, the nose with mupirocin (Bactroban) ointment and the skin by washing with 1% chlorhexidine wash for 5 days.

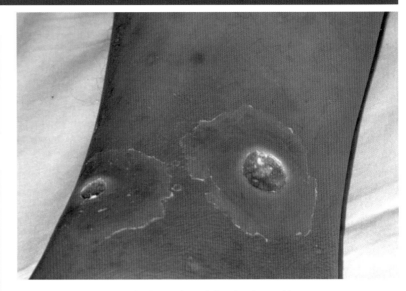

Fig. 7.34 Ecthyma: punched-out ulcers following insect bites

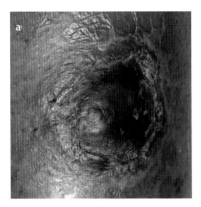 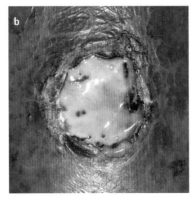

Fig. 7.33 Ecthyma: (a) with crust on surface; (b) with crust removed to reveal pus

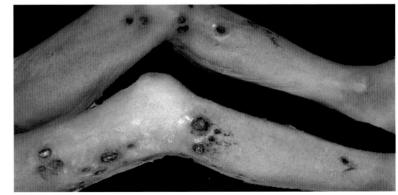

Fig. 7.35 Multiple lesions of ecthyma on legs in a patient with PVL +ve *S. aureus*

ACUTE ECZEMA

Acute eczema clinically presents with tiny vesicles that burst to produce erosions, exudate and crusts. It may be due to an acute flare of chronic atopic eczema (*see* p. 236), or an allergic contact dermatitis. It may be difficult to distinguish from impetiginised eczema (*see* p. 107). A common mistake is to assume that weeping eczema is infected and treat it with antibiotics rather than topical steroids.

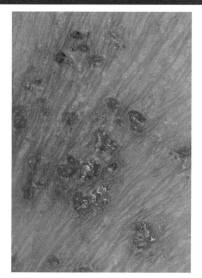

Fig. 7.37 Acute eczema: broken vesicles

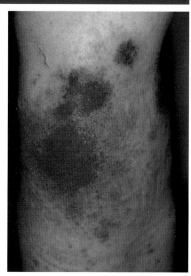

Fig. 7.38 Acute eczema with erosions and exudate

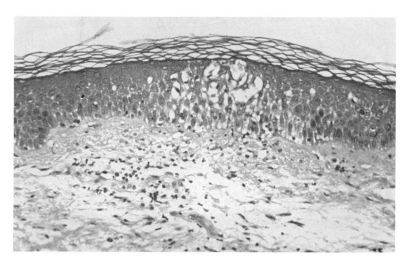

Fig. 7.36 Histology of acute eczema showing vesicles within the epidermis

DISCOID ECZEMA (WET TYPE)

Discoid eczema presents as well-defined, coin-shaped (nummular) plaques. The wet type is made up of coalescing erosions with exudate on the surface. The exudate dries to form crusts. There may be one or a number of lesions (*see* also p. 243).

TREATMENT: ACUTE ECZEMA

It is no good trying to apply creams or ointments to an exuding rash, because they are not able to penetrate the skin. First, dry up the exudate with an astringent such as Burow's solution (aluminium acetate) or diluted potassium permanganate solution (1:10 000), *see* p. 30. The latter should be a light-pink colour (*see* Fig. 2.01, p. 30). Either put the solution in a bath or bowl and soak the affected area or soak a towel or flannel in the solution and apply it to the affected area for 10 minutes four times a day. After soaking, dry the skin with a towel and then apply a potent[UK]/group 2–3[USA] steroid ointment. If a contact allergy is suspected, refer the patient for patch testing once the rash has settled.

Face, Trunk and Limbs
Acute erythematous rash
Generalised rash (>50% body surface)

GENERALISED RASH (>50% body surface)

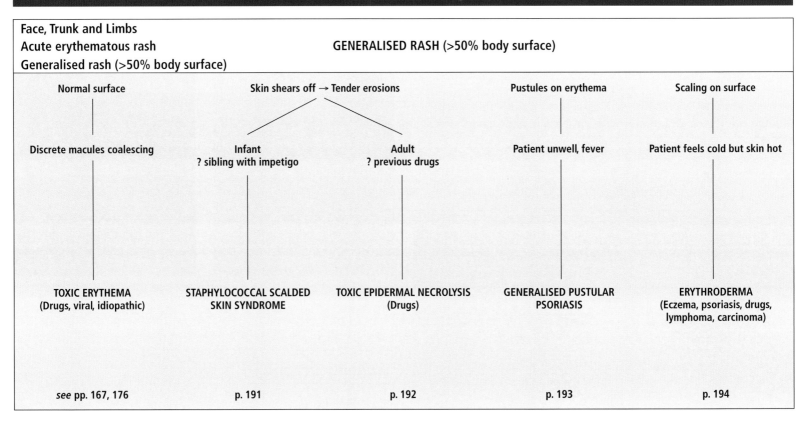

| Normal surface | Skin shears off → Tender erosions | | Pustules on erythema | Scaling on surface |

Discrete macules coalescing | Infant ? sibling with impetigo | Adult ? previous drugs | Patient unwell, fever | Patient feels cold but skin hot

TOXIC ERYTHEMA (Drugs, viral, idiopathic)

STAPHYLOCOCCAL SCALDED SKIN SYNDROME

TOXIC EPIDERMAL NECROLYSIS (Drugs)

GENERALISED PUSTULAR PSORIASIS

ERYTHRODERMA (Eczema, psoriasis, drugs, lymphoma, carcinoma)

see pp. 167, 176   p. 191   p. 192   p. 193   p. 194

STAPHYLOCOCCAL SCALDED SKIN SYNDROME

This is an infection due to phage type 71 *S. aureus*, which produces a toxin that causes a split in the upper part of the epidermis. It occurs almost entirely in infants and young children. The skin becomes red and very tender (like a scald) and then peels off. It often begins in the flexures but usually spreads to involve the whole body. The child will be screaming with pain. The source of infection is often an older sibling with impetigo, infected eczema or scabies.

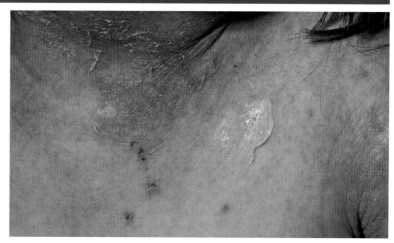

Fig. 7.40 Staphylococcal scalded skin syndrome in a young child

TREATMENT: STAPHYLOCOCCAL SCALDED SKIN SYNDROME

Treatment is flucloxacillin elixir 62.5 mg (children under age 2) or 125 mg (age over 2 years) every 6 hours for 7 days. The pain will stop almost immediately but the skin peeling takes longer to stop due to persistence of the toxin. Other children in the family may require treatment for impetigo or infected eczema at the same time.

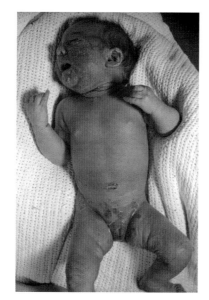

Fig. 7.39 Staphylococcal scalded skin syndrome

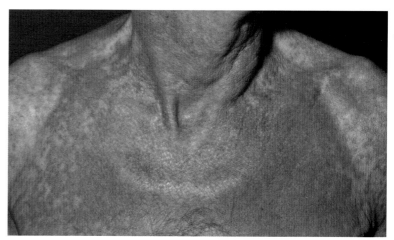

Fig. 7.41 Toxic erythema: the skin is just red, with no evidence of skin peeling or systemic upset

TOXIC EPIDERMAL NECROLYSIS

This is an uncommon but serious skin disease in which the whole of the epidermis dies and shears off. It is most commonly due to drugs:

- allopurinol
- carbamazepine
- phenytoin
- thiacetazone.
- barbiturates
- NSAIDs
- sulphonamides

However, it can also occur in patients with a lymphoma or HIV infection. In some cases no cause is found.

The **prognosis of toxic epidermal necrolysis** can be very poor, especially if large amounts of skin are lost. The following scoring system will help determine the prognosis. Score one point for each of the following features:

- age >40
- cancer or HIV
- loss of >30% skin
- urea >10 mM/L.
- heart rate >120
- blood sugar >14 mM/L
- bicarbonate <20 mM/L

Mortality: score 0–1 = 3%; score 3 = 35%; score >5 = 90%

TREATMENT: TOXIC EPIDERMAL NECROLYSIS

Stop the suspected drug. The extensive skin loss will need to be treated just like a burn and admission to a burns unit or intensive care unit is essential. Surgical debridement is not necessary, as only the epidermis is shed. *Survival depends on good management with replacement of fluids and electrolytes lost through the skin, prevention of infection and septicaemia, and careful handling of the patient's skin, which tends to tear off easily.*

Early treatment with large doses of intravenous immunoglobulin (2 g/kg body weight given daily for 3–4 days) may be life saving. The immunoglobulins inhibit Fas-mediated epidermal cell death and allow the epidermis to recover. Systemic steroids do not help and may be harmful.

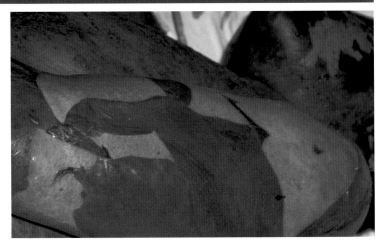

Fig. 7.42 Toxic epidermal necrolysis: the whole epidermis is shearing off

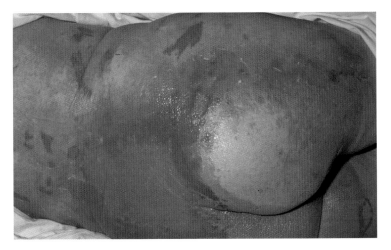

Fig. 7.43 Toxic epidermal necrolysis

GENERALISED PUSTULAR PSORIASIS

This acute, serious and unstable form of psoriasis is often precipitated by withdrawal of systemic or very potent topical steroids. Sheets of erythema studded with tiny sterile pustules come in waves associated with fever (*see* Figs. 7.44, 45, 46) and general malaise. This is the main reason why psoriasis should not be treated with either topical or systemic steroids.

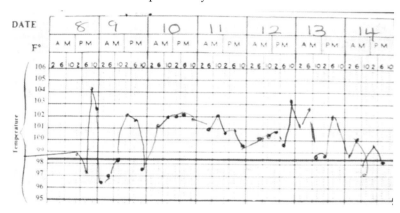

Fig. 7.44 Temperature chart for patient with generalised pustular psoriasis

TREATMENT: GENERALISED PUSTULAR PSORIASIS

This is a dermatological emergency and carries a significant mortality. The patient should be admitted to hospital for bed rest and sedation. Initially the skin will be treated with emollients (e.g. equal parts white soft paraffin and liquid paraffin[UK]/ petrolatum[USA]). The patient should be nursed under a 'space blanket' to prevent hypothermia. The associated fever is not due to infection, so there is no need for antibiotics. Both topical and systemic steroids are contraindicated. If the patient fails to improve on the aforementioned measures, systemic treatment will be needed with methotrexate or ciclosporin.

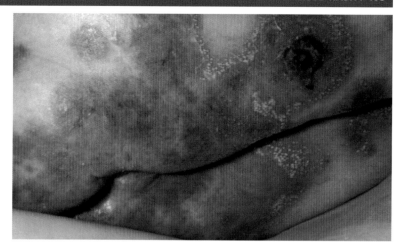

Fig. 7.45 Generalised pustular psoriasis

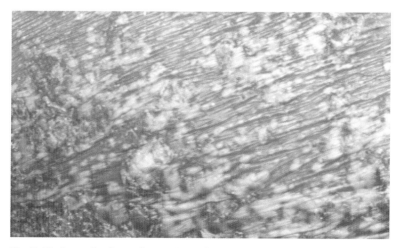

Fig. 7.46 Generalised pustular psoriasis: sheets of shallow pustules on an erythematous background

ERYTHRODERMA (EXFOLIATIVE DERMATITIS)

Erythroderma is the term used when >90% of the body's surface is red and scaly. It can be caused by:

- eczema
- psoriasis
- a drug reaction, e.g. due to:
  - allopurinol
  - barbiturates
  - captopril
  - carbamazepine
  - chlorpromazine
  - chloroquine
  - cimetidine
  - gold
  - isoniazid
  - nalidixic acid
  - phenytoin
  - sulphonamides
- Sézary syndrome (cutaneous T-cell lymphoma, *see* p. 231)
- an underlying carcinoma.

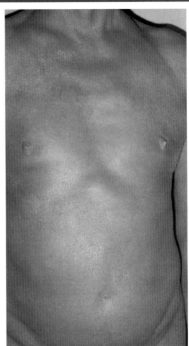

Fig. 7.48 Erythroderma due to carcinoma of the pancreas

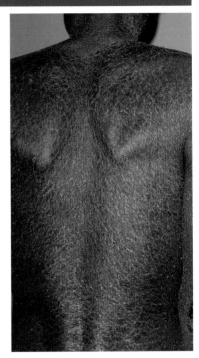

Fig. 7.49 Erythroderma in black skin

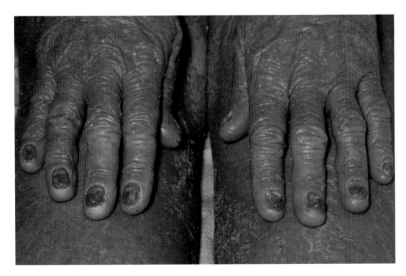

Fig. 7.47 Sézary syndrome

TREATMENT: ERYTHRODERMA

These patients should be managed in hospital, both to find the cause and to prevent hypothermia, congestive cardiac failure or renal failure. Initially the skin should be treated with emollients such as white soft paraffin[UK]/petrolatum[USA]. Specific causes should be treated, e.g. psoriasis can be treated with methotrexate, or eczema with topical steroids. Stop any drugs and look for an underlying carcinoma or lymphoma.

Chronic erythematous lesions on trunk and limbs

8

Trunk and limbs
Chronic erythematous rash
Normal surface
No pustules (pustules present, *see* p. 201)

MULTIPLE SMALL PAPULES (<5 mm)
(For single papules *see* p. 213)

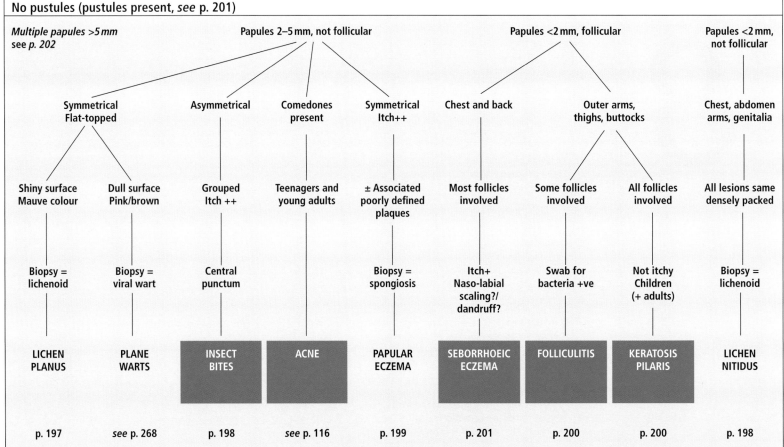

Multiple papules >5 mm
see p. 202

Papules 2–5 mm, not follicular

Papules <2 mm, follicular

Papules <2 mm, not follicular

Symmetrical Flat-topped — Asymmetrical — Comedones present — Symmetrical Itch++

Chest and back — Outer arms, thighs, buttocks — Chest, abdomen arms, genitalia

Shiny surface Mauve colour — Dull surface Pink/brown — Grouped Itch ++ — Teenagers and young adults — ± Associated poorly defined plaques

Most follicles involved — Some follicles involved — All follicles involved — All lesions same densely packed

Biopsy = lichenoid — Biopsy = viral wart — Central punctum — Biopsy = spongiosis

Itch+ Naso-labial scaling?/ dandruff? — Swab for bacteria +ve — Not itchy Children (+ adults) — Biopsy = lichenoid

LICHEN PLANUS — PLANE WARTS — INSECT BITES — ACNE — PAPULAR ECZEMA — SEBORRHOEIC ECZEMA — FOLLICULITIS — KERATOSIS PILARIS — LICHEN NITIDUS

p. 197 — *see* p. 268 — p. 198 — *see* p. 116 — p. 199 — p. 201 — p. 200 — p. 200 — p. 198

LICHEN PLANUS

The lesions in lichen planus are small mauve, flat-topped, shiny papules, which sometimes have white streaky areas on the surface (Wickham's striae). The most characteristic place to look for the rash is on the flexor aspect of the wrist, but it is usually widespread on the trunk and limbs, and may occur at sites of trauma (Köebner phenomenon). Some lesions may become plaques. Although it is very itchy, scratch marks are not usually seen. As the rash gets better the colour of the papules change from mauve to brown (see Fig. 1.65, p. 14). It is uncommon in children. The buccal mucosa may be involved, with a white, lace-like, streaky pattern (see Fig. 6.19, p. 149). The rash tends to last 9–18 months before disappearing. There may be some residual post-inflammatory hyperpigmentation for a time. In pigmented skin the rash tends to become hyperpigmented with a characteristic bluish-black colour (see Fig. 8.06). Lichen nitidus is a variant where the papules are less than 2 mm in diameter (see Fig. 8.04).

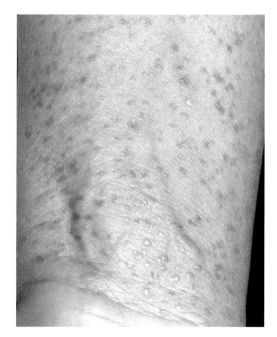

Fig. 8.01 Lichen planus: flat-topped shiny papules on flexor aspect of wrist

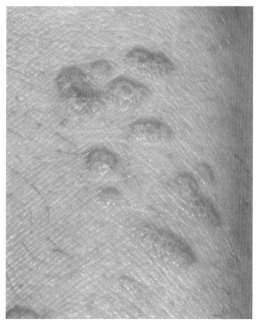

Fig. 8.02 Lichen planus: Wickham's striae

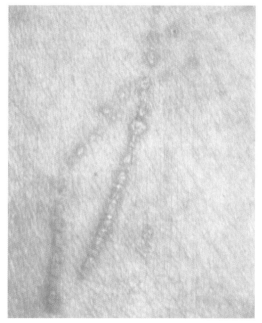

Fig. 8.03 Lichen planus: Köebner phenomenon

TREATMENT: LICHEN PLANUS

Topical treatment will not make the rash go away any quicker, but the application of a potent[UK]/group 2–3[USA] topical steroid will control the itching.

Patients with extensive blistering (bullous) or severe erosive mucous membrane lichen planus may require treatment with systemic steroids and should be referred urgently to a dermatologist

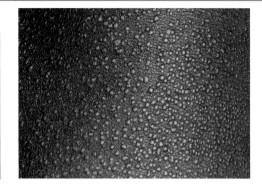

Fig. 8.04 Lichen nitidus

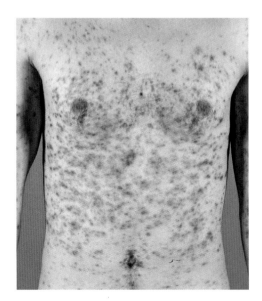

Fig. 8.05 Lichen planus: the rash may become hyperpigmented as it gets better

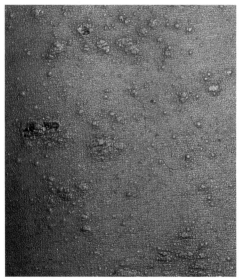

Fig. 8.06 Lichen planus in pigmented skin

INSECT BITES (PAPULAR URTICARIA)

Insect bites present as itchy papules with a central punctum. If there are groups or rows of three or four bites, think of flea bites. Single very large lesions on the face or hands are suggestive of bedbugs, particularly where new lesions are found each morning. Numerous other insects can also bite humans. Usually the patient is not able to identify the insect involved. Sometimes large blisters follow insect bites.

TREATMENT: INSECT BITES

Most patients will have acquired flea bites from an infestation in the home. Cats and dogs catch fleas from other pets and bring them into the home, mostly during the summer but at other times of the year during spells of warm weather. Humans can be bitten by fleas, which live on cats and dogs throughout the adult stage of their life cycle. Fleas lay eggs on their cat or dog host, which will drop to the ground and undergo several life cycle stages before reaching adulthood, when they can return to the host and feed. If no animal host is available they may remain on furniture, bedding or carpets for months.

To get rid of animal fleas, use both a drug that kills adult fleas, such as Frontline (fipronil) or Advocate (imidacloprid), as a monthly topical treatment on the pet and an insect development inhibitor, such as Program (lufenuron), for the larval stages. These are available from veterinary surgeons.

It may also be necessary to spray areas of the house such as carpets, sofas and pet bedding, where eggs will have fallen, with a suitable product such as Indorex, which contains permethrin, piperonyl butoxide and pyriproxyfen.

Insect repellents

Mosquitos can be discouraged from biting by using an insect repellent. DEET (N,N-diethyl-m-toluamide) is the most effective insect repellent available at the moment, but it can cause irritation on the skin and should not be used around the eyes. It is available as a lotion, stick or spray. Lotions are generally cheaper than sticks or sprays. All are equally effective if they are applied often enough. Aerosols and sprays last 1–2 hours; liquids, lotions, creams and pump sprays last 2–3 hours. Gels and sticks last 4 hours. In children the insect repellent is applied to clothing near to the exposed skin, rather than on the skin itself so there will be no local irritation and no risk of the child getting it in his or her eyes.

PAPULAR ECZEMA

Eczema may sometimes present as papules that remain discrete rather than coalescing into poorly defined plaques. It can be difficult to diagnose. A biopsy may be necessary to distinguish it from folliculitis.

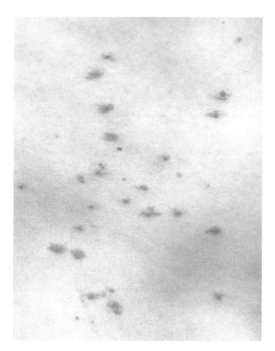

Fig. 8.07 Flea bites: grouped papules with intervening skin normal

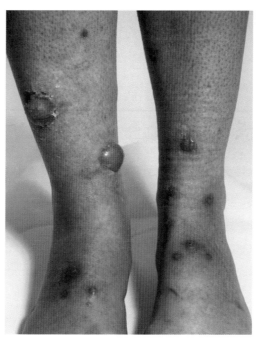

Fig. 8.08 Large blisters on the lower leg from flea bites

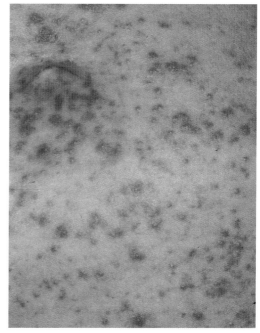

Fig. 8.09 Papular eczema

KERATOSIS PILARIS

Erythematous follicular papules develop on the upper arms and thighs. It is distinguished from folliculitis, as it is rough to the touch. Also, all follicles are involved and there are no pustules (*see* p. 324).

FOLLICULITIS

Inflammation of hair follicles is very common. One (*see* Fig. 7.29, p. 185) or several follicles may be involved. Pustules are often present. It is usually due to *Staphylococcus aureus*, particularly if the patient also has eczema. Folliculitis can be caused by, or made worse by, the application of greasy ointments, tar preparations or plasters on the skin. The wearing of oily overalls may precipitate folliculitis of the thighs (**oil acne**).

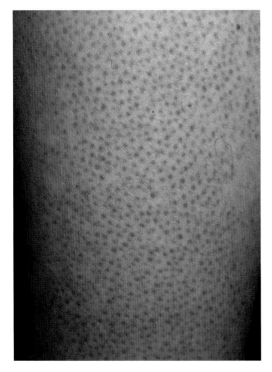

Fig. 8.10 Keratosis pilaris on thigh: erythematous follicular papules that are rough to the touch

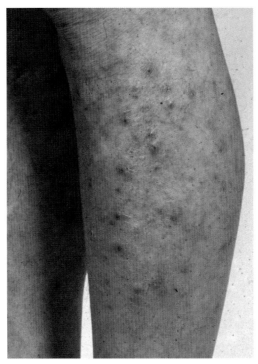

Fig. 8.11 Folliculitis infection of hair follicles on lower leg in a patient with atopic eczema

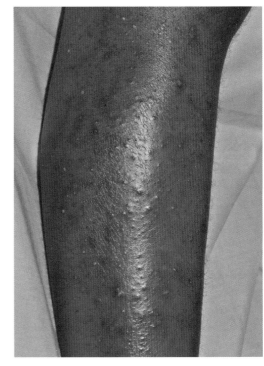

Fig. 8.12 Folliculitis in black skin caused by the application of greasy ointments

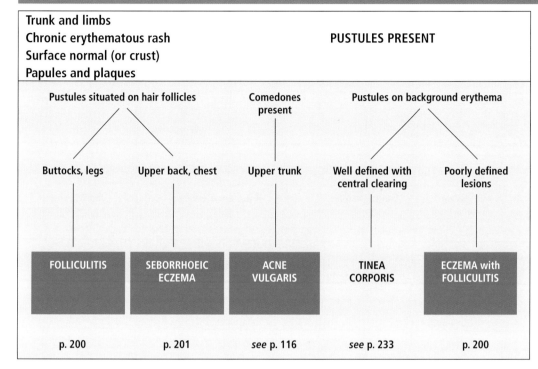

Trunk and limbs
Chronic erythematous rash
Surface normal (or crust)
Papules and plaques

PUSTULES PRESENT

Pustules situated on hair follicles · Comedones present · Pustules on background erythema

Buttocks, legs · Upper back, chest · Upper trunk · Well defined with central clearing · Poorly defined lesions

FOLLICULITIS · SEBORRHOEIC ECZEMA · ACNE VULGARIS · TINEA CORPORIS · ECZEMA with FOLLICULITIS

p. 200 · p. 201 · *see* p. 116 · *see* p. 233 · p. 200

SEBORRHOEIC ECZEMA (PITYROSPORUM FOLLICULITIS)

On the trunk, seborrhoeic eczema may present as extensive follicular papules and pustules that are caused by overgrowth of pityrosporum yeast in the follicles (**pityrosporum folliculitis**, *see* Fig. 8.13). This rash tends to come and go. The diagnosis is made by the association with typical seborrhoeic eczema on the face (*see* p. 135) and scalp (*see* p. 89). For treatment *see* p. 136.

TINEA CORPORIS

Tinea uncommonly presents with pustules on a background of erythema. Think of it when the lesions are unilateral or asymmetrical. The diagnosis is made by taking swabs for bacteriology (to exclude secondarily infected eczema), and mycology scrapings that will confirm a dermatophyte fungus (*see* p. 233).

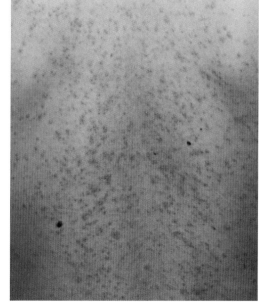

Fig. 8.13 Pityrosporum folliculitis: papules and pustules on the back or chest; look for seborrhoeic dermatitis at other sites

Face, trunk and limbs
Chronic erythematous rash
Macules, small patches and plaques
Normal surface (or slight scale)

MULTIPLE LESIONS (all >5 mm and <2 cm)
(Multiple large plaques >2 cm, *see* p. 208)
(Single/few large papules and nodules, *see* p. 213)

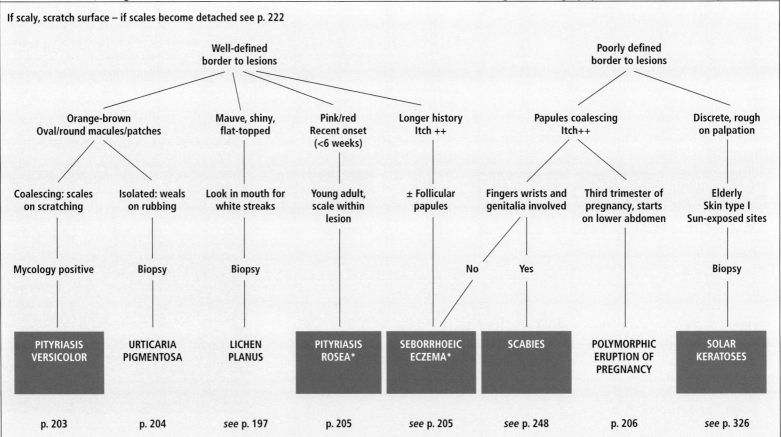

If scaly, scratch surface – if scales become detached see p. 222

Well-defined border to lesions

- **Orange-brown** Oval/round macules/patches
  - Coalescing: scales on scratching
    - Mycology positive
    - **PITYRIASIS VERSICOLOR** — p. 203
  - Isolated: weals on rubbing
    - Biopsy
    - **URTICARIA PIGMENTOSA** — p. 204
- **Mauve, shiny, flat-topped**
  - Look in mouth for white streaks
    - Biopsy
    - **LICHEN PLANUS** — *see* p. 197
- **Pink/red Recent onset (<6 weeks)**
  - Young adult, scale within lesion
    - **PITYRIASIS ROSEA*** — p. 205
- **Longer history Itch ++**
  - ± Follicular papules
    - **SEBORRHOEIC ECZEMA*** — *see* p. 205

Poorly defined border to lesions

- **Papules coalescing Itch++**
  - Fingers wrists and genitalia involved — No
  - Yes
    - **SCABIES** — *see* p. 248
  - Third trimester of pregnancy, starts on lower abdomen
    - **POLYMORPHIC ERUPTION OF PREGNANCY** — p. 206
- **Discrete, rough on palpation**
  - Elderly Skin type I Sun-exposed sites
    - Biopsy
    - **SOLAR KERATOSES** — *see* p. 326

*If patient unwell, has lymphadenopathy and lesions on palms and soles, think of secondary syphilis, *see* p. 207.

PITYRIASIS VERSICOLOR

The word pityriasis means 'bran-like' and here means a scaly rash; versicolor means different colours. Pityriasis versicolor is a scaly rash of different colours. In different individuals it may be white, orange brown or dark brown. The lesions are small, less than 1 cm in diameter, usually round and always scaly when scratched. Some may join together to form larger lesions or confluent plaques. It is a disease of young adults and occurs predominantly on the upper trunk. It is due to an infection with a yeast, *Pityrosporum orbiculare*, which we all have on our skin as a harmless commensal. Under certain conditions, the yeast produces hyphae and becomes pathogenic. It is then known as *Malassezia globosa*. The depigmentation is due to inhibition of tyrosinase by dicarboxylic acids produced by the pityrosporum yeast leading to suppression of melanin production.

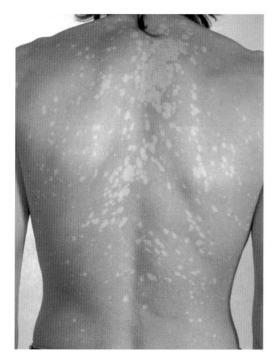

Fig. 8.14 Pityriasis versicolor, white variety

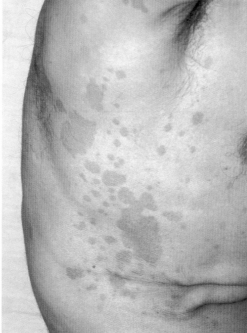

Fig. 8.15 Pityriasis versicolor, orange-brown variety

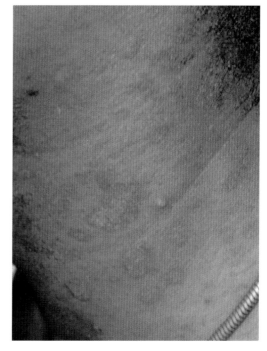

Fig. 8.16 Pityriasis versicolor in black skin, dark-brown variety

Most people with the rash have picked up the pathogenic form of the organism from someone else with it when on holiday in a warm climate; it is possible to transform your own commensal organisms if you are on steroids or other immunosuppressive therapy.

The orange-brown variety can be confused with pityriasis rosea, but the diagnosis can be easily confirmed by scraping off the scales, mixing them with a mixture of equal parts of 20% potassium hydroxide solution and Parker blue-black ink. The organism takes up the blue colour of the ink and shows both spores and hyphae ('spaghetti and meatballs', *see* Fig. 8.17).

TREATMENT: PITYRIASIS VERSICOLOR

If the rash is localised, use an imidazole cream such as clotrimazole twice a day for 2 weeks. If it is extensive then a single dose of oral ketaconazole 400 mg works well. An alternative is itraconazole 100 mg/day for 5 days. Griseofulvin and terbinafine do *not* work.

It is important to tell the patient that any hypopigmented areas will look the same after treatment. It usually takes 3 months for the pigment to return to normal. Patients with the orange-brown or dark-brown variety will look normal immediately after treatment.

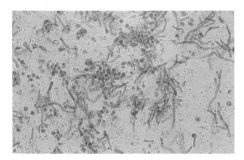

Fig. 8.17 Direct microscopy of scale in pityriasis versicolor ('spaghetti and meatballs')

URTICARIA PIGMENTOSA

This rare condition is due to increased mast cells in the skin. Orange-brown pigmented macules and small patches appear in children and young adults. The lesions may coalesce to form larger patches. The surface is not scaly but on rubbing a weal appears (Darier's sign), due to release of histamine from the mast cells. Most patients are asymptomatic but do not like the appearance of the rash; some patients may itch. Systemic symptoms of histamine release (flushing, headaches, dyspnoea, wheeze, diarrhoea or syncope) are extremely rare.

Avoid any mast cell degranulating agents (aspirin, alcohol, morphine, codeine). Antihistamines (both H_1- and H_2-antagonists) can be tried. If the patient is itching, PUVA therapy (*see* p. 61) is helpful and the tan it produces will mask the rash.

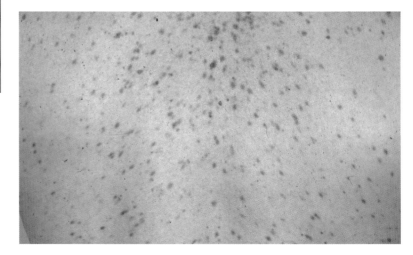

Fig. 8.18 Urticaria pigmentosa

PITYRIASIS ROSEA

This condition is a viral infection due to the human herpesvirus-7. It occurs in otherwise fit and healthy children or young adults, and lasts about 6 weeks. First a single oval, scaly plaque 2–3 cm in diameter appears on the trunk or on a limb. This is the 'herald patch', which can sometimes be misdiagnosed as ringworm. A few days later, the rest of the rash appears. It consists of two different kinds of lesions: first, petaloid lesions, which are similar to the herald patch but smaller in size and consisting of oval pink scaly macules or plaques where the scale is just inside the edge of the lesion; second, small, pink follicular papules. If the herald patch is on the trunk, the rest of the rash is confined to the vest and pants area, and the individual lesions follow Langer's lines, giving a 'Christmas tree' pattern. Look at the hands for evidence of **scabetic burrows**, especially if the rash is particularly itchy at night (*see* p. 248).

(*see* p. 248).

TREATMENT: PITYRIASIS ROSEA

It is usually asymptomatic and needs no treatment other than reassurance that it is harmless and will get better on its own in about 6 weeks. If it is particularly itchy you can use a simple moisturiser or 1% hydrocortisone cream twice a day.

SEBORRHOEIC ECZEMA

On the trunk, **seborrhoeic dermatitis** may present as petaloid plaques over the sternum (Fig. 8.22) and central back, extensive follicular papules and pustules (pityrosporum folliculitis, *see* p. 201) or a pityriasis rosea-like rash. The clue to the diagnosis is that it has been present for more than 6 weeks and there is other evidence of seborrhoeic eczema such as scaling around the nasolabial folds (*see* p. 135) and on the scalp (*see* p. 89). For treatment *see* p. 136.

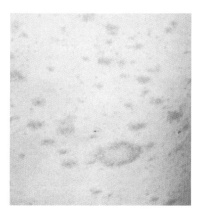

Fig. 8.19 Pityriasis rosea: herald patch with numerous petaloid and papular lesions

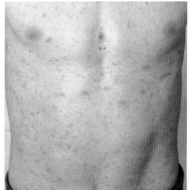

Fig. 8.20 Pityriasis rosea showing 'Christmas tree' distribution, petaloid and follicular lesions

Fig. 8.21 Pityriasis rosea showing scale within a petaloid lesion

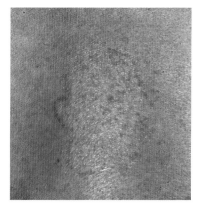

Fig. 8.22 Seborrhoeic eczema, petaloid lesions in the centre of the back

POLYMORPHIC ERUPTION OF PREGNANCY (PRURITIC URTICARIAL PAPULES AND PLAQUES OF PREGNANCY)

This is a common rash (about 1:150 pregnancies) that usually occurs in the third trimester of the first pregnancy. It is a very itchy condition, which starts on the abdomen. It is made up of urticated papules, plaques and sometimes vesicles. It clears up within 2–3 weeks of delivery and does not reoccur in subsequent pregnancies. The baby is not affected. It needs to be distinguished from prurigo of pregnancy (*see* p. 252) and the more serious pemphigoid gestationis.

Table 8.01 Features of polymorphic eruption of pregnancy and pemphigoid gestationis

Polymorphic eruption	Pemphigoid gestationis (*see* p. 256)
Common	Very rare
Urticated papules, vesicles, plaques	Tense vesicles and bullae
Cause unknown	Antibodies to basement membrane
Very itchy	Very itchy
Usually primigravida	Reoccurs in each pregnancy
Occurs third trimester	Second and third trimester
Clears 2–3 weeks after delivery	May take weeks to months to clear
Baby not affected	Baby may be born with same rash

TREATMENT: POLYMORPHIC ERUPTION OF PREGNANCY

Apply a moderately potent[UK]/group 4–5[USA] topical steroid cream twice a day to relieve the itching. Occasionally an oral antihistamine will also be needed, such as chlorphenamine (Piriton) 4–8 mg every 4 hours (maximum of 24 mg in 24 hours). If these measures fail to work, oral prednisolone 20–30 mg/day for 5 days, and tapered off over 2 weeks, is safe and effective carried out in liaison with an obstetrician.

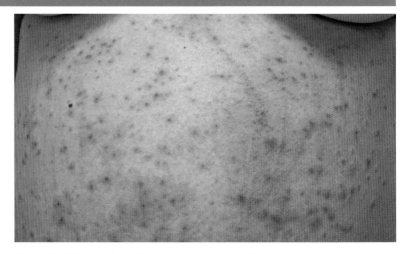

Fig. 8.23 Polymorphic rash of pregnancy over abdomen

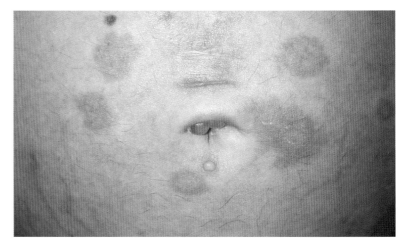

Fig. 8.24 Pemphigoid gestationis: plaques and blisters on abdomen; the rash may look like erythema multiforme

SECONDARY SYPHILIS

Secondary syphilis occurs about 6 weeks after a primary infection with *Treponema pallidum*. The skin lesions are preceded by a flu-like illness and painless lymphadenopathy. The rash is very variable and may consist of macules, papules, pustules and plaques ranging in colour from pink to mauve, orange to brown. There are often lesions on the palms and soles (*see* Figs 8.28 and 8.29), patchy alopecia and flat warty lesions on the genitalia (*see* Fig. 11.02, p. 353) and perianal skin. The diagnosis can be confirmed by demonstrating *T. pallidum* on dark ground microscopy (*see* Fig. 11.04, p. 353), and a positive VDRL test, which distinguishes it from all the other non-itchy rashes on the skin.

For treatment *see* p. 354.

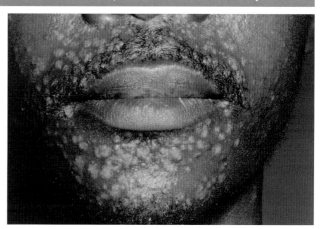

Fig. 8.27 Secondary syphilis: lesions around the mouth

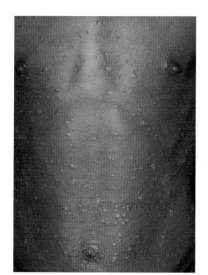

Fig. 8.25 Secondary syphilis: papular rash on black skin

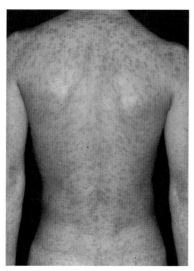

Fig. 8.26 Secondary syphilis: pityriasis rosea-like rash on trunk

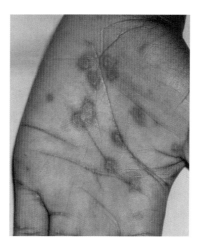

Fig. 8.28 Secondary syphilis lesions on palm

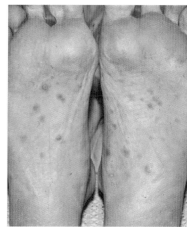

Fig. 8.29 Secondary syphilis lesions on soles

Trunk and limbs
Chronic erythematous rash/multiple lesions
Normal surface
Large patches and plaques (>2 cm)

LARGE LESIONS (>2 cm): NORMAL SURFACE

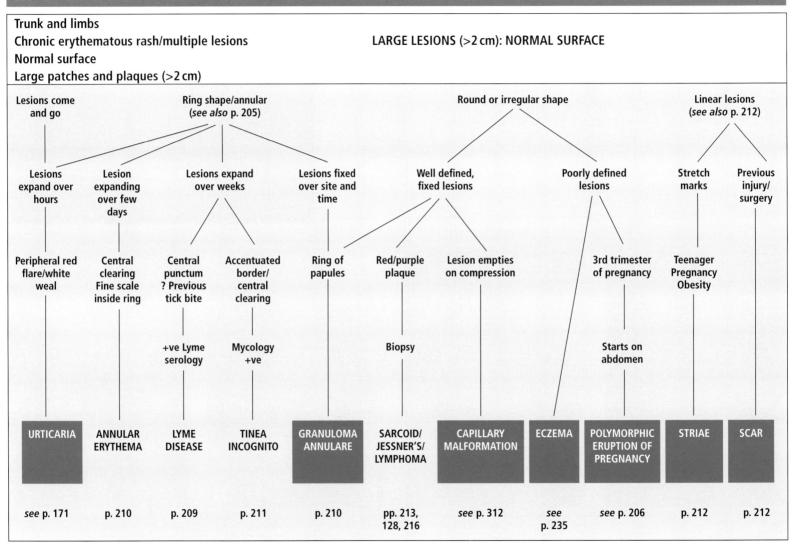

Causes of annular lesions

With normal surface:

- annular erythema (*see* p. 210)
- erythema chronicum migrans (Lyme disease)
- erythema multiforme (*see* p. 174)
- granuloma annulare (*see* p. 210)
- Jessner's lymphocytic infiltrate (*see* p. 128)
- urticaria (*see* p. 171).

With crust or scale:

- annular psoriasis (*see* p. 225)
- discoid eczema (*see* p. 243)
- porokeratosis (*see* p. 326)
- pityriasis rosea (*see* p. 205)
- tinea corporis (*see* p. 233)

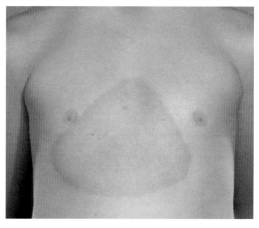

Fig. 8.30 Erythema chronicum migrans (Lyme disease)

LYME DISEASE

A single lesion of gradually expanding erythema (**erythema chronicum migrans**) with or without a central punctum is likely to be Lyme disease, especially if the patient has been walking in an area where ticks are common. It is due to a tick bite, which transmits a spirochaete (*Borrelia burgdorferi*) into the skin. Outbreaks of Lyme disease tend to occur in late May and early June, when the ticks leave the ground vegetation to feed on their animal hosts (deer and sheep). They may wander onto humans walking through the countryside.

If treatment is delayed, patients can go on to develop arthritis (initially intermittent swelling of large joints and later a chronic erosive arthritis), meningoencephalitis, facial nerve palsy and heart problems (conduction defects, myocarditis and pericarditis) weeks or months later. If suspected the diagnosis can be confirmed by finding antibodies to the spirochaete in the patient's serum. There should be a fourfold rise in antibody titre over 2–3 weeks. The antibody (ELISA, enzyme-linked immunosorbent assay) test can be performed at your local hospital.

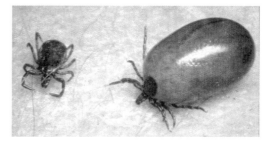

Fig. 8.31 Tick before (left) and after (right) feeding

TREATMENT: LYME DISEASE

Doxycycline 100 mg bid, amoxicillin 500 mg tid or cefuroxime 250 mg bid for 14 days is the treatment of choice. In children under the age of 12, give phenoxymethylpenicillin (Penicillin V) 50 mg/kg body weight per day in divided doses instead. If children are allergic to penicillin, they can be given erythromycin 50 mg/kg body weight per day in divided doses for 10–14 days.

ANNULAR ERYTHEMA

This describes areas of erythema that are annular or figurate in shape. Over a period of days the areas of erythema gradually expand or change. The lesions are often scaly just inside the spreading edge. In most instances no cause can be found, but very rarely some patients may have an underlying neoplasm (lymphoma or leukaemia). No treatment is available unless there is an underlying cause.

GRANULOMA ANNULARE

Granuloma annulare can present in one of three ways.

1. Small pink papules that join together to form rings. There is never any scale on the surface, so it should not be confused with tinea. It is usually seen on the dorsum of hands, elbows and knees, but it can occur anywhere.
2. A flat pink or mauve patch often seen on the thighs, upper arms, trunk or dorsum of the foot (see Fig. 8.36).
3. A generalised asymptomatic macular rash with no surface change (a biopsy is usually needed for diagnosis).

Localised granuloma annulare is not associated with diabetes mellitus; three-quarters of cases of generalised granuloma annulare are.

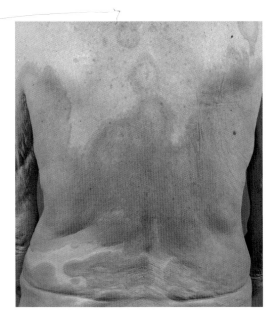

Fig. 8.32 Widespread annular erythema

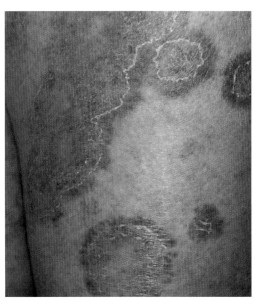

Fig. 8.33 Annular erythema showing scale within ring

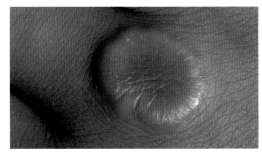

Fig. 8.34 Granuloma annulare: annular ring on dorsum of hand

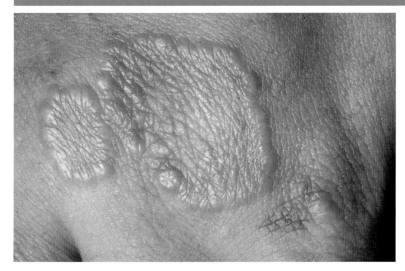

Fig. 8.35 Granuloma annulare on back of the hand

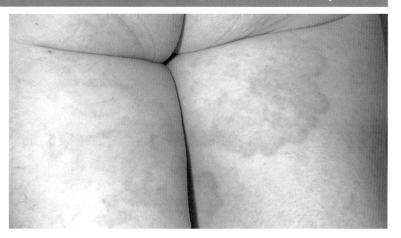

Fig. 8.36 Granuloma annulare: patch of erythema on back of thigh; note this is never scaly so should not be confused with tinea (*see* Figs. 8.37, 8.51, 8.74 and 8.75)

TREATMENT: GRANULOMA ANNULARE

If it is asymptomatic, which it usually is, the patient can be reassured that it is harmless and will eventually go away on its own. It may take quite a long time – months or even years rather than weeks. If it is painful, injection of triamcinolone 5–10 mg/mL intralesionally will stop the pain and may make it go away.

TINEA INCOGNITO

Tinea incognito develops when tinea corporis (ringworm) is inadvertently treated with topical steroids. This alters the clinical appearance so that the lesions have no appreciable scale, and may be distributed symmetrically. Nevertheless, scraping the edge will reveal fungus. Stop applying the steroid and for treatment *see* p. 233.

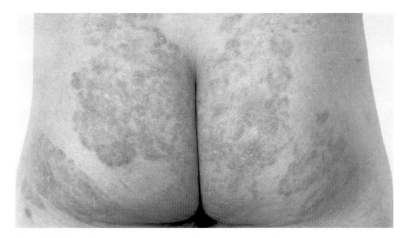

Fig. 8.37 Tinea incognito: symmetrical and non-scaly plaques due to treatment of tinea with steroids – mycology will be positive

LINEAR LESIONS

Linear lesions occur in the following.

With a normal surface

- Striae or stretch marks (*see* Fig. 8.38).
- Surgical scars:
  — normal, keloid or hypertrophic (*see* p. 214)
  — sarcoid can occur in old scars (*see* p. 213).
- Köebner phenomenon – when due to a scratch will be linear, e.g. in psoriasis, lichen planus, plane warts (*see* Fig. 8.03, p. 197).
- Along the line of blood vessels or lymphatics:
  — thrombophlebitis: inflammation of superficial veins
  — lymphangitis: inflammation of lymphatics associated with cellulitis (*see* p. 373)
  — sporotrichosis: deep fungal infection in which nodules occur along the course of a lymphatic vessel (*see* p. 410).
- Larva migrans – larvae leave a serpiginous track (*see* p. 428).
- Linear morphoea (*see* p. 80).
- Dermatomyositis – erythema over metacarpals and along fingers (*see* p. 132).

With a scale or warty surface

- Köebner phenomenon – psoriasis and plane warts.
- Present from birth or early childhood down the length of a limb or around the side of the trunk:
  — epidermal naevus (*see* p. 317)
  — inflammatory linear verrucous epidermal naevus
  — lichen striatus.

With blistering, exudate or erosions

- Linear contact dermatitis from external agents:
  — phytophotodermatitis due to sunlight and plant sap brushed onto the skin (*see* p. 182)

  — allergic contact dermatitis due to plant sap (*see* p. 182)
  — Berloque dematititis due to sunlight and psoralen (from cosmetics) in contact with skin.
- Dermatomal – herpes zoster (*see* p. 179).
- Dermatitis artefacta – self-inflicted (*see* p. 260).

STRIAE

Linear red/purple plaques occur commonly on the thighs and lumbosacral regions in teenagers. With time they flatten off and become atrophic. Similar lesions occur on the abdomen and breasts in pregnancy, and in the flexures in patients on systemic steroids or using potent topical steroids. No treatment will get rid of them.

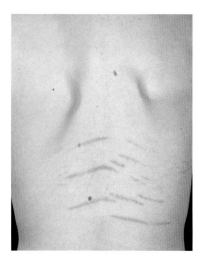

Fig. 8.38 Striae: linear stretch marks on the back of a teenager

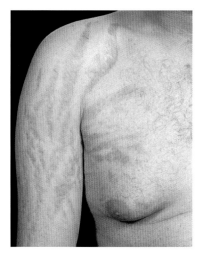

Fig. 8.39 Striae in patient with psoriasis who has used excessive topical steroids

Trunk and limbs
Chronic erythematous lesions
Normal surface
Nodules

NODULES AND LARGE PAPULES
(All lesions >5 mm – normal surface)

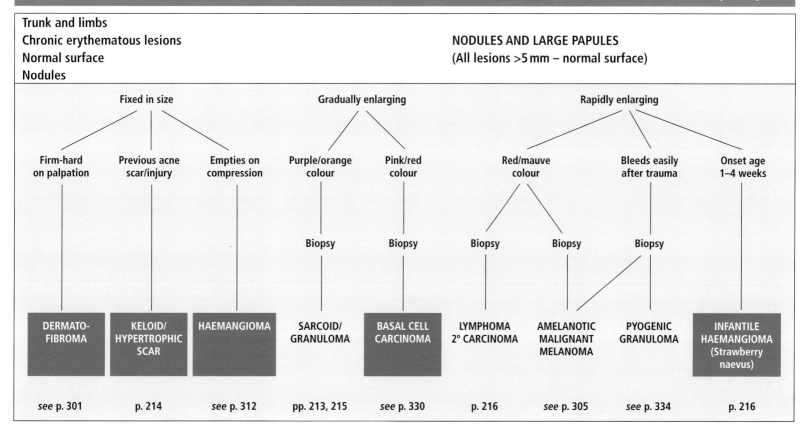

SARCOID

Multiple mauve/purple papules or plaques on the trunk and limbs may be due to sarcoid, especially if old scars are affected. Sarcoid can present with very different features – papules, plaques or even hypopigmented patches. The clinical appearance can be very varied. For this reason, any rash where there is no surface change needs to be biopsied to establish the histological diagnosis. Skin histology is usually diagnostic but you will also need to X-ray the chest, check the eyes and do a serum calcium to confirm the diagnosis. If there is evidence of sarcoid elsewhere, referral to a chest physician is advised.

TREATMENT: SARCOIDOSIS

Whether or not you treat the skin lesions will depend on whether there is sarcoid elsewhere. Topical steroids are not of any help. Systemic steroids work well but cannot be justified for skin lesions alone (the side effects [*see* p. 51] may outweigh the benefits). If the lesions are not visible and do not itch, the patient may be prepared to put up with it. Methotrexate 10–25 mg (*see* p. 52) once a week may be used as an alternative to systemic steroids.

KELOID AND HYPERTROPHIC SCARS

Hypertrophic scars are an overgrowth of scar tissue confined to the site of injury, while keloid scars grow out beyond the original site of injury. The commonest sites for keloid scarring are on the front of chest, around the shoulders, on the earlobes (*see* p. 162) and at the back of the scalp (*see* p. 96).

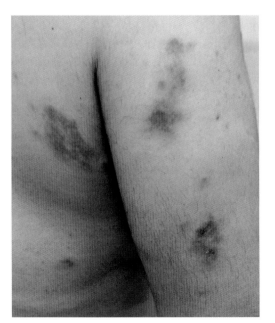

Fig. 8.40 Plaque of sarcoidosis on the back and arm; the colour gives a clue to diagnosis but a biopsy needs to be done to confirm this

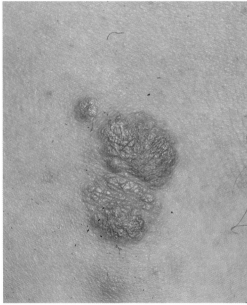

Fig. 8.41 Close-up of sarcoid papule and plaques

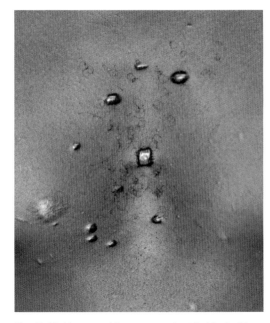

Fig. 8.42 Hypertrophic scars on chest in black skin secondary to acne

TREATMENT: KELOID SCARS

Injection of triamcinolone 10 mg/mL directly into the scar will flatten it off and reduce the red colour. Use a 25-gauge needle rather than a smaller one, because considerable pressure is needed to get the triamcinolone into the scar. Repeat every 4–6 weeks until the scar is flat. The resulting scar will be atrophic with obvious telangiectasia. You will need to warn the patient about this. An alternative is Haelan (fludroxycortide) tape applied daily to the scar for up to 6 months.

Silicone gel has been shown to be effective, especially in preventing keloids developing after surgery at high-risk sites. Various formulations from gels to sheets are available over the counter.

The pulse dye laser will improve the pruritus and erythema of scars but will not reduce the thickness. Re-excision of the scar is contraindicated but sometimes this may work if, following surgery, you inject triamcinolone around the wound or irradiate it within 24 hours with superficial X-rays (1–3 fractions of 7 Gy).

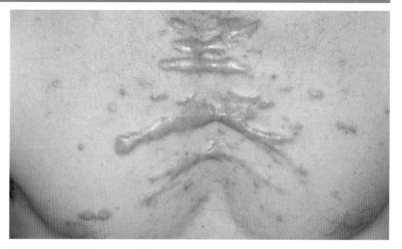

Fig. 8.43 Keloid scars secondary to acne

GRANULOMATOUS INFILTRATES IN THE SKIN

A granuloma is strictly a histological term referring to a collection of monocytes, macrophages, epithelioid and giant cells in the dermis. It occurs in response to a persistent irritant such as a foreign body (lipid, oil, glass fibre, talc, silica, metals) or infection (tuberculosis, leprosy, atypical mycobacterium, fungi). Quite often no obvious cause for a granuloma is found. Clinically, granulomas are indurated nodules, orange to purple in colour with a normal surface. They tend to grow very slowly. Diagnosis is made by skin biopsy for histology and culture looking for atypical mycobacteria (incubate at <30°C), tuberculosis or fungi. A foreign body can be identified on histology by using polarised light. Treat any infection (atypical mycobacteria, *see* p. 410; tuberculosis, *see* p. 128; leprosy, *see* p. 283; fungus, *see* p. 47) and surgically excise foreign bodies.

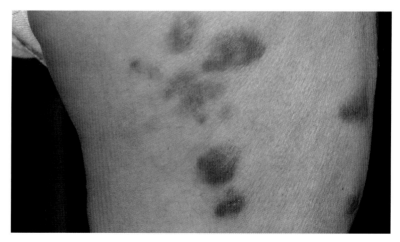

Fig. 8.44 Granulomas secondary to insulin injections in the thigh; a lymphoma would look the same – a biopsy is necessary to confirm the diagnosis

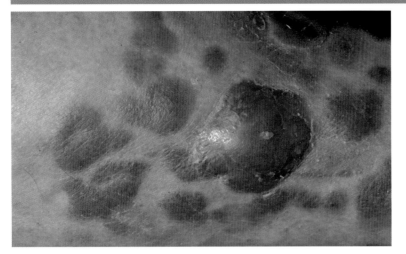

Fig. 8.45 B-cell lymphoma on calf

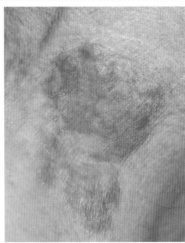

Fig. 8.46 Metastatic breast carcinoma on the neck

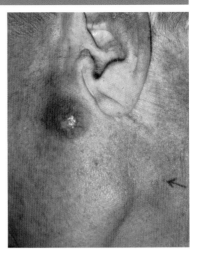

Fig. 8.47 Amelanotic melanoma on cheek with enlarged lymph gland in neck (indicated with arrow)

LYMPHOMA, CARCINOMA, SARCOMA, AMELANOTIC MELANOMA

A cutaneous B-cell lymphoma usually presents as a rapidly growing red/purple indurated nodule with no surface changes. There may be one or several lesions, and in many instances is not associated with an internal lymphoma; a full systemic workup is necessary, however. Cutaneous B-cell lymphoma nodules on the leg have a particularly poor prognosis and need early histological identification. Cutaneous T-cell lymphoma can mimic eczema or psoriasis (*see* p. 231).

Lymphoma, granuloma, metastatic carcinoma in the skin, a soft tissue sarcoma or an amelanotic malignant melanoma can all look the same, presenting as nodules or indurated plaques with no surface change (because the epidermis is usually unaffected). Diagnosis can only be made by skin biopsy.

INFANTILE HAEMANGIOMA (STRAWBERRY NAEVUS)

An accurate history of when it occurred is vital in making the correct diagnosis for vascular lesions in childhood. A lesion present at birth is a **vascular malformation**, and these will never resolve. The commonest is the capillary malformation (port wine stain, *see* p. 127).

Haemangiomas occur after birth and the commonest is the strawberry naevus (infantile haemangioma). These red nodules are quite unmistakable. They

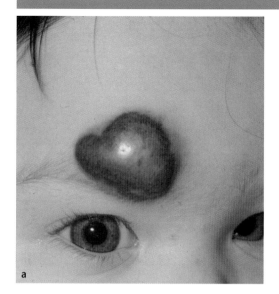 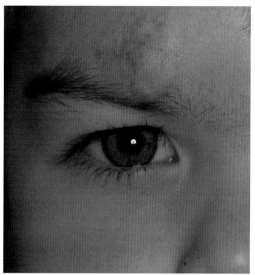 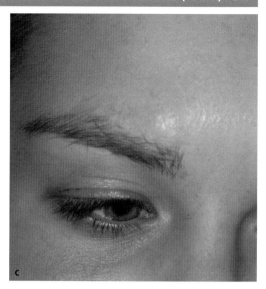

Fig. 8.48 (a) Infantile haemangioma at age of 14 months; (b) same patient at age of 5 years; (c) same patient at age of 13 years

are not present at birth but appear during the first 4 weeks of life. They grow quite quickly up to the age of 12–24 months, and then they gradually and spontaneously involute. During this phase the colour becomes blue/purple, and as the nodule shrinks the overlying skin becomes slightly flaccid. Most lesions resolve completely by the age of 10 years (70% by 7 years, 90% by 9 years), but may leave some residual flaccidity of the skin. The main problem is a cosmetic one, but if traumatised, haemorrhage and ulceration can occur. Very rarely platelet consumption can occur causing thrombocytopenia (Kasabach–Merritt syndrome). If the child has multiple strawberry naevi or an odd segmental presentation (e.g. craniofacial/sacral), refer for investigation to exclude systemic haemangiomatosis.

Treatment: Infantile haemangioma

Most lesions will resolve spontaneously so they should be left alone to do so. Treatment is only needed if very large or when there are complications such as bleeding, thrombosis or interference with function (e.g. eyesight, eating, airway obstruction, defecation). Treatment with propranolol 1–2 mg/kg/day with feeds for up to 12 months will rapidly resolve the lesion. This is initially administered as an inpatient by a dermatologist or paediatrician. Side effects include bradycardia, heart failure, hypotension, cardiac conduction disorders, bronchospasm, weakness and fatigue, disturbed sleep, and hypoglycaemia. Blood pressure and heart rate are monitored weekly in the community. Topical β-blockers such as 0.1% timoptol gel applied five times daily for 6 months can also be used in cases of poor response to oral propranolol.

Trunk and limbs
Chronic erythematous rash
Scaly surface
Plaques: single or few

SINGLE OR FEW SCALY PLAQUES

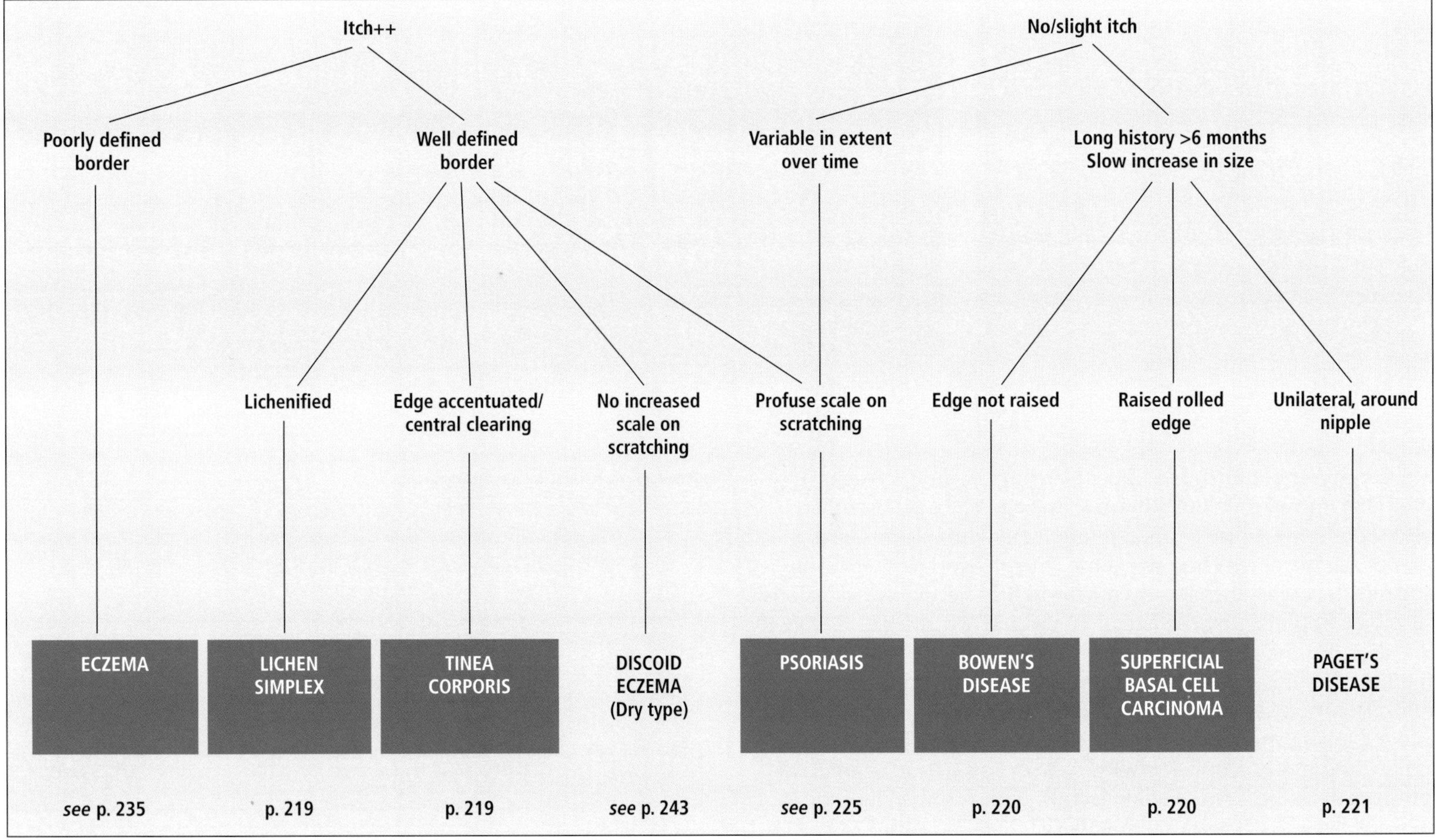

Itch++

No/slight itch

Poorly defined border

Well defined border

Variable in extent over time

Long history >6 months
Slow increase in size

Lichenified

Edge accentuated/ central clearing

No increased scale on scratching

Profuse scale on scratching

Edge not raised

Raised rolled edge

Unilateral, around nipple

| ECZEMA | LICHEN SIMPLEX | TINEA CORPORIS | DISCOID ECZEMA (Dry type) | PSORIASIS | BOWEN'S DISEASE | SUPERFICIAL BASAL CELL CARCINOMA | PAGET'S DISEASE |

see p. 235   p. 219   p. 219   *see* p. 243   *see* p. 225   p. 220   p. 220   p. 221

LICHEN SIMPLEX

Lichen simplex is a well-defined itchy plaque with increased skin markings on the surface (lichenification) due to persistent scratching. The commonest sites are the occiput, ankles, elbows and genitalia. Single or multiple sites may be involved.

TREATMENT: LICHEN SIMPLEX

If the patient stops scratching it will get better, but this is often easier said than done. The patient may need to look at the circumstances in his or her life that are causing him or her to scratch and deal with or come to terms with them.

Apply a very potent[UK]/group 1[USA] topical steroid such as 0.05% clobetasol propionate (Dermovate[UK]/Temovate[USA]) bid, or Haelan tape daily. This will reduce the itching. Once this has happened, reduce the strength of the steroid to a moderately potent[UK]/group 4–5[USA] one. If topical steroids do not work, try an occlusive bandage Zipzoc (left in place for a week at a time).

TINEA CORPORIS (RINGWORM)

Ringworm of the body is due to dermatophyte fungi, which live on keratin, so the clinical picture is of one or more pink, scaly plaques, which gradually extend outwards and heal from the centre, forming a ring (*see* p. 233).

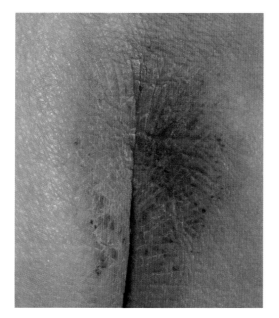

Fig. 8.49 Lichen simplex on sacrum

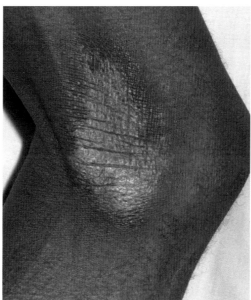

Fig. 8.50 Lichen simplex on elbow

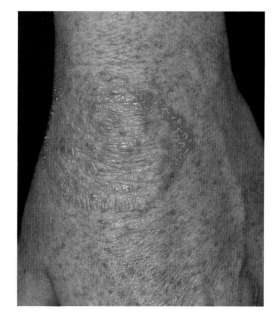

Fig. 8.51 Tinea corporis on dorsum of hand

SUPERFICIAL BASAL CELL CARCINOMA

On the trunk, basal cell carcinomas often spread superficially and slowly over several years, presenting as a flat, scaly plaque (*see* Fig. 8.52). The edge of the lesion is just like a basal cell carcinoma elsewhere with a slightly raised, rolled edge; this can be seen more easily if the skin is put on the stretch (*see* Fig. 1.81, p. 16). The centre of the lesion may be scaly and can be confused with Bowen's disease, or even eczema. A biopsy will distinguish between them.

TREATMENT: SUPERFICIAL BASAL CELL CARCINOMA

If the lesion is small, excision is the best option. Lesions bigger than 2 cm or where excision is difficult can be treated with the following:

- imiquimod 5% (Aldara) cream five times a week for 6 weeks; if the inflammatory reaction is very severe, stop treatment to allow it to settle down, and recommence at three times a week, to complete a total of 6 weeks' treatment (*see* also Fig. 9.72, p. 291)
- photodynamic therapy using methyl aminolevulinate (Metvix) cream and a red light source (*see* p. 63).

Both produce an inflammatory reaction leading to resolution of the lesion.

BOWEN'S DISEASE

Bowen's disease is an intraepidermal squamous cell carcinoma (in situ). It presents as a fixed red, scaly plaque that looks like psoriasis or eczema. It does not respond to treatment with topical steroids but gradually expands in size over many months. It can occur on any sun-exposed site but characteristically occurs on the lower legs. Multiple lesions are common. Change to an invasive squamous cell carcinoma is uncommon and only occurs after many years.

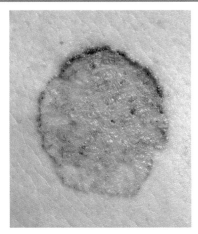

Fig. 8.52 Superficial basal cell carcinoma with 'rolled' edge

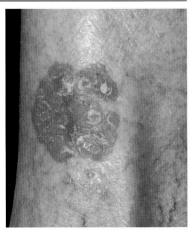

Fig. 8.53 Bowen's disease: plaque on lower leg looking like psoriasis

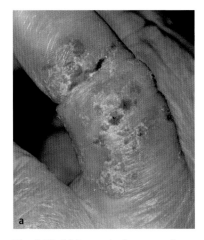

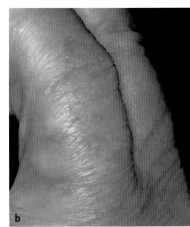

Fig. 8.54 (a) Bowen's disease on finger; (b) after 4 weeks' treatment with 5-fluorouracil cream

TREATMENT: BOWEN'S DISEASE

The options for treatment include:

- cryotherapy
- 5-fluorouracil (Efudix^UK/Effudex^USA) cream bid for 4 weeks
- imiquimod (Aldara) cream three times a week for 12 weeks (*see* pp. 34, 291)
- photodynamic therapy (*see* p. 63)
- curettage and cautery
- excision.

Which you choose will depend on the size and site of the lesion, what facilities are available and the convenience of the patient. Only curettage and excision will give you histology unless a biopsy is taken first. Care should be taken on the lower legs because all these options can lead to leg ulceration.

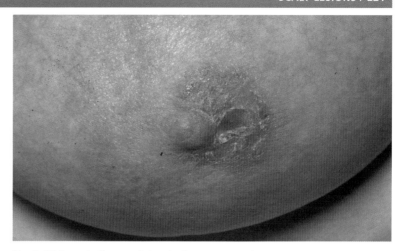

Fig. 8.55 Paget's disease of the nipple

PAGET'S DISEASE OF THE NIPPLE

This is due to invasion of the skin around the nipple by malignant cells derived from an intraductal carcinoma. There is a unilateral red, scaly plaque surrounding the nipple with or without crusting. It gradually increases in size and is often mistaken for eczema. The fact that it is unilateral and does not respond to topical steroids should alert you to the diagnosis, which can be confirmed by a skin biopsy. Patients should be referred to a breast surgeon.

ECZEMA OF THE NIPPLE AND AREOLA

Eczema of the areola and nipple is much more common than Paget's disease and may or may not be associated with atopic eczema. A red, scaly, itchy rash confined to the nipple and areola of one or both breasts is quite common in teenagers and young women particularly in Africans. Treatment is the same as for eczema elsewhere (*see* p. 239).

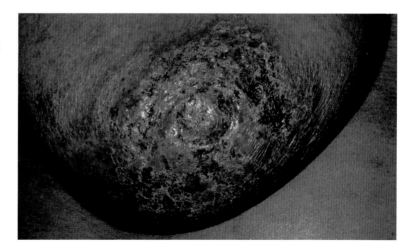

Fig. 8.56 Eczema on and around nipple

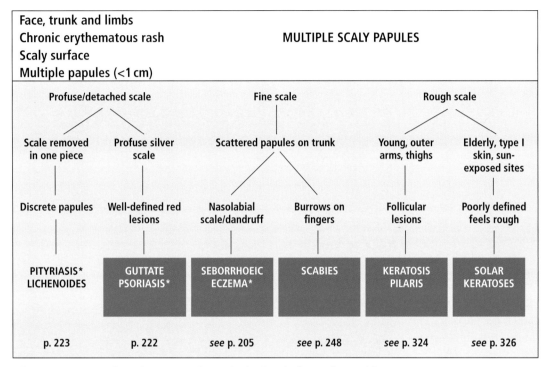

Face, trunk and limbs
Chronic erythematous rash
Scaly surface
Multiple papules (<1 cm)

MULTIPLE SCALY PAPULES

Profuse/detached scale | Fine scale | Rough scale

Scale removed in one piece | Profuse silver scale | Scattered papules on trunk | Young, outer arms, thighs | Elderly, type I skin, sun-exposed sites

Discrete papules | Well-defined red lesions | Nasolabial scale/dandruff | Burrows on fingers | Follicular lesions | Poorly defined feels rough

PITYRIASIS* LICHENOIDES | GUTTATE PSORIASIS* | SEBORRHOEIC ECZEMA* | SCABIES | KERATOSIS PILARIS | SOLAR KERATOSES

p. 223 | p. 222 | see p. 205 | see p. 248 | see p. 324 | see p. 326

*If the patient is unwell, has lesions on palms and soles, lymphadenopathy, consider secondary syphilis (see pp. 207, 353).

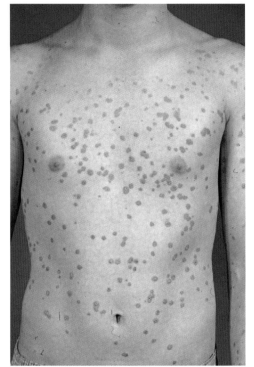

Fig. 8.57 Guttate psoriasis

GUTTATE PSORIASIS

This is an acute form of psoriasis that appears suddenly 10–14 days after a streptococcal sore throat. The individual lesions are typical of psoriasis, being bright red and well demarcated with silvery scaling, but all the lesions are uniformly small (0.5–1 cm in diameter). The rash may be very widespread, appearing more or less overnight. It gets better spontaneously after 2–3 months.

It may be the first manifestation of psoriasis or it may occur in someone who has had psoriasis for years. It differs from small plaque psoriasis because there is no variation in size of the lesions. Since it is usually not itchy, it can be confused with pityriasis rosea and secondary syphilis (see pp. 205 and 207). For treatment see p. 230.

PITYRIASIS LICHENOIDES

This rash is rarely recognised by non-dermatologists. The **chronic form** consists of widespread small, red-brown, scaly papules, from which the scale can be 'picked off' in one piece (the 'mica scale'). It occurs mainly in children and young adults and lasts for several months. It often improves in the sun.

The **acute form** presents as necrotic papules, erosions or ulcers, and it may heal with scarring. The more typical chronic scaly lesions may also be present. The diagnosis of pityriasis lichenoides is made by histology, which shows a cutaneous vasculitis.

TREATMENT: PITYRIASIS LICHENOIDES

This responds well to ultraviolet light. In the summer the patient can get out into the sunshine and expose the affected skin for half an hour each day. Alternatively, narrowband ultraviolet light (UVB) three times a week for 6–8 weeks clears it up. Rarely PUVA treatment needs to be given (see p. 61). Tetracycline 500 mg qid or lymecycline 408 mg daily for 3 weeks may work well in adults.

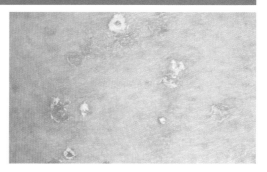

Fig. 8.59 Pityriasis lichenoides chronica: close-up of mica scale

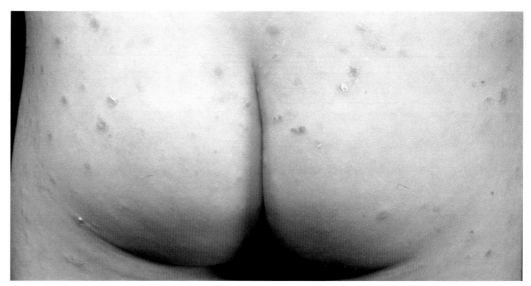

Fig. 8.60 Pityriasis lichenoides chronica: scaly papules

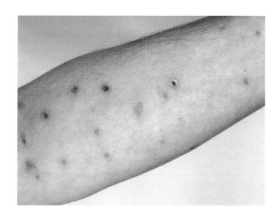

Fig. 8.58 Pityriasis lichenoides acuta: small necrotic papules

Face, trunk and limbs
Chronic erythematous rash
Scaly surface
Multiple plaques

MULTIPLE SCALY PLAQUES (>1 cm)

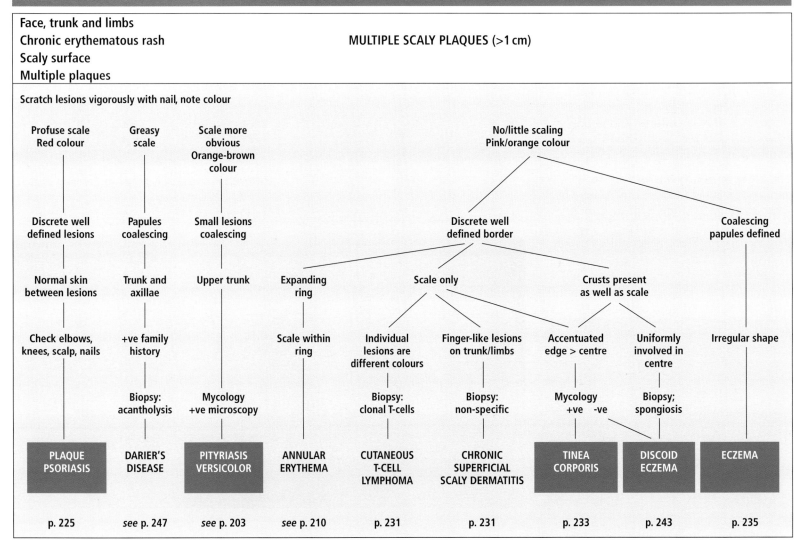

Scratch lesions vigorously with nail, note colour

Profuse scale Red colour	Greasy scale	Scale more obvious Orange-brown colour		No/little scaling Pink/orange colour		
Discrete well defined lesions	Papules coalescing	Small lesions coalescing		Discrete well defined border		Coalescing papules defined
Normal skin between lesions	Trunk and axillae	Upper trunk	Expanding ring	Scale only	Crusts present as well as scale	
Check elbows, knees, scalp, nails	+ve family history		Scale within ring	Individual lesions are different colours / Finger-like lesions on trunk/limbs	Accentuated edge > centre / Uniformly involved in centre	Irregular shape
	Biopsy: acantholysis	Mycology +ve microscopy		Biopsy: clonal T-cells / Biopsy: non-specific	Mycology +ve -ve / Biopsy; spongiosis	
PLAQUE PSORIASIS	**DARIER'S DISEASE**	**PITYRIASIS VERSICOLOR**	**ANNULAR ERYTHEMA**	**CUTANEOUS T-CELL LYMPHOMA** / **CHRONIC SUPERFICIAL SCALY DERMATITIS**	**TINEA CORPORIS** / **DISCOID ECZEMA**	**ECZEMA**
p. 225	see p. 247	see p. 203	see p. 210	p. 231 / p. 231	p. 233 / p. 243	p. 235

CHRONIC PLAQUE PSORIASIS

Psoriasis is a common chronic, inflammatory skin disease that affects about 2% of the population worldwide. The inheritance of psoriasis is probably controlled by several genes, so that the occurrence within families is variable. It is characterised by rapid turnover of epidermal cells so that the keratin is immature and therefore scaly. This is a result of abnormalities in both innate and adaptive immunity. Psoriasis was thought to be a Th1-mediated disease, because of a predominance of Th1 pathway cytokines, such as tumour necrosis factor-α (TNF-α), interferon gamma (IFN-γ), interleukin–2 (IL-2) and IL-12 in psoriatic plaques. However, in the last few years, a far more complex interplay has been demonstrated, where IL-23 secreted by dendritic cells activates Th17 T-cells to produce IL-17A and IL-17F, which drive the keratinocyte proliferation seen in psoriasis. Increased levels of vascular endothelial growth factor from activated lymphocytes causes vascular dilation and hyperplasia, while mast cells secrete large amounts of TNF-α, IFN-γ and IL-8, recruiting the large numbers of neutrophils seen in plaques. Neutrophils then further recruit and activate T lymphocytes and the cycle continues, which the new biologic therapies aim to block.

Psoriasis can occur at any age but most often begins between the ages of 15 and 25 years. The clinical features can be explained by the pathology (*see* Fig. 8.61). The lesions are bright red in colour, have clearly defined borders (edges) and a silvery scale. The scale becomes more obviously silvery when scratched (*see* Figs 1.45 and 1.46, p. 11), comes off easily and may make a mess on the floor.

Characteristically the lesions are symmetrical, commonly affecting the elbows, knees, sacral area and lower legs, but any part of the skin can be involved, including the scalp and nails. Most patients only have a few plaques but psoriasis can become very extensive. A small proportion will have involvement of their joints as well (psoriatic arthropathy). The severity of the psoriatic arthropathy is often unrelated to the extent of the skin involvement.

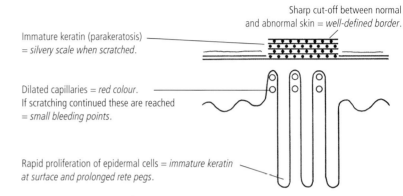

Immature keratin (parakeratosis) = *silvery scale when scratched.*

Sharp cut-off between normal and abnormal skin = *well-defined border.*

Dilated capillaries = *red colour.*
If scratching continued these are reached = *small bleeding points.*

Rapid proliferation of epidermal cells = *immature keratin at surface and prolonged rete pegs.*

Fig. 8.61 Correlation of pathology of psoriasis with physical signs

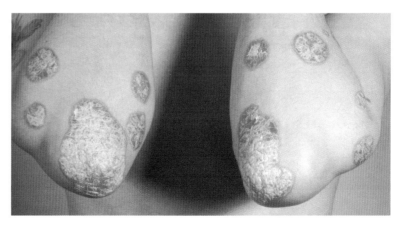

Fig. 8.62 Plaque psoriasis on elbows

TREATMENT: PLAQUE PSORIASIS

Assess the following.

a. The *extent* of body coverage, and the number and size of lesions as this will determine the type of treatment required (*see* Table, p. 227).

b. The disease *severity* using these simple descriptive terms: clear, nearly clear, mild, moderate, severe, very severe.

c. *Quality of life* issues: the physical, social and psychological impact (i.e. any arthritis, depression or work issues). You might want to use a quality of life questionnaire to assess this and progress after treatment.

d. Any *co-morbidities* such as cardiovascular risk (if psoriasis severe).

Adopt a stepladder approach: try the first option and move down the list if the initial option is not effective.

TREATMENT OPTIONS

- Emollients and salicylic acid ointment BP are useful for softening scale.
- Vitamin D_3 analogues are more effective than emollients and useful if used frequently and regularly.
- Tar and dithranol are messy and are rarely used these days.
- Topical steroids are very effective, but strong ones need to be used for *short periods only*; unfortunately, relapse or even rebound (psoriasis worsens afterwards) is generally the rule. Combination with a vitamin D_3 analogue may reduce steroid side effects.
- 0.1% Protopic ointment or a topical retinoid (0.05% tazarotene) can be tried.
- Sun exposure and holidays will help if possible.
- Extensive psoriasis will need the help of a dermatologist at a specialist centre.

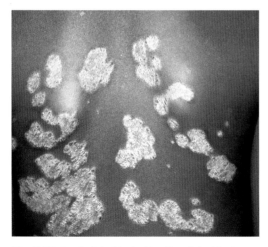

Fig. 8.63 Psoriasis in black skin: the clinical features are exactly the same as in white skin

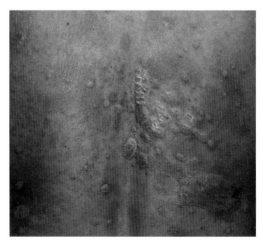

Fig. 8.64 Psoriasis showing post-inflammatory hyperpigmentation and some erythema on the active areas

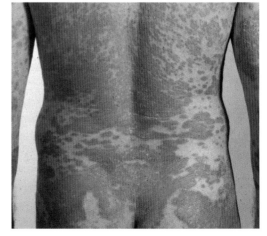

Fig. 8.65 Widespread psoriasis that requires ultraviolet light treatment or systemic therapy

Summary of treatment of psoriasis

	Few localised plaques (<2% surface area)	Large plaques (2%–10% surface area)	Guttate psoriasis or widespread small plaques	Widespread plaques (>10% surface area)
General practice choice	1. Emollients 2. Keratolytics 3. Vitamin D_3 analogue 4. Dithrocream, Miconal short contact therapy 5. Potent topical steroid (max 4 weeks only) ± salicylic acid (Diprosalic ointment)	1. Vitamin D_3 analogue 2. Vitamin D_3 analogue and steroid combination (e.g. Dovobet) alternating with an emollient every 2 weeks 3. Protopic ointment especially for the face	1. Emollients 2. Tar cream (e.g. Exorex lotion – *not cream*) 3. Recreational sun exposure	Refer to specialist for: 1. narrowband UVB 2. day treatment with tar or dithranol (if available) 3. PUVA 4. systemic treatment, e.g. methotrexate or ciclosporin 5. biologics, which should be given if the above fail to control the disease
Specialist's alternative	Retinoid (tazarotene) gel or cream	Narrowband UVB therapy Dithranol in Lassar's paste or crude coal tar ointment – either of these combined with UVB as a day treatment	Narrowband UVB phototherapy	

Keratolytics and moisturisers

Many patients are content to reduce the scaling of psoriasis with emollients containing urea or lactic acid (Lacticare, Calmurid), or salicylic acid ointment BP (2%).

Vitamin D$_3$ analogues

- Calcitriol (Silkis) ointment: apply once daily
- Calcipotriol[UK]/calcipotriene[USA] (Dovonex) ointment: apply twice a day
- Tacalcitol (Curatoderm) ointment: apply once daily

These are the first-line treatment for most patients with psoriasis because they are not messy to use. The main problem is that they do not clear psoriasis, usually only reducing the scaling and thickness of the plaques. To be at all effective they must be applied twice daily regularly. They can irritate the skin of the face and flexures (calcitriol less so than the others).

Dithranol[UK]/anthralin[USA]

Dithranol[UK]/anthralin[USA] is rarely used because it stains skin (*see* Fig. 8.69) and clothing and can irritate normal skin. In selected individuals with a few plaques it can be applied using the **short contact method**. In this method Dithrocream[UK]/Drithocreme[USA] is applied by rubbing it carefully on to the individual plaques. Leave it on for 30 minutes and then wash off with soap and water. If no irritation occurs, the strength of dithranol cream can be increased every 2–3 days from 0.1% to 0.25%, to 0.5%, to 1.0% and finally to 2%. When the psoriatic plaques go brown (*see* Fig. 8.69), stop using the treatment. The brown colour fades after 7–10 days.

Alternatively, 1% and 3% Micanol cream, or Psorin ointment can be used.

The application of dithranol in **Lassar's paste** in a hospital or clinic setting (*see* p. 230) will clear psoriasis in about 3 weeks. It is time-consuming and messy, but in some instances it can lead to prolonged periods of remission.

Coal tar

For very superficial or very numerous small plaques of psoriasis, tar is easier to use than dithranol because it can be rubbed all over the skin without taking any special care. For superficial plaques use a proprietary cream containing coal tar solution (*see* p. 34). For thicker plaques, crude coal tar can be used. This is very messy and is usually used in a day care unit or as an inpatient (*see* p. 230).

Vitamin D$_3$ analogue and topical steroid

A vitamin D$_3$ analogue can be combined with a potent[UK]/group 2–3[USA] topical steroid, either each applied separately (vitamin D$_3$ analogue in the morning and steroid in the evening) or as Dovobet gel or ointment (calcipotriol + betamethasone). The combination is more effective than the vitamin D$_3$ analogue alone, and using the combination probably diminishes steroid side effects. It should not be used for more than 4 weeks at a time because of the long-term side effects of topical steroids (*see* p. 33). A steroid-free interval of 2 weeks (using a moisturiser or vitamin D$_3$ analogue) should be maintained between treatments.

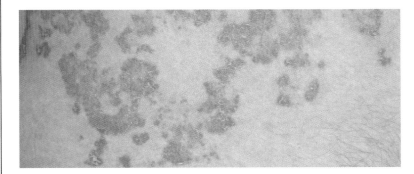

Fig. 8.66 Psoriasis treated with topical steroids: plaques have become flat with little scale but they still are red

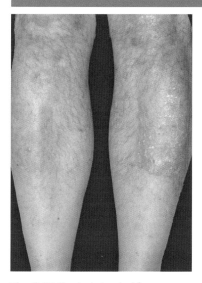

Fig. 8.67 Psoriasis treated for 4 weeks with Dovobet gel (right leg) and Dovonex ointment (left leg): the plaque on the right leg is flatter and less scaly than on the left

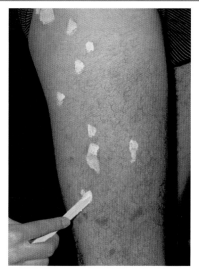

Fig. 8.68 Dithranol in Lassar's paste being applied to plaques with a spatula in Ingram's regimen

Topical steroids

The use of topical steroids in psoriasis is controversial. They are effective in clearing psoriasis without being messy, and are thus the mainstay of treatment in Europe and the United States, but they are used less often in the United Kingdom. There is no doubt that *very potent* topical steroids, if used extensively, can result in worsening of psoriasis when the treatment is stopped (rebound) or even generalised pustular psoriasis. They will also cause all the other side effects of topical steroids (*see* p. 33).

The problem is how to use them without running into problems. We would recommend the following options.

- Use steroids in the potent group on the body and the moderate potency group on the face.
- Use at any one site for a maximum of 4 weeks, after which they should be not be used for a further 2 weeks – use a moisturiser.
- If the psoriasis rebounds or relapses quickly then other treatments need to be considered. If maintenance treatment is needed, restrict this to two applications a week (weekend treatment).
- Restrict the amount of steroid to 100 g per week.

Sun exposure

Recreational sun exposure, provided that burning is avoided, will generally be beneficial.

Fig. 8.69 Staining of hands following application of dithranol: when the stain remains on the surface, this means that the exfoliation caused by psoriasis has ceased and therefore the psoriasis will have resolved – the stain takes up to 4 weeks to resolve

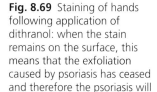

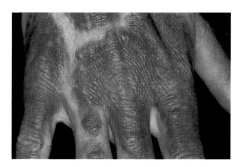

Topical retinoids and immunosuppressants

A topical retinoid such as 0.05% or 0.1% tazarotene gel or cream (Zorac[UK]/Tazorac[USA]) applied twice a day works by modifying abnormal epidermal differentiation. It can be effective but, like all topical retinoids, it produces marked skin irritation. Applying it once daily can reduce this. It is a useful treatment for a few isolated plaques.

0.1% tacrolimus (Protopic) ointment can also be tried for stable plaques, especially on the face.

TREATMENT: GUTTATE AND SMALL PLAQUE PSORIASIS

Guttate psoriasis will clear in 2–3 months. If it is itchy use an emollient.

Ultraviolet light therapy (*see* p. 60) is very effective but requires attending a hospital or clinic three times a week. For those who cannot do this, a tar cream is the most useful treatment.

Refined coal tars (coal tar solution/liquor picis carbonis[UK]/liquor carbonis detergens[USA]) mixed with a moderately potent steroid ointment can be effective.

TREATMENT: EXTENSIVE PLAQUE PSORIASIS

Ultraviolet light therapy

Narrowband ultraviolet light therapy or PUVA are effective treatments for extensive larger plaque psoriasis, but the lifetime dose of treatment should be restricted (*see* pp. 60–1).

Day care or inpatient treatment: Ingram's or Goerckerman's regimen

1. **Tar bath**: the patient soaks in a bath containing 20–30 mL of a tar emulsion (Balnatar, Lavatar[USA], Polytar, Zetar[USA]) for 10–15 minutes. While in the bath the scales can be rubbed off with a soft brush.
2. **Ultraviolet light therapy**: after getting out of the bath and patting dry the skin, the patient is exposed to a sub-erythema dose of narrowband UVB (*see* p. 60).
3a. **Ingram's regimen**: dithranol[UK]/anthralin[USA] in Lassar's paste is applied carefully to each psoriatic plaque (*see* Fig. 8.68) and left on for 24 hours. Over a 3- to 4-week period the concentration of dithranol is gradually increased. Start with 0.1% dithranol and increase daily by increments of 0.1% up to 1% and then by increments of 1% up to 10%. Talcum powder is applied to the surface of the paste to stop it being smudged. The body is covered with Clinifast/Tubifast to prevent staining of clothes and bedding. The paste needs to be removed the next day with arachis oil or liquid paraffin.

3b. **Goerckerman's regimen**: 2% crude coal tar in white soft paraffin or Lassar's paste is applied to the psoriasis and covered by a tubular dressing. The strength of tar is increased to 20% gradually over a 3- to 4-week period. A treatment of 2% or 5% crude coal tar in Lassar's paste is a very effective treatment for psoriasis of the face.
4. The next morning (or later that day for day treatment) the paste is cleaned off with arachis oil or liquid paraffin[UK]/petrolatum[USA]. Tar ointment can be removed with ordinary soap and water.

Repeat the process daily until the psoriasis has cleared. It is usually possible to clear psoriasis in 3–4 weeks by these methods.

TREATMENT: PSORIASIS – SYSTEMIC THERAPY

Patients who fail to respond to topical therapy or narrowband UVB, or those who frequently relapse or have very extensive disease, require systemic treatment. The following are available:

- PUVA (*see* p. 61)
- methotrexate (*see* p. 52)
- acitretin (*see* p. 49)
- ciclosporin (*see* p. 53)
- hydroyxcarbamide (hydroxyurea, *see* p. 55)
- fumaric acid esters (*see* p. 55).

These all have serious side effects so should only be initiated by a dermatologist.

Intolerance or failure of systemic treatment are indications for the use of **biologic agents** (*see* p. 56), monoclonal antibodies that target TNF-α, IL-12, IL-23 and IL-17:

- infliximab
- adalimumab
- etanercept
- ustekinumab.

These are extremely expensive but can be very effective, especially when other agents have failed. In time, when the price becomes more reasonable and their long-term effects are known, their use will increase.

CHRONIC SUPERFICIAL SCALY DERMATITIS (DIGITATE DERMATITIS)

This is a pink, scaly rash with oblong or finger-shaped plaques around the trunk. The surface has a fine 'cigarette paper' wrinkling. It is usually asymptomatic. It differs from cutaneous T-cell lymphoma in that the lesions are all the same colour and a biopsy will show eczema and not a lymphoma.

TREATMENT: SUPERFICIAL SCALY DERMATITIS

If it itches, narrowband UVB phototherapy will stop the itching temporarily, but it will not make the rash go away. It is given two to three times a week for 6–8 weeks. Topical steroids tend not to work.

CUTANEOUS T-CELL LYMPHOMA (MYCOSIS FUNGOIDES)

A T-cell lymphoma is usually confined to the skin. It presents as itchy, red, scaly patches (*see* Figs 8.71a & b) that may mimic either eczema or psoriasis. The main differentiating feature is that individual lesions are of different colours, so that some patches are pink, others red or orange brown. The patches become more indurated to form plaques (*see* Fig. 8.72). These stages of cutaneous T-cell lymphoma may persist for many years.

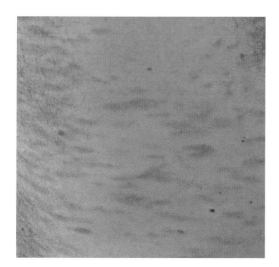

Fig. 8.70 Chronic superficial scaly dermatitis: note finger-like patches

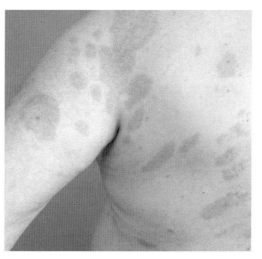

Fig. 8.71a Cutaneous T-cell lymphoma: patch stage

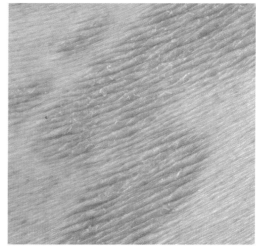

Fig. 8.71b Close-up of cutaneous T-cell lymphoma, patch stage

Late in the course of the disease, tumours develop (*see* Fig. 8.73) from the plaques. The disease may then spread to other organs of the body and become more aggressive. Progression is, however, very variable. The diagnosis is confirmed by skin biopsy and polymerase chain reaction to show that the abnormal cells are monoclonal.

TREATMENT: CUTANEOUS T-CELL LYMPHOMA

All patients should be referred to a dermatologist for confirmation of the diagnosis. In the plaque stage the options are:

- a moderately potent[UK]/group 4–5[USA] topical steroid ointment or cream – this may be all that is needed for many years; it will alleviate the itching and keep the patient comfortable
- PUVA (*see* p. 61) given twice weekly for 8–10 weeks may make the rash go away for a period of months or years.

Once tumours have developed, radiotherapy or chemotherapy will be needed.

For disseminated disease, bexarotene (a retinoid variant), electron beam therapy to the whole body, extracorporeal photophoresis, monoclonal antibodies and various chemotherapy regimens are used at specialist centres as required.

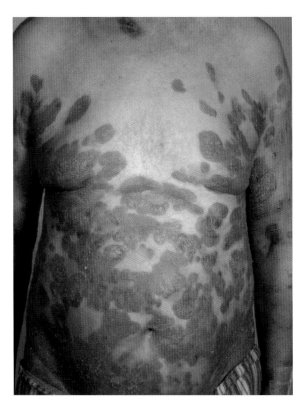

Fig. 8.72 Cutaneous T-cell lymphoma: plaque stage

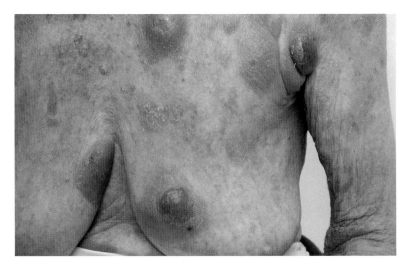

Fig. 8.73 Cutaneous T-cell lymphoma: tumour stage

TINEA CORPORIS (RINGWORM)

Ringworm of the body is due to dermatophyte fungi of the *Microsporum*, *Trichophyton* and *Epidermophyton* species. Dermatophytes live on keratin, so the clinical picture is of one or more pink, scaly papules or plaques, which gradually extend outwards healing from the centre and forming a ring. You should always consider the diagnosis in any unilateral or asymmetrical red, scaly rash whether or not it is annular in shape. It is a mistake to consider all annular rashes as tinea. What should alert you to the diagnosis is that the lesions tend to be asymmetrical (*see* Fig. 5.54, p. 136).

TREATMENT: TINEA CORPORIS

Since the infection is in the keratin layer on the surface of the skin, topical treatment works better than systemic therapy. The options are:
- an imidazole cream applied twice a day for 2 weeks
- terbinafine (Lamisil) cream applied daily for 7 days.

It is acceptable practice to treat a scaly rash that you think is due to a fungal infection with an antifungal cream *provided* you first take scrapings to be sent for mycology (*see* p. 20) where the fungal hyphae can be visualised by direct microscopy and cultured. The patient can be followed up after 4 weeks when the result of the mycology is known. If the mycology is negative and the rash no better you should reconsider the diagnosis.

It is bad practice to treat scaly rashes with antifungal-steroid combinations to 'hedge your bets'. The steroid may make the fungal infection worse, and eczema will respond better to a topical steroid alone.

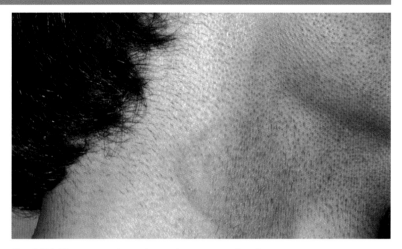

Fig. 8.74 Tinea corporis on the neck: note annular plaque

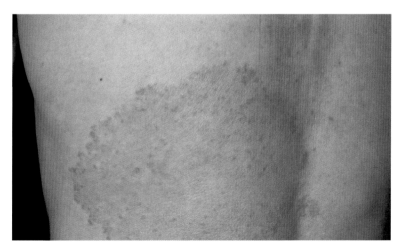

Fig. 8.75 Tinea corporis on the back: note the well-defined border

Face, trunk and limbs
Chronic eczema

CHRONIC ECZEMA

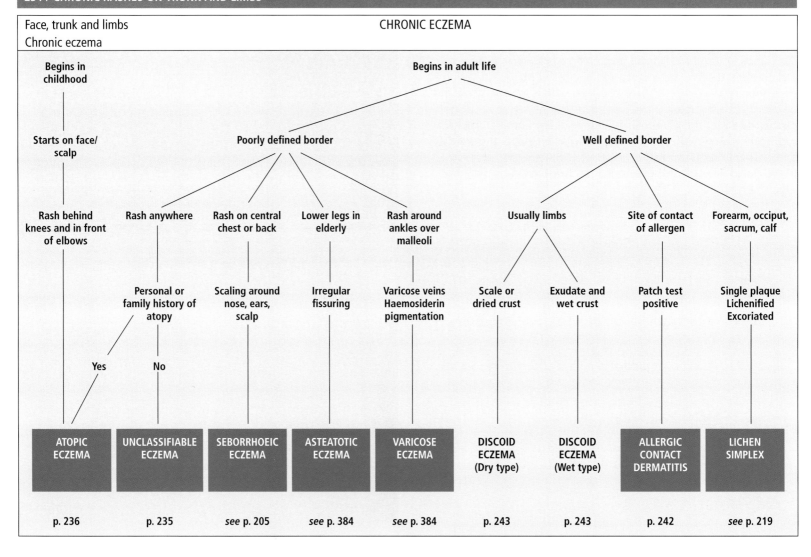

Begins in childhood

Starts on face/ scalp

Rash behind knees and in front of elbows

Yes

ATOPIC ECZEMA

p. 236

Rash anywhere

Personal or family history of atopy

No

UNCLASSIFIABLE ECZEMA

p. 235

Begins in adult life

Poorly defined border

Rash on central chest or back

Scaling around nose, ears, scalp

SEBORRHOEIC ECZEMA

see p. 205

Lower legs in elderly

Irregular fissuring

ASTEATOTIC ECZEMA

see p. 384

Rash around ankles over malleoli

Varicose veins Haemosiderin pigmentation

VARICOSE ECZEMA

see p. 384

Well defined border

Usually limbs

Scale or dried crust

DISCOID ECZEMA (Dry type)

p. 243

Exudate and wet crust

DISCOID ECZEMA (Wet type)

p. 243

Site of contact of allergen

Patch test positive

ALLERGIC CONTACT DERMATITIS

p. 242

Forearm, occiput, sacrum, calf

Single plaque Lichenified Excoriated

LICHEN SIMPLEX

see p. 219

CHRONIC ECZEMA/DERMATITIS

In this book the term eczema is used for the endogenous eczemas. For those due to external factors the word dermatitis is used. In the United States the term dermatitis is used for both endogenous and exogeneous causes.

The word *eczema* comes from a Greek word meaning to bubble through (*see* Fig. 7.36, p. 189), and the hallmark of eczema (or dermatitis) is the presence of vesicles. In practice, vesicles are only seen in acute eczema (*see* Fig. 8.76), but the patient will often tell you that small blisters have been present in the past, and the remains of these are seen as small pinhead-size crusts (*see* Fig. 7.37, p. 189).

Chronic eczema is diagnosed by identifying the typical morphological features of eczema. What you normally see is an itchy, poorly defined erythematous scaly rash. It is distinguished from psoriasis by being much less vivid in colour (usually a nondescript pink), with poorly defined edges and less obvious scale. Scaling is present but does not become either more obvious or silvery in colour when scratched. Persistent scratching, leads to thickening of the skin, with increased skin markings (lichenification, *see* Fig. 8.81).

Any symmetrical eczema on the trunk and limbs that does not fit any of the recognisable patterns (i.e. atopic, seborrhoeic, discoid, varicose, hand and foot) is called unclassifiable eczema.

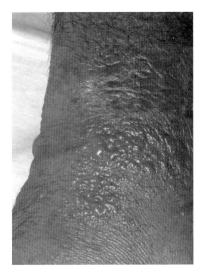

Fig. 8.76 Acute eczema with vesicles and erosions

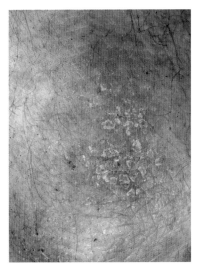

Fig. 8.77 Chronic eczema: poorly defined pink, scaly rash

Fig. 8.78 Chronic eczema in pigmented skin, brown not pink

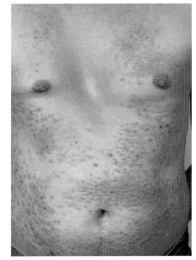

Fig. 8.79 Lichenified eczema

ATOPIC ECZEMA

Atopy means an inherited predisposition to eczema, asthma or hay fever, and atopic individuals may have one or all of these manifestations. It is becoming recognised that an inherited defective skin barrier is important in its cause. The protein filaggrin helps bind keratin fibres in the stratum corneum, and this protein has been found to be defective in atopic eczema. The result of this is that corneocytes are deformed, natural moisturising factors are reduced and an increase in skin pH promotes inflammation. The defective barrier then results in loss of water, dryness of the skin and penetration of irritants and allergens such as house dust mites, pollen and bacteria. The developing immune system in infants becomes unbalanced with Th-2 lymphocytes and cytokines predominating over Th-1 cells. A vicious circle develops where the inflammation reduces the barrier, allowing penetration of irritants and allergens (especially bacteria), which causes further inflammation. Autoimmunity and the production of IgE antibodies is likely to be a by-product of these factors.

The eczema usually begins between the ages of 3 and 12 months (asthma at age 3–4 years and hay fever in the teens) on the scalp and face, and may or may not spread to involve the rest of the body. When children get older it may localise in the flexures, particularly the popliteal and antecubital fossae. It is very itchy so excoriations and lichenification (*see* Fig. 8.81) may be seen, and if children rub rather than scratch, the nails may become very shiny. 50% of such children will also have ichthyosis (also associated with a filaggrin defect) with dry skin and increased skin markings on the palms and soles. In 90% of children the eczema will clear

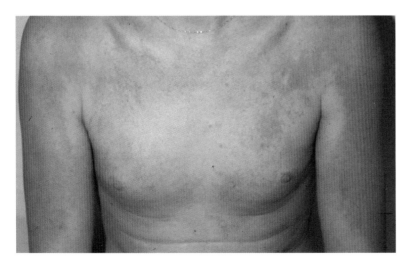

Fig. 8.80 Atopic eczema in an adult: note the symmetrical, pink, poorly defined rash – there is little scale, but it is present if you look carefully

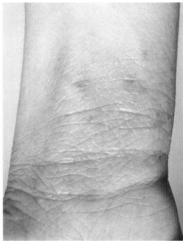

Fig. 8.81 Lichenification on flexor aspect of the wrist

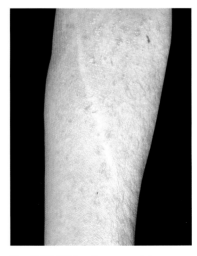

Fig. 8.82 White dermographism

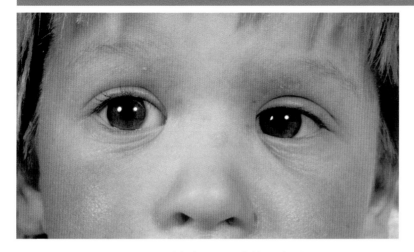

Fig. 8.83 Atopic eczema on a child's face: note folds under the eyes

spontaneously by puberty, but in a small minority it will persist into adult life or become active again later. A few of these will have very extensive and troublesome eczema. Less commonly, atopic eczema may develop in adult life.

In adults a diagnosis of atopic eczema can be made if there is a history of infantile eczema, or if they also have or have had asthma, hay fever, ichthyosis, increased skin markings on the palms (*see* Fig. 8.85) and soles, or white dermographism (stroke gently with your fingernail through an area of eczema: after 30 seconds a white line appears, *see* Fig. 8.82). A history of atopic eczema, asthma or hay fever in the immediate family (parents, siblings, children) is further evidence of atopy.

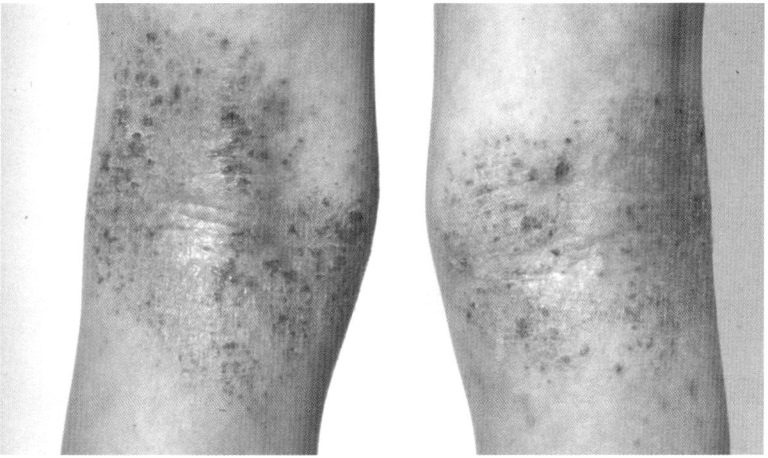

Fig. 8.84 Atopic eczema localised to the popliteal fossae

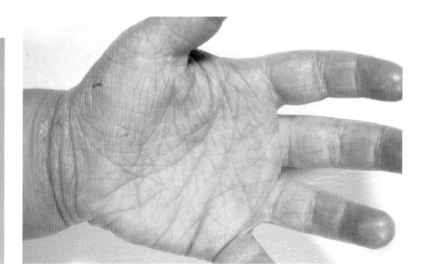

Fig. 8.85 Increased skin markings on the palm in a child with ichthyosis vulgaris

TREATMENT: ATOPIC ECZEMA

Prevention of atopic eczema

As it is now recognised that the primary cause of atopy in children is a defective skin barrier, it is critical to apply moisturisers frequently, especially in infants with a strong family history of atopy. Irritants such as soap, bubble baths and prolonged immersion in water need to be avoided. The patient should bathe using one of the dispersible bath oils (*see* Table 2.01b, p. 27) for 10 minutes daily. Secondary skin infections can be prevented by cleansing the skin with a low concentration of antiseptic (e.g. Dermol shower/wash/lotion).

Once eczema starts to develop it is *very important to treat it immediately* with topical steroids. The benefit from the reduction of the inflammation far outweighs any perceived risk from topical steroids. Proactive treatment with a twice weekly application of a topical calcineurin inhibitor (e.g. tacrolimus 0.03%) or a moderately potent[UK]/group 4–5[USA] topical steroid ointment to previously affected skin has been shown to reduce the occurrence of acute flares of eczema.

Allergy and eczema

Although patients with atopic eczema have elevated IgE levels to foods, grass pollen, cats and house dust mites, these allergies do not affect the severity of the eczema. Prick testing is unhelpful because of multiple false positives. A positive specific RAST test also does not mean that the allergen is the cause of the eczema. The only way to be sure is to avoid the allergen for a week (which will result in improvement in the eczema) *and* then to reintroduce it again to establish a rapid relapse in the eczema.

Food allergy (cows' milk, egg, soya, peanut) may also affect children with eczema, but this will result in acute urticaria or angio-oedema rather than worsening of the eczema. Some children under age 3 also have gastro-intestinal symptoms with a good history of a dietary trigger. This food intolerance may be temporary, and reintroducing the item several months later may be possible.

Airborne allergens cause asthma and hay fever, but these are immediate reactions – runny nose, swollen eyes, sneezing or wheezing. Environmental allergens (cats, house dust mite) are difficult to avoid, and a positive reaction is generally unhelpful.

Treatment plan

Consider the following when planning treatment of atopic eczema.
1. Use emollients routinely for moisturising, bathing and washing.
2. If the eczema is weeping – dry it up with an astringent such as potassium permanganate or aluminium acetate solution (*see* p. 30).
3. For the eczema itself – treat with a topical steroid potent enough to quickly control the eczema, and then reduce frequency of application and potency to maintain control.
4. Immune-modulators are useful as steroid sparing or proactive treatment.
5. If the patient is awake at night – use a sedative antihistamine.
6. If there is infection – use a systemic antibiotic for a week only. Do not use topical antibiotics or steroid-antibiotic mixtures.
7. Wrapping eczematous skin is useful in controlling acute flare ups or in preventing excessive scratching in young children.
8. Other considerations – clothing, reduction in house dust mite, stress.
9. UV phototherapy (*see* p. 60) or systemic agents such as ciclosporin (*see* p. 53–4) or azathiaprine (*see* p. 54) may be necessary if the above fail to control the disease. These can be provided by dermatologists.

1. Complete emollient therapy

The use of emollients on dry and eczematous skin is an important part of the treatment and prevention of atopic eczema. Emollients should be used liberally and frequently for moisturising, washing and bathing, even if the skin is clear. Everything that goes on the skin should be emollient based so that the skin barrier is repaired and maintained. Numerous emollients are available (*see* Table 2.01a, p. 26), and how greasy these need to be is often a matter of patient choice or trial and error. The drier the skin, the more greasy the moisturiser needs to be. Lighter (cream) emollients can be used for daytime or summer, and heavier (ointment based) emollients used at night and in winter. Patients should be offered a leave-on emollient, a product to wash with (soap must be avoided) and a bath emollient. The patient can be offered product testers to find which suit him or her best.

Bathing: soaking in a lukewarm bath for 10–15 minutes every day is helpful provided 10–20 mL of one of the dispersible bath oils has been added (*see* p. 27). Emollient shower/wash formulations (e.g. Doublebase shower gel, E45 wash cream, QV gentle wash) or Epaderm cream should be used instead of soap, detergents or bubble bath, but these *should not be used as a leave-on emollient*. Aqueous cream is best avoided as it contains sodium lauryl sulphate, which is a skin irritant.

Moisturisers should also be applied to the skin after getting out the bath, while the skin is still warm and moist. Apply the moisturiser starting at the neck, and smoothing (not rubbing) it in downwards on the trunk, arms and legs. The moisturiser should be applied first, and left on for 20 minutes before applying a topical steroid.

Humectants such as glycerol, urea, polyethylene glycol and lactic acid are often added to emollients as they can increase the horny layer's capacity to retain water (*see* p 26). Some products such as Doublebase Dayleve and Oilatum cream contain film-forming agents that form an additional protective layer over the surface of the skin, helping to reduce water loss and penetration of irritants and allergens.

Antiseptics. Emollients which contain antiseptic products such as chlorhexidine and benzalkonium chloride (Dermol cream, Eczmol cream) may help to reduce bacterial colonisation and infection, which can exacerbate eczema. However these agents may be irritant so need to be used with caution.

Antipruritics such as lauromacrogols have properties of a mild topical anaesthetic and have an antipruritic effect (Balneum Plus cream, E45 Itch Relief cream).

Allergen-free products such as ointments or products containing no preservative (e.g. Emollin spray) are useful in patients who are allergic to them. Emollient sprays are useful in elderly patients who have difficulty in reaching areas of skin (back, lower legs).

2. Astringents

Astringents (*see* p. 30) dry up exudate by coagulating protein. Soak the affected areas in one of these solutions by applying moistened gauze swabs or by emersion in a bath or hand basin.

3a. Topical steroids

Topical steroid ointments are still the mainstay of treatment for atopic eczema. Patients or parents are often afraid of using topical steroids because of the widespread publicity about side effects. Failure to treat active eczema will cause more harm to the patient by allowing allergens to penetrate the defective cutaneous barrier.

You will need to explain that there are different strengths of steroids (*see* p. 32). Start with 1% hydrocortisone ointment applied daily on the face and skin folds, and on the trunk and limbs use a moderately potent[UK]/group 4–5[USA] topical steroid ointment. Short courses (5 days) of potent[UK]/group 2–3[USA] steroids for an acute flare may be necessary to get the eczema under control quickly, and for lichenified or thickened plaques.

By using a steroid with the appropriate potency to quickly control the eczema and continuing treatment until completely clear will reduce the likelihood of a rebound flare. Then taper therapy to alternate days before reducing to *proactive treatment*: twice weekly applications of a topical steroid to previously affected skin for up to a month. This has been shown to reduce flares of eczema and improve the quality of life. Continuous long term use of potent steroids on the face and body folds must be avoided, and a topical calcineurin inhibitor may be used instead (*see* p. 240).

Ointments work much better than creams, since the grease forms an occlusive barrier preventing evaporation of water and delivers the steroid more effectively to the skin. They are best applied after a bath. First apply a moisturiser all over, and after 20 minutes the topical steroid can be rubbed into the eczematous areas.

It is important to give the patient enough ointment, and to monitor the amount being used (too little may be as bad as too much). To cover the whole body surface twice a day, infants will need approximately 10 g a day (70 g/week); a 7-year-old, 20 g a day (140 g/week); and adults, 30 g a day (210 g/week) – see fingertip units p. 32. A record of the amount of steroid prescribed and used (ask the patient or parent to bring back used tubes) will be helpful in monitoring this. Using too little steroid may be as relevant as using too much.

4. Topical immune-modulators

These drugs work by blocking the molecular mechanisms of inflammation in the skin (*see* p. 34). Two drugs are available: 0.1% and 0.03% tacrolimus (Protopic) ointment and 1% pimecrolimus (Elidel) cream. Both can cause a burning/stinging sensation when first used, which stops after about 20 minutes and disappears altogether after a few days. Use in the following situations:
- proactive (preventative) treatment twice weekly to previously affected areas
- patients with facial, periocular or neck eczema
- patients who have not responded, are using too much or too strong a steroid, or who have developed steroid side effects
- patients with poor compliance with topical steroids because they are afraid of the side effects
- patients with perioral dermatitis (*see* p. 115) or rosacea (*see* p. 122) which has been triggered by topical steroids
- patients in whom you would otherwise be considering systemic treatment.

5. Antihistamines

Sedative antihistamines are useful if the child is not sleeping at night and is keeping the family awake. They will not stop the itching, but if given in adequate dosage the child will sleep through the night. Start with 5 mL of promethazine (Phenergan 5 mg/5 mL) or alimemazine (7.5 mg/5 mL) elixir which should be given around 6pm in the evening. Double the dose each night until the child sleeps until morning. Alimemazine forte is available as 30 mg/5 mL. Children surprisingly can tolerate much higher doses than adults. Neither is addictive and both are quite safe.

In adults, start with 10 mg of promethazine, hydroxyzine or alimemazine and double the dose as necessary until the patient sleeps through the night. Non-sedative antihistamines (*see* p. 49) are ineffective in treating eczema. They can be tried if sedative antihistamines produce unacceptable drowsiness, or during the day.

6. Treatment of secondary infection

If the eczema becomes suddenly worse, infection with *S. aureus* may be the cause. There will be associated pustules or yellow crusting. This is best treated with a systemic antibiotic such as flucloxacillin 125–500 mg qid (or erythromycin if allergic to penicillin) for one week only. Do not use topical antibiotics or topical steroid–antibiotic mixtures, as these are often ineffective and are likely to cause an allergic contact dermatitis.

If the pustules are umbilicated consider eczema herpeticum (*see* p. 109). In this condition, the lesions often are painful and the patient miserable. Treatment is with an antiviral agent (*see* p. 180).

7. Wrapping techniques

Localised wrapping or occlusion will cool, soothe and protect from scratching inflamed, excoriated or lichenified skin. Zinc impregnated bandages (Zipzoc, Fig. 8.86) or dressings (PB7, Icthopaste) can be applied overnight or left on for longer periods. Because the zinc paste is sticky, it will need to be covered by a tubular bandage or secondary dressing.

Generalised wrapping with a suit consisting of long sleeved vest, leggings, socks and mittens (Fig. 8.87) is useful for treating widespread itching and eczema. It prevents scratching and the occlusion provided by the garment allows better penetration of the moisturiser. The affected areas of skin are treated with a topical steroid ointment, and then the whole body surface is covered with a suitable emollient (*see* p. 26). These garments can be washed and used several times. They are available made of viscose (Acti-Fast, Comfifast, Easifast, Skinnies, Tubifast) or silk (Dermasilk, Dreamskin, Skinnies). The advantage of silk is that it is cooler, requires less moisturiser on the skin, and does not wear out, but it is more expensive.

Wet wrapping is very effective in bringing a generalised flare of eczema in children and adults under control quickly. It cools the skin, improves moisturisation, prevents scratching and reduces the need for topical steroids. Two layers of the therapeutic suits (as above) are put on following application of moisturiser and topical steroid. The layer adjacent to the skin is moistened with luke-warm water, squeezed dry and then a second *dry* layer is put on over this. Many children do not like it initially, but once put on the skin feels so much better that they can feel the benefit. Parents can spray water onto the inner layer to keep it moist. On removal, if the garment sticks to the open eczematous areas, it should be soaked off in a bath.

Table 8.02 Information sheet and prescription for child with atopic eczema

Rx			
1.	Leave on emollient (light cream)	_____	500 g
	apply frequently to all dry or inflamed areas during the day		
	AND/OR		
1b.	Leave on emollient (heavy oint)	_____	500 g
	apply all over after bathing and leave on overnight		
2.	Wash product	_____	500 mL
	to be used instead of soap, rub onto skin and wash off		
3.	Bath emollient	_____	250 mL
	add to bath water, soak daily for 10–15 minutes		
4a.	Topical steroid for the face	1% hydrocortisone oint	60 g
4b.	Moderately potent topical steroid for the body _____ oint		200 g
	apply steroids daily for 2 weeks or until clear. Then apply alternate days for 2 weeks, and thereafter only twice weekly up to a month.		
5.	Potent topical steroid	_____ oint	30 g
	apply daily for up to 5 days if eczema flares up, then revert to moderately potent steroid (4b)		
6.	Sedating antihistamine:	promethazine elixir	(200 mL)
	OR	promethazine/hydroxyzine tablets	10 mg ×56
	take 5 mL or 10 mg around 6pm in the evening, increase dose until sleeping through the night, reduce dose if morning drowsiness		
7.	Elasticated viscose garments	_____	4 sets
	long sleeved vest / leggings / mittens / socks		
	Put on after applying moisturisers and steroid ointment.		
	Either *apply single layer dry,*		
	Or *moisten first layer with luke warm water, squeeze dry, and put on a second **dry** layer over it.*		

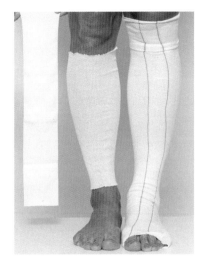

Fig. 8.86 Zipzoc. On left as removed from packaging which can be applied directly to skin (right leg), and then covered with blue line tubifast (left leg).

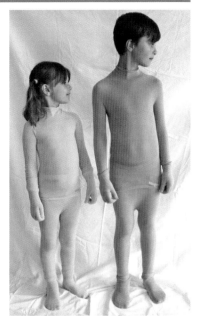

Fig. 8.87 Skinnies, viscose suits in blue or pink worn for wrapping; they are seamless and non-irritant available on prescription (for sizes *see* skinniesuk.com).

Table 8.02 lists the items that should be prescribed for a patient with atopic eczema. It is suggested that *this table can be reproduced* and given to the patient as instructions of what to use where. Fill in the product recommended on the blue line.

For suggestions: 1. emollients *see* Table 2.01a, p. 26;

2. wash products and 3. bath emollients, *see* Table 2.01b, p. 27,

4. and 5. topical steroids, *see* Table 2.02, p 32,

7. *see* BNF section A5.8.3

Recommended quantities that should be prescribed are listed on the right.

7. Other considerations

Cotton clothing worn next to the skin is comfortable, while wool is irritating. Reduction in contact with house dust or pets may be beneficial. The following measures will help to reduce levels of house dust mite.

- Vacuum all household carpets (especially around skirting boards), fabrics, and sofas daily.
- Remove dust regularly with a wet duster or damp mop.
- Laminated floor coverings are preferable to carpet in the bedroom as they can be damp mopped.
- Duvet and pillows should have synthetic fillings. Use mattress and pillow covers. Bedding and night clothing should be made of cotton.
- Keep humidity levels to around 50%. Dry air will dry the skin. Humid air encourages mould and house dust growth. A dehumidifier can be used to remove excess moisture. If the air is too dry, place a bowl of water under the radiator.

Keep pets out of the bedroom particularly at night and do not allow them to sleep on the bed. Only avoid contact with animals if definite improvement away from them (and relapse on re-exposure) can be demonstrated.

Where possible stress at school or work needs to be tackled. Patient and parent support can be provided by specialised dermatological nurses, the local dermatology department or the National Eczema Society.

ALLERGIC CONTACT DERMATITIS

A well-defined plaque of eczema may be due to contact with an allergen such as nickel in buckles or jean studs, colophony in elastoplast or chrome in leather straps. Creams containing parabens, antibiotics, antihistamines or even a topical steroid may also cause an allergic dermatitis (*see also* pp. 106 & 415). The patient will need to be patch tested (*see* p. 21) by a dermatologist with a special interest in contact dermatitis to interpret positive patch tests, some of which may not be relevant. Any allergens thought to be causing the dermatitis will need to be avoided. In theory avoidance results in a cure, although in practice this is not always the case. The dermatitis is treated with a potent[UK]/group 2–3[USA] topical steroid ointment.

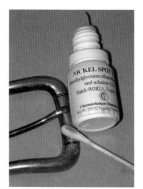

Fig. 8.88 Nickel testing kit: a drop of dimethylglyoxime and a drop of ammonia on a cotton wool bud rubbed onto the buckle stains pink

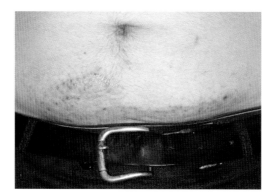

Fig. 8.89 Allergic contact dermatitis to a nickel belt buckle

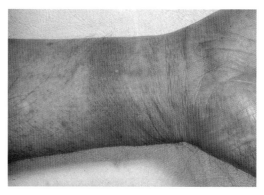

Fig. 8.90 Allergic contact dermatitis to chrome in watch strap: the leather has been chrome tanned

DISCOID (NUMMULAR) ECZEMA

This differs from other forms of eczema in that it presents as well-demarcated round, oval or annular red, scaly plaques. It can be wet or dry. The wet type consists of plaques made up of numerous vesicles that break to produce exudate (*see* Fig. 8.91) and crust (*see* Fig. 8.92) on the surface. The dry type is similar but has scale (*see* Fig. 8.94) on the surface. In young adults the commonest site is the dorsum of hands and fingers. In older individuals it is more usual on the lower legs. Some patients with atopic eczema, allergic contact dermatitis or unclassifiable eczema also have discoid plaques of eczema. Do not confuse it with tinea (*see* p. 233) just because it is round.

TREATMENT: DISCOID ECZEMA

- In the wet form, dry up the exudate with potassium permanganate or aluminium acetate soaks (*see* p. 30).
- Use a moisturiser regularly on the dry type.
- In both then use a potent[UK]/group 2–3[USA] topical steroid ointment applied twice a day. The response is variable – sometimes discoid eczema can be quite resistant to treatment or it can relapse quickly on stopping topical steroids.
- Resistant cases will need to be referred to a dermatologist.

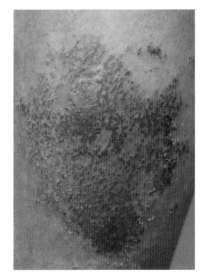

Fig. 8.91 Wet discoid eczema

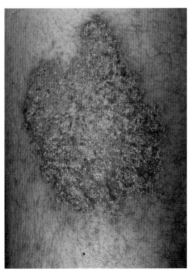

Fig. 8.92 Crust on surface of discoid eczema

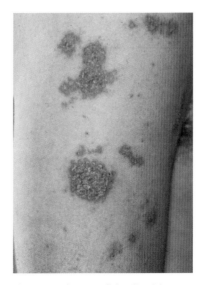

Fig. 8.93 Plaques of dry discoid eczema

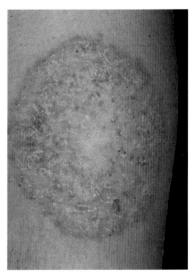

Fig. 8.94 Large plaques of dry discoid eczema on arm

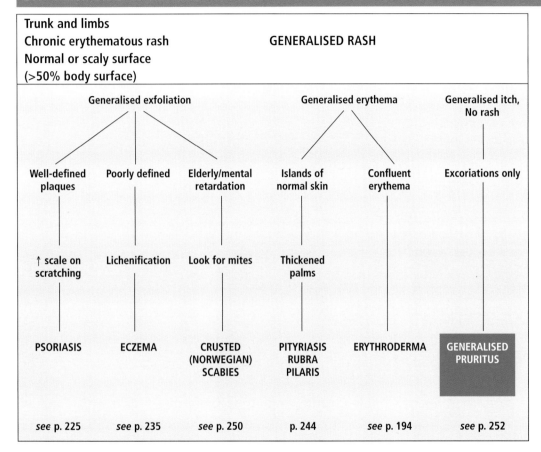

Trunk and limbs
Chronic erythematous rash   **GENERALISED RASH**
Normal or scaly surface
(>50% body surface)

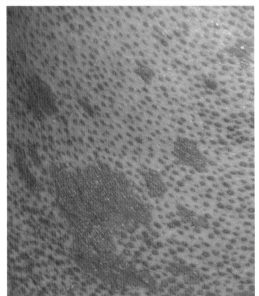

Fig. 8.95 Pityriasis rubra pilaris

PITYRIASIS RUBRA PILARIS

Pityriasis rubra pilaris is a rare condition of unknown cause. Red macules appear around follicles and gradually coalesce to areas of widespread erythema. Characteristically there are islands of spared normal skin. The palms and soles become hyperkeratotic and orange in colour and the nails thickened and discoloured distally.

TREATMENT: PITYRIASIS RUBRA PILARIS

The majority of cases resolve spontaneously in 1–3 years. Treatment with a systemic retinoid such as acitretin 0.75 mg/kg or isotretinin 1 mg/kg will hasten this (see p. 49). Topical steroids are not effective but emollients are useful.

Trunk and limbs
Chronic erythematous rash
Surface crust, excoriations
Widespread papules/plaques/small erosions
No blisters present, small erosions (<1 cm) only

CRUST AND EXCORIATIONS – no blisters

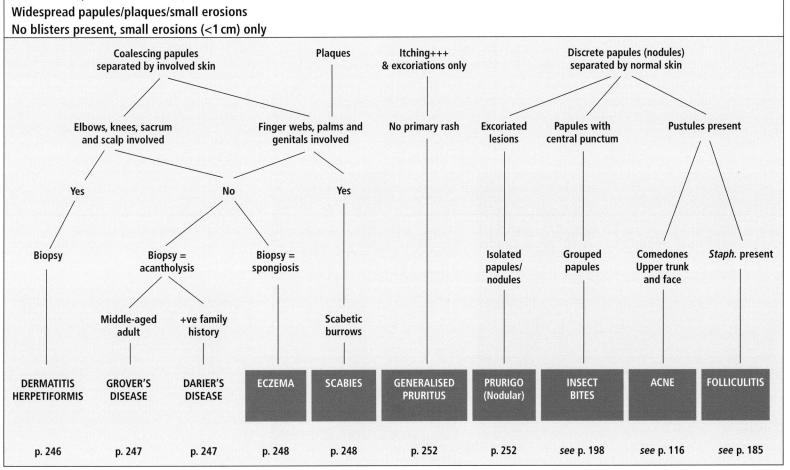

| Coalescing papules separated by involved skin | | Plaques | Itching+++ & excoriations only | Discrete papules (nodules) separated by normal skin |

Elbows, knees, sacrum and scalp involved — Finger webs, palms and genitals involved — No primary rash — Excoriated lesions — Papules with central punctum — Pustules present

Yes — No — Yes

Biopsy — Biopsy = acantholysis — Biopsy = spongiosis — Isolated papules/ nodules — Grouped papules — Comedones Upper trunk and face — *Staph.* present

Middle-aged adult — +ve family history — Scabetic burrows

| DERMATITIS HERPETIFORMIS | GROVER'S DISEASE | DARIER'S DISEASE | ECZEMA | SCABIES | GENERALISED PRURITUS | PRURIGO (Nodular) | INSECT BITES | ACNE | FOLLICULITIS |

| p. 246 | p. 247 | p. 247 | p. 248 | p. 248 | p. 252 | p. 252 | *see* p. 198 | *see* p. 116 | *see* p. 185 |

DERMATITIS HERPETIFORMIS

This is a disease classically of young adults and it presents with severe itching, particularly at night. Grouped vesicles in the distribution of psoriasis (elbows, knees, sacrum, scalp) are quickly scratched away to leave pink excoriated papules and plaques. It is unusual to see blisters and the rash can be confused with eczema. It is an important, if uncommon, disease because it is associated with a gluten enteropathy.

The diagnosis can be confirmed by finding:
- tissue transglutaminase IgA/IgG (tTG), anti-gliadin or anti-endomysial antibodies in the blood.
- a subepidermal blister containing polymorphs on skin biopsy.
- deposits of IgA in the upper dermis on immunofluorescence of normal skin.
- subtotal villous atrophy (as in coeliac disease) on jejunal biopsy.

TREATMENT: DERMATITIS HERPETIFORMIS

Initial treatment with dapsone, 50–150 mg daily is required. This will stop the itching within a few hours and is usually dramatic. Check a full blood count before starting dapsone, because it causes haemolysis of red blood cells. This normally occurs within a few days of starting treatment, so the blood count should be repeated after one week. Most patients will show some haemolysis and methaemoglobinaemia. The side effects can be minimised by giving cimetidine 400 mg tid with the dapsone.

A gluten-free diet will eradicate the IgA from the dermal papillae in 9–12 months and the itching will then stop. Although not pleasant, patients should be encouraged to stick to a gluten-free diet so that the dapsone may be stopped and to prevent the long-term risk of small bowel lymphoma from developing (the risk is the same as for coeliac disease).

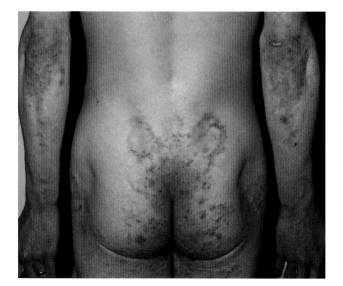

Fig. 8.96 Typical distribution of dermatitis herpetiformis

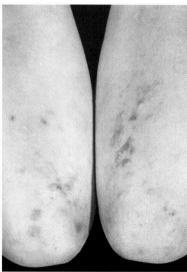

Fig. 8.97 Dermatitis herpetiformis: excoriated papules on elbows

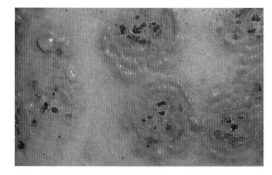

Fig. 8.98 Dermatitis herpetiformis: typical grouped small vesicles on trunk

GROVER'S DISEASE (ACANTHOLYTIC DERMATOSIS)

This is a very itchy rash that occurs on the trunk (usually middle-aged men). It is made up of itchy papules with an eroded surface. Individual papules are discrete and usually 2–3 mm in size. The rash lasts from 2 weeks to many months and tends to remit and relapse. Diagnosis is established by skin biopsy, which shows acantholysis (loss of cohesion) of the epidermal cells. Treatment is unsatisfactory, but it is worth trying anti-itch/anaesthetic emollients (Balneum plus cream, E45 itch cream) and a moderately potent topical steroid.

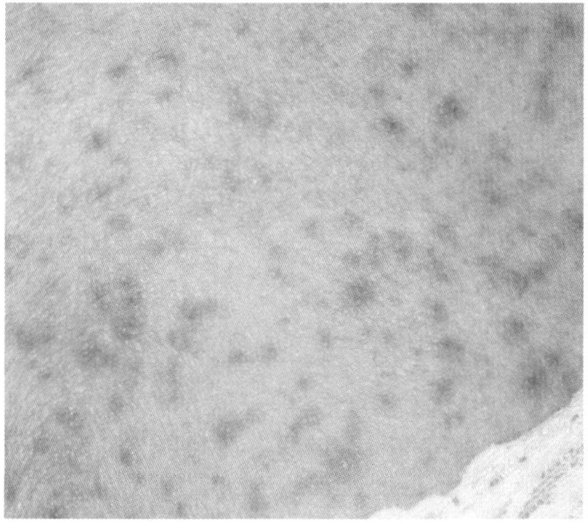

DARIER'S DISEASE

This rare condition is inherited as an autosomal dominant trait. The rash consists of follicular papules that coalesce into plaques affecting the trunk, upper arms, face and flexures. The surface is covered with a yellow-brown, greasy crust. A skin biopsy is diagnostic. Other changes are longitudinal ridging of the nails with V-shaped notches at the ends (*see* Fig. 14.07, p. 438), pits on the palms and soles, and plane wart-like papules on the dorsum of the hands and feet.

TREATMENT: DARIER'S DISEASE

For localised areas use 0.025% retinoic acid cream or a topical steroid–antibiotic mix twice a day. For extensive disease use acitretin 0.5–1 mg/kg/day which will need to be prescribed by a dermatologist. Photodynamic therapy can also be helpful in some patients.

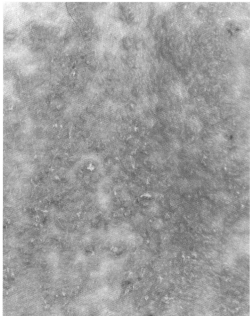

Fig. 8.101 Close-up of follicular papules of Darier's disease

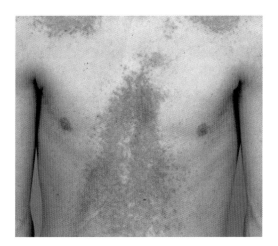

Fig. 8.100 Typical distribution of Darier's disease

Fig. 8.99 Close-up of Grover's disease: eroded papules on chest

SUBACUTE ECZEMA

The physical signs of eczema are the result of inflammation of the skin. In the acute phase, vesicles and exudate are seen in the epidermis (spongiosis, *see* p. 189). Once the acute phase has settled, any exudate dries, causing crusting and erosions. We call this subacute eczema. Intense itching results in excoriations and erosions. These physical signs can also occur in any very itchy rash (generalised pruritus, dermatitis herpetiformis), when there is breakdown of the epidermis (acantholysis – Darier's disease, Grover's disease, pemphigus), or with non-specific inflammation of the epidermis (scabies or eczematous drug rash). In all these conditions blisters are unlikely to be seen.

Intact blisters will be seen if the blistering occurs at the dermo-epidermal junction (pemphigoid) or is intraepidermal on the palms and soles where the stratum corneum is thickened (pompholyx eczema). For types of eczema and treatment, *see* p. 234.

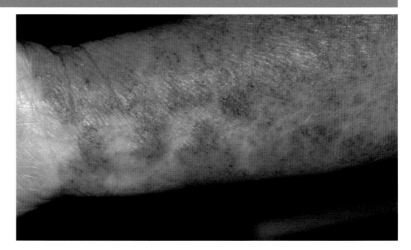

Fig. 8.102 Subacute eczema: erosions and crusts

SCABIES

Scabies is an infestation with the human scabies mite *Sarcoptes scabiei*. It is transmitted by prolonged skin-to-skin contact with someone who has it (usually by lying next to someone in bed all night or by holding hands). A fertilised female has to be transferred for infestation to take place. She will then find a place to lay her eggs (a burrow). Between 4 and 6 weeks later a secondary hypersensitivity rash occurs. This is characterised by intense itching, particularly at night. The rash is made up of excoriated papules scattered over the trunk and limbs but sparing the face (except in infants). The diagnosis is confirmed by finding one or more burrows (often there are fewer than 10 in total to be found). These are linear S-shaped papules, 3–5 mm in length and usually along the sides of the fingers or on the front of the wrists.

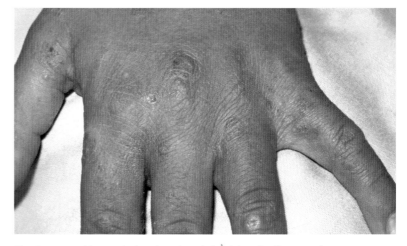

Fig. 8.103 Scabies: typical rash on hands involving the finger webs

Less commonly they can be found along the sides of the feet, around the nipples, on the buttocks or on the genitalia. There is almost always a rash on the hands and, in males, papules on the penis and scrotum. Other members of the family or sexual partners may also be itching. Scabies in developing countries can be associated with an increased incidence of streptococcal infection complications such as glomerulonephritis and rheumatic fever. Although scratching and skin damage makes colonisation with *Staphylococcus* and *Streptococcus* more likely, it is probable that the scabies mite itself may play a part in allowing these streptococcal antigens to damage the kidney or heart.

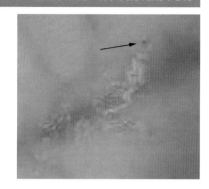
Fig. 8.105 Dermoscopy of scabetic burrow showing the 'jet contrail' sign: the mite is a small black dot at the head of the jet stream (indicated by arrow) in this picture and in Fig. 8.106.

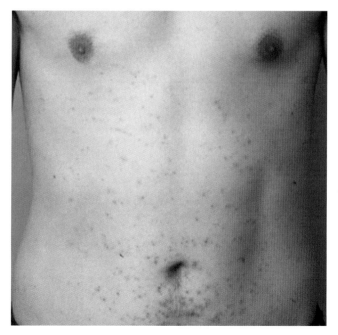
Fig. 8.104 Scabies: rash on trunk

Fig. 8.106 Scabies burrow

Fig. 8.107 (left) Scabies mite and egg (×350)

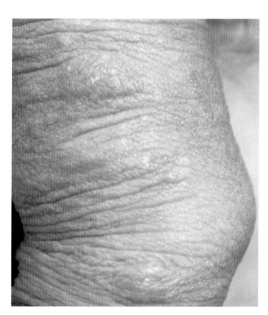
Fig. 8.108 (above) Scabies: penile papules

TREATMENT: HUMAN SCABIES

It is essential to treat not only the patient but also anyone else who has been in close contact, even if they are asymptomatic. In practice this means all individuals living in the same house and any sexual partner(s). If there are children in the family, grandparents, aunts and uncles, babysitters, neighbours and anyone else who has been holding the children will also need treating.

The idea of treatment is to kill all stages of the life cycle of the scabies mite (eggs, larvae, nymphs and adults) at the same time. A single treatment of 5% permethrin cream (Lyclear[UK]/Elimite[USA]) or 0.5% malathion lotion (Derbac-M) can be used. The cream or lotion is applied to the whole body surface except the face and scalp (including the skin between the fingers and toes, under the finger nails, the genitalia and the soles of the feet). Treatment is applied at night before the patient goes to bed and left on for 24 hours. The whole family and other contacts should be treated at the same time. Twenty-four hours later the patient can have a bath and wash the scabicide off. The patient should then change his or her underwear, pyjamas and the sheets on his or her bed. The clothes should be washed and ironed to kill any wandering acari, although in practice it is very unlikely that any will be left alive at this stage. There is no need to go to elaborate means to fumigate the house or bedding. 15 g of permethrin cream or 30 mL of malathion lotion will be needed for a single application (for an adult), so you can work out how much to prescribe for the whole family. Any residual itching can be treated with calamine lotion or crotamiton (Eurax) cream twice a day.

Treatment failure in scabies is due to:
- the scabicide not being applied over the whole body
- the contacts not being treated
- the wrong diagnosis.

A similar rash without any burrows can be due to **animal scabies**, where mites are found on the pet (usually a dog) and the diagnosis is confirmed by brushing the animal's fur on to a sheet and sending the brushings to the local microbiology laboratory to identify the mites. Treat the pet for scabies rather than the human contact.

CRUSTED (NORWEGIAN) SCABIES

This is an infestation with the human scabies mite in an individual with lowered immunity, mental retardation or sensory loss. The host response is abnormal leading to the presence of thousands of mites all over the skin. These are shed into the environment, eventually infecting other people. Thick hyperkeratotic scale occurs on palms, soles, flexures and under the nails. Eventually a widespread scaly rash occurs all over the body – this is often misdiagnosed as eczema. The diagnosis usually comes to light when those in contact with the patient develop an itchy rash (which is diagnosed as ordinary scabies). To confirm the diagnosis remove some of the thick scale from the patient and/or collect up scales and other debris from the bed, and examine under the microscope. Numerous eggs, larvae, nymphs and adult mites will be seen.

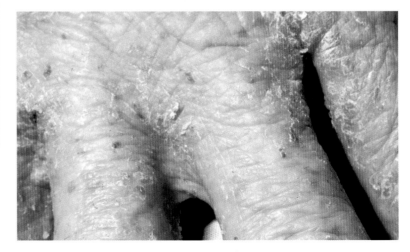

Fig. 8.109 Norwegian scabies: rash on back of hands looks like eczema

TREATMENT: CRUSTED SCABIES

TREATMENT IN AN OLD PEOPLE'S HOME

1. Identify the patient with crusted (Norwegian) scabies.
2. Identify a single room where he or she can be isolated and empty that room of all furniture and soft furnishings apart from a bed. Clean the room thoroughly and wash the floor and walls with a suitable detergent. Make up the bed with freshly washed and ironed bedding.
3. Treat the patient with permethrin (Lyclear) cream as a single application all over (including the face and scalp). Crusted scabies does not respond well to ivermectin.
4. After treatment put the patient into the cleaned single room.
5. The home should be closed to new residents and visitors until steps 6–9 have been carried out.
6. Explain to the staff (whether or not they have had direct physical contact with the patient) what is happening. Explain that the patient has Norwegian scabies and that whether or not they are itching they will almost certainly have caught it and will need treatment. Explain that the variety they have caught is ordinary scabies and not the very infectious kind that the patient has. Explain that they are only infectious to very close contacts, i.e. immediate family or those with whom they share a bed.
7. To remove any mites from the environment wash and iron all bedding, curtains and other soft furnishings in the patient's bedroom and any public rooms that he or she has used. Wash or spray the floors, walls and other hard surfaces in all the rooms where he or she has been with 1% lindane emulsion.
8. Explain what is happening to the other residents and tell them that they will not be able to go out or have visitors until they have been treated. Treat them once with 5% permethrin cream over the whole of the skin except the face and scalp. Leave it on the skin for 24 hours.
9. All staff and their husbands, wives, boyfriends, girlfriends and children must be treated with permethrin cream as directed on p. 250. Ivermectin tablets (200 µg/kg) given as a single dose is a convenient alternative for everyone apart from the patient with crusted scabies.
10. Once steps 6–9 on this list have been done, the home can be reopened to visitors.

BODY LICE

Body lice live and lay their eggs in the seams of clothing, but they need to bite humans to obtain their blood. The adult louse is 2–4 mm in length. Body lice thrive when humans are not able to wash and iron their clothes (which would kill the lice). Lice are mainly seen in vagrants but are also seen in refugee camps or in war situations. Infestation is spread by sharing bedding, clothing or by very close contact. You will not find the lice on the patient's skin – look along the seams of his or her clothing to find the lice and nits.

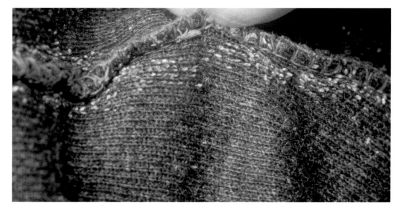

Fig. 8.110 Body louse on seam of clothing, with nits scattered along the seam

TREATMENT: BODY LICE

> Since the lice live off the body, there is no need to treat the patient. Clothing should be hot washed and tumble dried, or dry-cleaned, ironed or burnt. The itching will stop once the lice have been removed.

GENERALISED PRURITUS

In most instances if someone is itching all over but no rash is seen other than excoriations no cause will be found, but it is important to exclude the conditions shown in Table 8.03.

In the elderly, generalised pruritus (**senile pruritus**) is quite common and may in part be due to drying out of the skin through too-frequent bathing or showering. There may be psychological issues, so look for evidence of depression, anxiety or emotional upset. Very often no cause can be found.

PRURIGO

Prurigo is a rash that is caused by the patient scratching and picking his or her skin. Sometimes just excoriations are seen, but often numerous discrete intensely itchy pink, mauve or brown excoriated papules or nodules occur (**nodular prurigo**). They heal to leave white scars that sometimes have very obvious follicular openings within them. Prurigo can sometimes be associated with eczema.

Prurigo of pregnancy is common, with secondary signs of scratching. It resolves at term. Check the liver function tests, since itching can be due to elevated bile salts in the blood, raising the possibility of **intrahepatic cholestasis of pregnancy**. In this condition, itching of the palms and soles is characteristic. It can be associated with abnormal clotting (treated with vitamin K) and foetal distress. Early delivery may be necessary.

Table 8.03 Systemic causes of generalised pruritus and investigations needed to rule them out

Systemic cause	Investigation
Anaemia, especially iron deficiency	Full blood count, serum iron and ferritin
Polycythaemia rubra vera (itching, especially in a hot bath)	Full blood count
Uraemia (also seen in 80% of patients on maintenance haemodialysis)	Urea and creatinine
Obstructive jaundice (may occur in patients with primary biliary cirrhosis before jaundice occurs)	Liver function tests; autoimmune profile
Thyroid disease, both hypo- and hyperthyroid	T4 and thyroid-stimulating hormone; autoimmune profile
Lymphoma, especially in young adults	Enlarged lymph nodes clinically and on chest X-ray
Carcinoma, especially in old age	Good history, full physical examination, chest X-ray, occult bloods, abdominal ultrasound and CAT scan
HIV/AIDS	HIV ELISA test
Body lice, likely in vagrants living rough (*see* p. 251)	Look for lice and nits in the seams of underwear
Delusions of infestation	*See* p. 254

TREATMENT: PRURITUS AND PRURIGO

Any specific cause found needs treating.

In the elderly, prescribe emollients. If no cause is found, treatment will need to be symptomatic. Try the following measures.

1. Start with 10% crotamiton (Eurax) cream twice a day.
2. If it does not help, use a moderately potent[UK]/group 4–5[USA] steroid ointment or cream.
3. If the topical steroids do not adequately control the itching and it is interfering with sleep, a sedative antihistamine such as alimemazine (10–20 mg) or promethazine (Phenergan, 25–50 mg) taken about an hour before going to bed may help. The patient will, of course, need to be careful about driving the next day.
4. In patients with uraemia or HIV infection, UVB therapy two to three times a week may help (see p. 60).
5. Other measures worth trying include doxepin cream or 0.5% menthol in aqueous/hydrophilic cream (Levomenthol).
6. If none of these measures help, you can try a tricyclic antidepressant such as amitriptyline 10 mg at night.

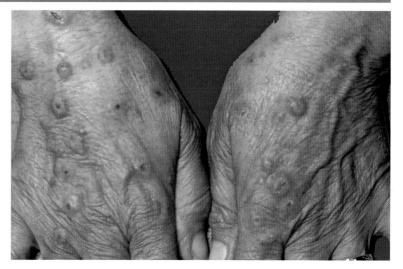

Fig. 8.111 Nodular prurigo on dorsum of hands

TREATMENT: NODULAR PRURIGO

In order to get this better the patient somehow has got to stop scratching and picking the skin. A potent[UK]/group 2–3[USA] topical steroid ointment applied twice a day may help control the itching. Fluandrenalone (Haelan) tape may be applied to individual lesions and left on for several days at a time. Sometimes a sedative antihistamine at night may be needed. If it is confined to the arms and legs, they can be wrapped up in an occlusive paste bandage (Ichthopaste or Zipzoc) covered with Tubifast for a week at a time. Unfortunately, when the bandages are taken off the patient will often begin to scratch again. Severe cases may need systemic steroids (prednisolone 30 mg for 2 weeks to break the itch–scratch cycle, and slowly reducing the dose by 5 mg per fortnight). Often this will work, although relapse may occur when the dose of steroid is reduced.

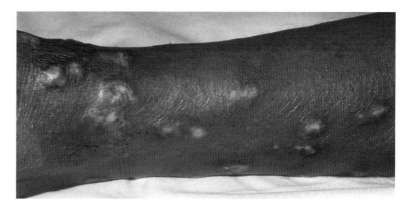

Fig. 8.112 Nodular prurigo in black skin

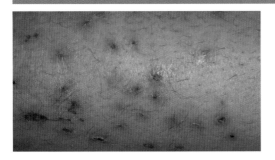

Fig. 8.113 Excoriations in a patient with pruritus: no underlying primary rash is seen

DELUSIONS OF INFESTATION

This is a psychiatric illness where the patient is convinced that parasites or mites are in his or her skin. The patient will complain of itching, or a crawling sensation. The skin shows multiple excoriated papules where the patient has tried to dig out the offending insect. Often he or she will present with a matchbox or container with bits of skin that have been scratched off as 'proof' of the infestation (*see* Fig. 8.115). When examined under the microscope no creatures are found. The patient may become quite angry with you if you do not take his or her complaint seriously. A similar condition called **Morgellons syndrome** is associated with the delusion that fibres are trapped in the skin, and the patient attempts to pick them out, resulting in the same clinical picture.

TREATMENT: DELUSIONS OF INFESTATION

Treatment is difficult, since it is almost impossible to convince the patient that the infestation is imagined. Referral to a psychiatrist generally is not helpful, but a combined dermatology and psychiatric clinic is. It is important to keep the patient's trust that you are trying to help cure the problem, otherwise the patient will not return for further appointments. To do this the possibility of infestation needs to be excluded by medical tests (such as mycology and bacteriology). The eventual aim is to persuade the patient to take an antipsychotic such as pimozide, which in most cases resolves the problem.

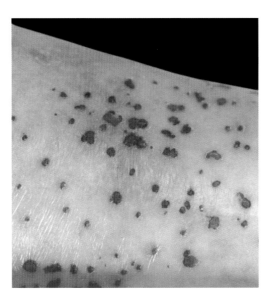

Fig. 8.114 Delusions of infestation: multiple excoriations with crusting

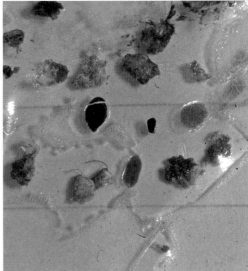

Fig. 8.115 'Matchbox sign': fragments of skin and crust brought by patient

Trunk and limbs
Chronic erythematous rash
Surface crust, exudate
Widespread vesicles, bullae and/or large erosions

BLISTERS and/or LARGE EROSIONS

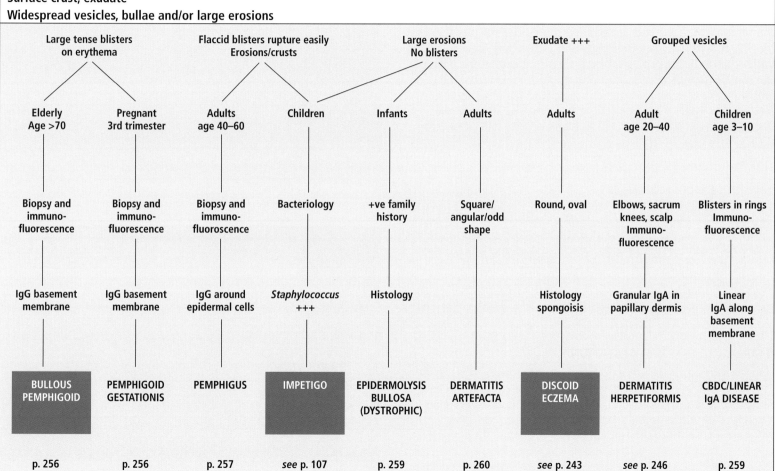

Large tense blisters on erythema		Flaccid blisters rupture easily Erosions/crusts		Large erosions No blisters		Exudate +++	Grouped vesicles	
Elderly Age >70	Pregnant 3rd trimester	Adults age 40–60	Children	Infants	Adults	Adults	Adult age 20–40	Children age 3–10
Biopsy and immuno-fluorescence	Biopsy and immuno-fluorescence	Biopsy and immuno-fluorescence	Bacteriology	+ve family history	Square/angular/odd shape	Round, oval	Elbows, sacrum knees, scalp Immuno-fluorescence	Blisters in rings Immuno-fluorescence
IgG basement membrane	IgG basement membrane	IgG around epidermal cells	*Staphylococcus* +++	Histology		Histology spongoisis	Granular IgA in papillary dermis	Linear IgA along basement membrane
BULLOUS PEMPHIGOID	**PEMPHIGOID GESTATIONIS**	**PEMPHIGUS**	**IMPETIGO**	**EPIDERMOLYSIS BULLOSA (DYSTROPHIC)**	**DERMATITIS ARTEFACTA**	**DISCOID ECZEMA**	**DERMATITIS HERPETIFORMIS**	**CBDC/LINEAR IgA DISEASE**
p. 256	p. 256	p. 257	*see* p. 107	p. 259	p. 260	*see* p. 243	*see* p. 246	p. 259

BULLOUS PEMPHIGOID

Bullous pemphigoid is an autoimmune disease that usually begins with a non-specific itchy rash that does not look quite right for either eczema or urticaria. Weeks or months later, blisters occur. The separation of the skin is at the dermo-epidermal junction (*see* Fig. 8.119), with localisation of IgG antibodies here (*see* Fig. 8.120). Antibodies to basement membrane are also found in the blood. The roof of the blister is made up of the full thickness of the epidermis, so blisters may become large and haemorrhagic and may remain intact for several days. It is often localised to one part of the body for a while, but like pemphigus will eventually become widespread. It is the commonest cause of blisters in the elderly.

TREATMENT: BULLOUS PEMPHIGOID

Localised areas can be treated with a potent[UK]/group 2–3[USA] topical steroid ointment or cream applied twice a day. Widespread blistering requires treatment with systemic steroids (e.g. prednisolone 30–40 mg day) until the blistering stops. The dose can then be reduced by 5 mg weekly down to 15 mg and then by 2.5 mg weekly. If blistering starts up again the dose is put up and a steroid-sparing agent such as azathioprine (up to 3 mg/kg in divided doses) is added. Long-term maintenance with around 5–10 mg of prednisolone is usually necessary.

PEMPHIGOID (HERPES) GESTATIONIS

This is a very rare condition occurring in pregnancy. It is a very itchy rash looking like either widespread erythema multiforme or bullous pemphigoid usually with periumbilical involvement. It needs to be differentiated from the much more common polymorphic eruption of pregnancy (*see* p. 206).

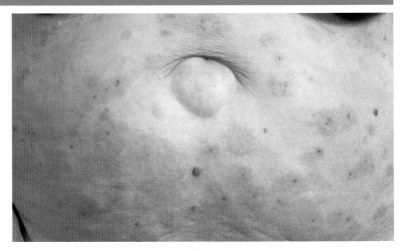

Fig. 8.116 Bullous pemphigoid: pre-bullous rash

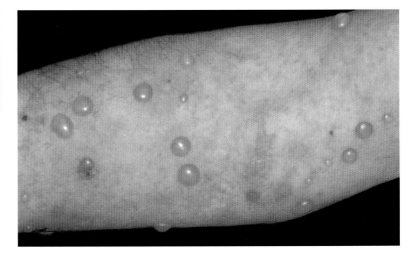

Fig. 8.117 Bullous pemphigoid: tense blisters on background erythema

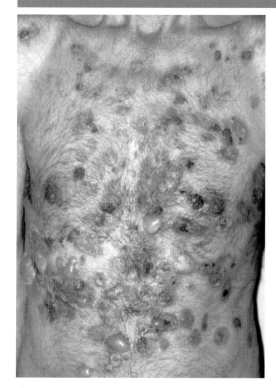

Fig. 8.118 Bullous pemphigoid: large blisters, some haemorrhagic, erosions and secondary crusting

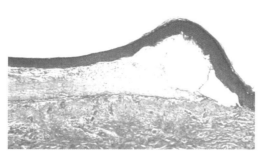

Fig. 8.119 Histology of bullous pemphigoid: blister at dermo-epidermal junction

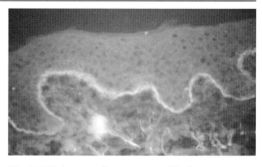

Fig. 8.120 Immunofluorescence of bullous pemphigoid: IgG antibodies localised to basement membrane

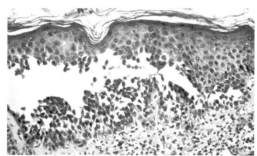

Fig. 8.121 Histology of pemphigus vulgaris: individual epidermal cells have separated from one another, causing a blister within the epidermis

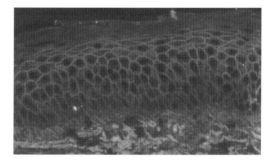

Fig. 8.122 Immunofluorescence of pemphigus vulgaris: IgG antibodies localised around individual epidermal cells

TREATMENT: PEMPHIGOID GESTATIONIS

Treatment with topical steroids is given if the patient is near term. If it occurs earlier and itching is intolerable, systemic steroids (prednisolone 30 mg/day) may be needed. The application of ice cubes or bags of frozen peas may also help the itching!

PEMPHIGUS VULGARIS

This is an autoimmune disease in which circulating IgG antibodies target desmosomal proteins (desmoglein 3 ± desmoglein 1). The epidermal cells come apart from one another (acantholysis) resulting in an intraepidermal blister. These are always very superficial so are unable to stay intact for very long. Therefore, you see mainly erosions and crusts. The blisters are never haemorrhagic. The skin shears easily if rubbed, producing an erosion (Nikolsky's sign, *see* Fig. 8.123). It most commonly begins with erosions in the mouth and it may be weeks or months before the telltale blisters appear on the skin. It may spread very rapidly and be life-threatening. Diagnosis is confirmed by histology (*see* Fig. 8.121), immunofluorescence (*see* Fig. 8.122), and high titres of serum antibodies.

PEMPHIGUS FOLIACEUS

Here the split is just below the granular layer so the blisters are very superficial. Clinically, widespread, crusted erosions on the face, scalp and upper trunk are seen. It is often misdiagnosed as seborrhoeic eczema, as no blisters are seen. It is less common than pemphigus vulgaris in Europe and the United Sates, but commoner in Africa and South America. Here the antigen is desmoglein 1. The diagnosis can be confirmed by skin biopsy and immunofluorescence.

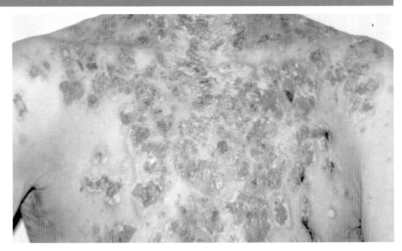

Fig. 8.124 Pemphigus vulgaris: flaccid blisters, erosions and crusts

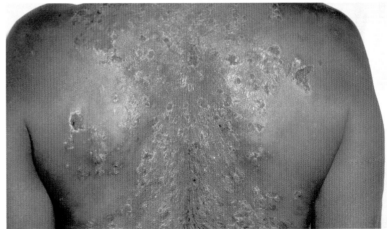

Fig. 8.125 Pemphigus foliaceus

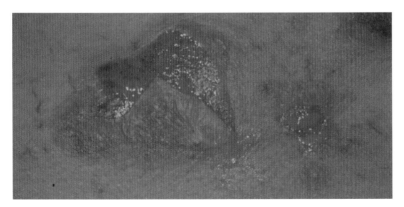

Fig. 8.123 Nikolsky's sign: skin shears off by tangential pressure

TREATMENT: PEMPHIGUS VULGARIS/FOLIACEUS

Immediate referral to hospital is recommended. Sometimes it is necessary to treat the patient in a burns unit if large areas of skin are eroded. Treatment is started with prednisolone 120 mg daily until the blisters stop. The dose is then gradually reduced to a maintenance dose of 5–10 mg a day.

What often happens is that the blisters dry up initially but once the dose is down to 50 mg a day, new blisters appear. Steroid-sparing agents such as azathioprine, ciclosporin or methotrexate may well be needed too. Complications caused by high-dose steroids or secondary infection can result in considerable morbidity.

Pemphigus foliaceus responds better to steroids and may eventually be controllable with topical steroids.

EPIDERMOLYSIS BULLOSA (DYSTROPHIC)

This is a group of inherited diseases where blisters and erosions appear in response to trauma. Dystrophic epidermolysis bullosa is due to a split below the epidermal basement membrane. Many patients do not survive the first 2 years of life (*see* Fig. 8.127), while others are disabled by the skin shearing off easily. Secondary scarring, milia formation, infection and binding together of fingers and toes can occur (*see* Fig. 13.54, p. 429). Patients will need referral to a dermatology department for confirmation of diagnosis by skin biopsy and electron microscopy.

TREATMENT: EPIDERMOLYSIS BULLOSA

Treatment is a wound care problem. Raw areas need to be dressed with a non-adherent dressing (*see* p. 46). The skin should be moisturised with emollients and protected from injury by hydrocolloid dressings. Shoes and clothing should not be allowed to rub. Pain and secondary infection need treatment, and genetic counselling and parent support will be necessary.

DEBRA, the international epidermolysis bullosa charity, has specialist trained nurses based out of London and Birmingham who cover the entire country and will see all newly suspected patients with epidermolysis bullosa. They will see the baby, perform a punch biopsy for specialist split skin histology and electronmicroscopy performed in London to identify the specific epidermolysis bullosa type and instigate the best dressing regimens with carers and family as required.

CHRONIC BULLOUS DISEASE OF CHILDHOOD

A rare disease of young children (usually begins age 3–5), with grouped blisters around the genitalia, umbilicus and on the face. It is not itchy and it gets better spontaneously after 3–4 years. Histology shows a subepidermal blister and on direct immunofluorescence a linear band of IgA is seen along the basement membrane of the epidermis.

Linear IgA disease is the adult version of chronic bullous disease of childhood. Usually the blisters occur in rings. Immunofluorescence and histology are the same.

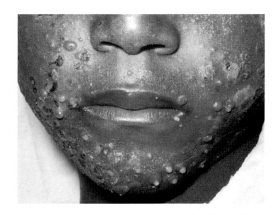

Fig. 8.126 Chronic bullous disease of childhood

TREATMENT: CHRONIC BULLOUS DISEASE OF CHILDHOOD/LINEAR IGA DISEASE

Oral dapsone 25–100 mg/day is given until it remits spontaneously. Check the full blood count regularly for haemolysis. Add cimetidine 400 mg tid if haemolysis or methaemoglobinaemia occurs.

DERMATITIS ARTEFACTA

These lesions are self-induced. The clue is that instead of being round or oval, like most naturally occurring rashes, they have straight sides – square, rectangular, triangular (*see* Fig. 1.84, p. 17). They occur anywhere that the patient can reach and damage the skin with fingernails, scissors, nail files, phenol, acids, household cleansers, and so forth. The open wounds exude serum then form crusts.

TREATMENT: DERMATITIS ARTEFACTA

This is very difficult to treat because the patient (often female) is not willing to admit to producing the lesion(s) or to the idea that treatment involves facing up to the problem or conflict in her life that is causing her to damage her own skin. If the lesions are occluded so that the patient cannot get at them, they will usually heal very quickly.

These patients need psychiatric help. Unfortunately, psychiatrists are not always interested in helping them. Direct confrontation usually leads to the patient seeking help elsewhere.

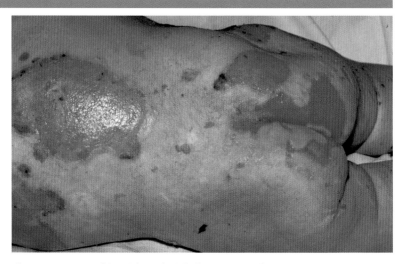

Fig. 8.127 Dystrophic epidermolysis bullosa in a newborn

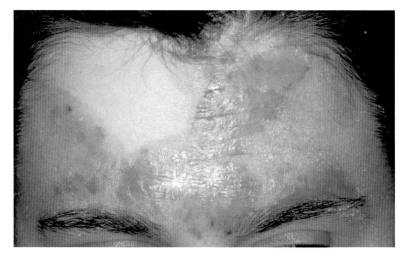

Fig. 8.128 Dermatitis artefacta: note straight rather than round margin to rash

Non-erythematous lesions

9

Face, trunk and limbs
Non-erythematous lesions
Normal surface
Skin coloured, pink

1. SKIN COLOURED (PINK): ISOLATED PAPULES

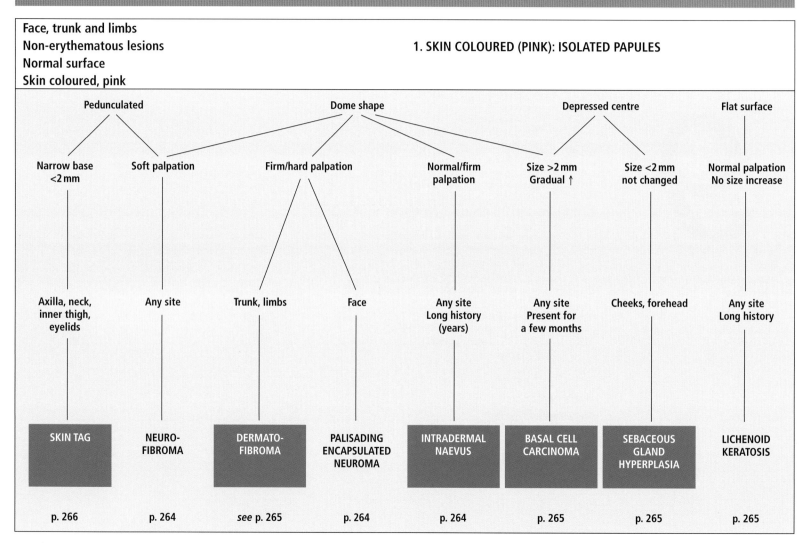

Pedunculated

Dome shape

Depressed centre

Flat surface

Narrow base
<2 mm

Soft palpation

Firm/hard palpation

Normal/firm
palpation

Size >2 mm
Gradual ↑

Size <2 mm
not changed

Normal palpation
No size increase

Axilla, neck,
inner thigh,
eyelids

Any site

Trunk, limbs

Face

Any site
Long history
(years)

Any site
Present for
a few months

Cheeks, forehead

Any site
Long history

SKIN TAG

**NEURO-
FIBROMA**

**DERMATO-
FIBROMA**

**PALISADING
ENCAPSULATED
NEUROMA**

**INTRADERMAL
NAEVUS**

**BASAL CELL
CARCINOMA**

**SEBACEOUS
GLAND
HYPERPLASIA**

**LICHENOID
KERATOSIS**

p. 266

p. 264

see p. 265

p. 264

p. 264

p. 265

p. 265

p. 265

Face, trunk and limbs
Non-erythematous lesions
Normal surface
Skin coloured, pink, yellow

2. SKIN COLOURED (PINK, YELLOW): MULTIPLE SIMILAR PAPULES

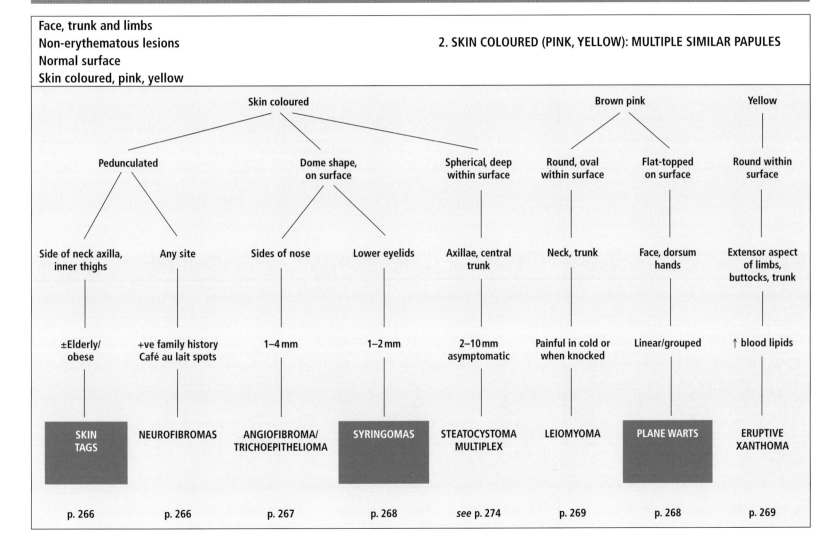

Skin coloured

Pedunculated

Side of neck axilla, inner thighs
±Elderly/ obese
SKIN TAGS
p. 266

Any site
+ve family history Café au lait spots
NEUROFIBROMAS
p. 266

Dome shape, on surface

Sides of nose
1–4 mm
ANGIOFIBROMA/ TRICHOEPITHELIOMA
p. 267

Lower eyelids
1–2 mm
SYRINGOMAS
p. 268

Spherical, deep within surface

Axillae, central trunk
2–10 mm asymptomatic
STEATOCYSTOMA MULTIPLEX
see p. 274

Brown pink

Round, oval within surface

Neck, trunk
Painful in cold or when knocked
LEIOMYOMA
p. 269

Flat-topped on surface

Face, dorsum hands
Linear/grouped
PLANE WARTS
p. 268

Yellow

Round within surface

Extensor aspect of limbs, buttocks, trunk
↑ blood lipids
ERUPTIVE XANTHOMA
p. 269

INTRADERMAL NAEVUS

This is a skin-coloured melanocytic naevus. All the naevus cells are in the dermis so pigment is no longer seen on the surface (*see* p. 303). It is a small, round, dome-shaped or papillomatous papule. Occasionally telangiectasia can be seen on the surface, but the lack of growth, long history and symmetrical dome shape distinguish it from a basal cell carcinoma. They are sometimes pedunculated, and can be difficult to distinguish from neurofibromas or skin tags. If necessary they can be removed by shaving them off flush with the skin, and cauterising the base with heat or aluminium chloride solution (Driclor, Anhydrol Forte).

PALISADING ENCAPSULATED NEUROMA

A palisading encapsulated neuroma is a fairly common asymptomatic, solitary, skin-coloured papule mainly found on the face. It has a distinctive histological appearance with a proliferation of Schwann cells and a large number of axons within a perineural-derived capsule. It is harmless and not associated with neurofibromatosis.

SOLITARY NEUROFIBROMA

These are dome-shaped or pedunculated soft papules that when pressed in the centre have a hole at the base (like a buttonhole). They are distinguished from intradermal naevi by being softer and usually larger (5–9 mm).

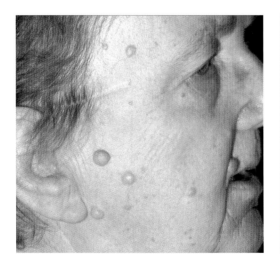

Fig. 9.01 Multiple intradermal naevi on the cheek and temple

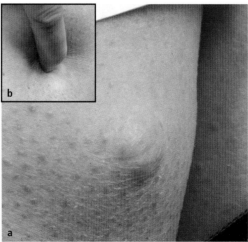

Fig. 9.02 (a) Solitary neurofibroma on buttock; (b) (inset) central pressure with a finger elicits a 'hole' or soft centre.

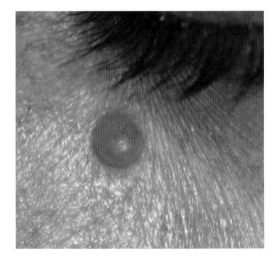

Fig. 9.03 Palisading encapsulated neuroma: easily confused with a basal cell carcinoma

DERMATOFIBROMA

Dermatofibromas are easily recognised clinically because they are always firm on squeezing between thumb and finger. They are pink or skin-coloured papules or nodules resulting from trauma such as an insect bite or foreign body (*see* p. 301).

BASAL CELL CARCINOMA

The early growth of a nodular basal cell carcinoma can look just like an intradermal naevus. However, if you look closely there is always telangiectasia over the surface (*see* p. 330). If in doubt, excise for histology.

SEBACEOUS GLAND HYPERPLASIA

This is a common benign lesion due to enlargement of sebaceous glands around a single hair follicle on the face. It is a small (2–5mm diameter), skin-coloured-yellow papule with telangiectasia running over the surface and a central punctum (the opening of the hair follicle). It is sometimes confused with a small basal cell carcinoma, since both occur on the face of middle-aged or elderly individuals. They can be removed by cautery under local anaesthetic.

LICHENOID KERATOSIS

This is a variety of a solar lentigo, which is a pink papule with a smooth surface. On histology a lichenoid infiltrate is present. It can be confused clinically with an early basal cell carcinoma.

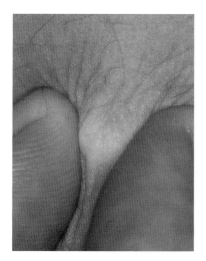

Fig. 9.04 Dermatofibroma

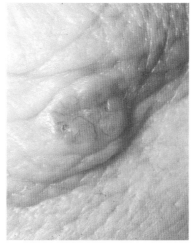

Fig. 9.05 Basal cell carcinoma: note pink colour with telangiectasia

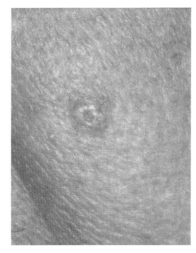

Fig. 9.06 Sebaceous gland hyperplasia

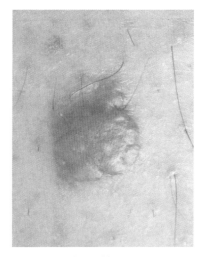

Fig. 9.07 Lichenoid keratosis

SKIN TAGS

These are small pedunculated, skin-coloured or brown papules around the neck, in the axillae or sometimes on the inner thighs. Single tags are commonly seen in the elderly on the eyelids.

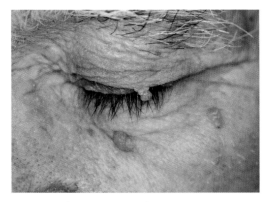

Fig. 9.08 Skin tags around the eyes

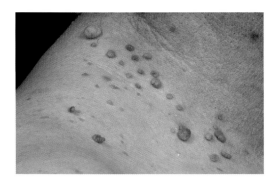

Fig. 9.09 Multiple skin tags around neck

TREATMENT: SKIN TAGS

If the patient wants them removed, snip the tag off with a pair of sharp scissors without any local anaesthetic. Bleeding is stopped with aluminium chloride (Driclor) , a silver nitrate stick or cautery. Alternatively, if they are very small, ablate with the hyfrecator.

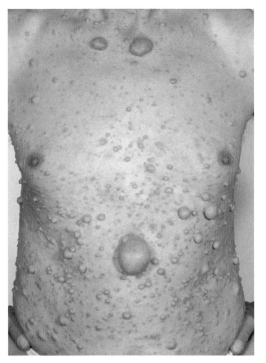

Fig. 9.10 Neurofibromatosis

NEUROFIBROMATOSIS (VON RECKLINGHAUSEN'S DISEASE)

Multiple skin-coloured, pink or red papules and nodules appear anywhere on the skin after puberty. If you press on the surface, the lesions are found to be soft with a hole at the base (like a buttonhole). They vary in size from 1–2 mm to several centimetres in diameter. Some are sessile, some pedunculated. The patient will also have multiple (more than five) café au lait patches (*see* p. 294) and axillary freckling. Lisch nodules (pigmented iris hamartomas) are seen on slit-lamp examination and help confirm the diagnosis. Various endocrine and neurological abnormalities can also be present. This condition is inherited as an autosomal dominant trait, the gene being on chromosome 17.

TREATMENT: NEUROFIBROMAS

Single lesions can be removed by excision or shave and cautery. It is impossible to remove all the lesions in von Recklinghausen's disease, but any particularly unsightly ones can be excised.

TRICHOEPITHELIOMA

Single or multiple translucent papules around the eyes or on the nasolabial folds appear after puberty. They look similar to angiofibromas but are not red and there is no telangiectasia on the surface. They are benign hair follicle tumours also known as **epithelioma adenoides cysticum**. They are inherited as an autosomal dominant trait.

TREATMENT: ANGIOFIBROMAS/TRICHOEPITHELIOMAS

A few lesions can be removed by shave and cautery under local anaesthetic. Widespread lesions present a problem. Extensive debridement can be tried using a carbon dioxide (CO_2) laser, shave or curettage and cautery under general anaesthetic. Unfortunately, there is a tendency for the lesions to recur.

ANGIOFIBROMAS (ADENOMA SEBACEUM)

These are multiple very firm, discrete, translucent papules with a telangiectatic surface affecting the nasolabial folds and spreading out onto the cheeks and chin.

They appear in early childhood (age 3–4) and are a sign of tuberous sclerosis (epiloa). **Tuberous sclerosis** is an autosomal dominant disorder affecting many organs. Other skin lesions are oval or ash leaf-shaped white patches (*see* Fig. 9.14), which are present from birth, the shagreen patch (a connective tissue naevus, *see* p. 270) and periungual and subungual fibromas (*see* Fig. 14.43 and 14.44, p. 449), which appear after puberty. Other features of the syndrome include mental retardation, epilepsy and occasionally tumours affecting the heart and kidneys.

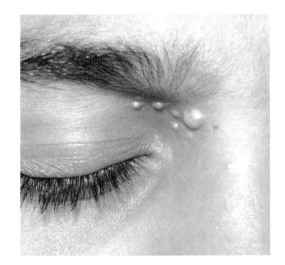

Fig. 9.11 Trichoepitheliomas

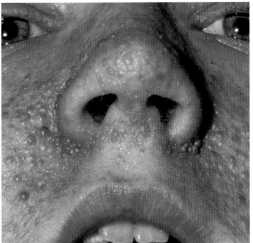

Fig. 9.12 Multiple angiofibromas in a patient with tuberous sclerosis

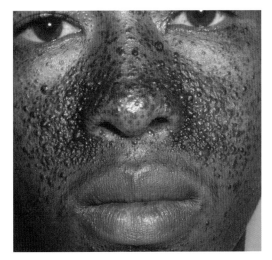

Fig. 9.13 Angiofibromas in black skin: same distribution as Fig. 9.12, different colour

SYRINGOMA

These small (1–5 mm), round, dome-shaped, translucent papules on the lower eyelids are very common and completely harmless. They are benign tumours of sweat glands that are inherited as an autosomal dominant trait. They appear after puberty. Cautery with a fine loop will ablate them. Rarely, multiple lesions may be seen elsewhere on the face and trunk.

PLANE WARTS

These are small, flat-topped papules but, unlike the papules of lichen planus, they are not shiny on the surface. They are not rough to the touch like common warts. They are skin coloured,

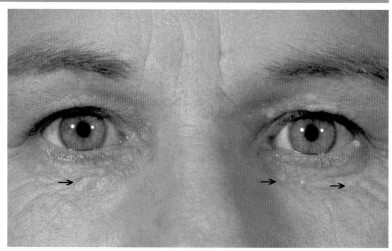

Fig. 9.15 Syringomas on lower eyelids in white skin

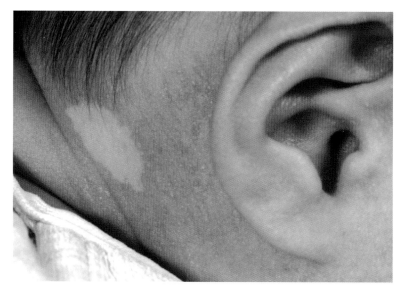

Fig. 9.14 Tuberous sclerosis: ash leaf macule behind the ear

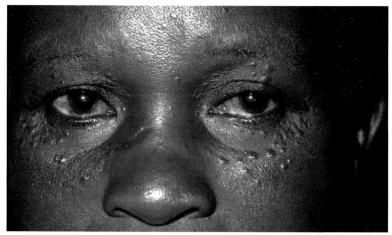

Fig. 9.16 Syringomas around eyes in black skin

pink or brown and may be found in straight lines at sites of trauma (Köebner phenomenon). They occur mainly in children, on the face and dorsum of the hands. Reassurance that they will eventually resolve spontaneously is usually all that is needed. You can try 5% salicylic acid ointment or a light freeze with liquid nitrogen (few seconds only) but treatment tends not to be very effective.

LEIOMYOMA

This is a benign smooth muscle tumour of the erector pili muscle. Multiple pink, red or brown papules are grouped together on the trunk or on a limb in young adults. They can be painful in the cold or when knocked, due to the smooth muscle contracting. Diagnosis is confirmed by skin biopsy. They can be removed by surgical excision if the lesions are not too large.

ERUPTIVE XANTHOMA

Eruptive xanthomas are yellow papules containing lipid deposits secondary to hypertriglyceridaemia. They commonly occur on the buttocks and extensor surface of limbs. Most of these patients are diabetic, so check the HbA1c as well as lipid levels. The lesions will clear once the underlying diabetes and hyperlipidaemia is treated.

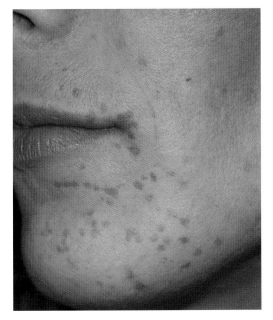

Fig. 9.17 Plane warts (*see* also Fig. 1.89, p. 17)

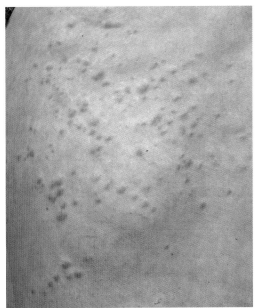

Fig. 9.18 Leiomyoma on side of chest

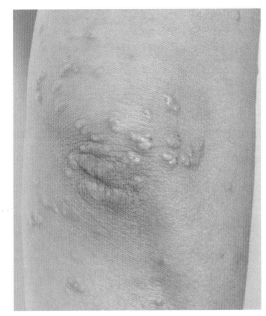

Fig. 9.19 Eruptive xanthomas

Non-erythematous lesions
Normal surface
Skin coloured, pink, yellow
Plaques

SKIN-COLOURED PLAQUES

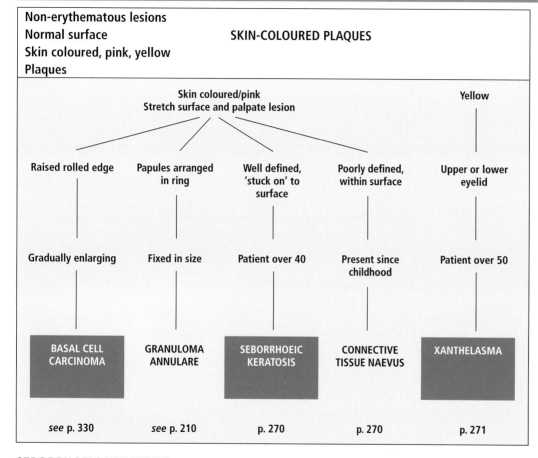

Skin coloured/pink
Stretch surface and palpate lesion

Yellow

Raised rolled edge	Papules arranged in ring	Well defined, 'stuck on' to surface	Poorly defined, within surface	Upper or lower eyelid
Gradually enlarging	Fixed in size	Patient over 40	Present since childhood	Patient over 50
BASAL CELL CARCINOMA	**GRANULOMA ANNULARE**	**SEBORRHOEIC KERATOSIS**	**CONNECTIVE TISSUE NAEVUS**	**XANTHELASMA**
see p. 330	*see* p. 210	p. 270	p. 270	p. 271

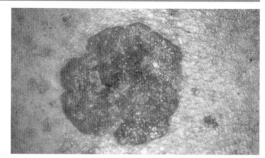

Fig. 9.20 Isolated seborrhoeic keratosis on lower leg

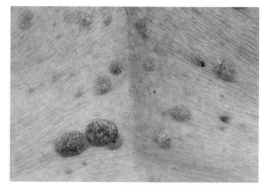

Fig. 9.21 Multiple skin-coloured seborrhoeic keratoses on back

SEBORRHOEIC KERATOSIS

The morphology of these lesions (*see* p. 320) is very varied depending on the skin type and degree of pigmentation. In fair-skinned individuals (skin types I and II) they commonly present as flat skin-coloured or pink plaques. Initially the surface may be quite smooth, although as they develop the surface may become papillomatous or scaly.

CONNECTIVE TISSUE NAEVUS

A connective tissue naevus is a birthmark consisting of a skin-coloured/yellowish plaque with a cobblestone surface. It may be an isolated naevus or part of tuberous sclerosis (*see* p. 267), called a shagreen patch.

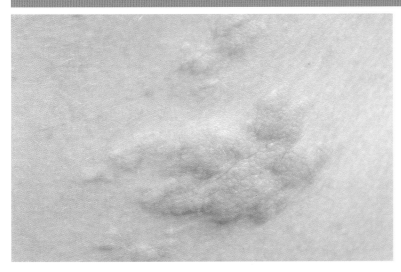

Fig. 9.22 Connective tissue naevus

XANTHELASMA

These are yellow, flat plaques usually found on the medial aspect of the eyelids. They are not necessarily associated with hyperlipidaemia.

TREATMENT: XANTHELASMA

Dip a cotton wool bud in a saturated solution of trichloracetic acid (TCA) and lightly paint the surface of the xanthelasma, making sure that it does not get onto normal skin. After a few seconds the surface goes white. Immediately smother the surface with surgical spirit – this quickly neutralises the acid. Any excess acid can also be washed away with copious amounts of water. The stinging caused by the acid should stop after just a few seconds. A week later the treated area scabs over and the skin will heal normally after about 6 weeks. Recurrences or residual areas can be retreated in the same way.

Alternatively, they can be removed by excision, or ablated by cautery or laser.

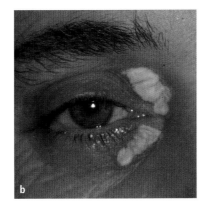
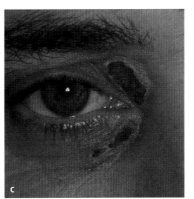
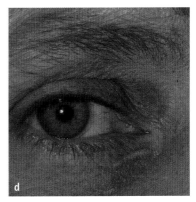

Fig. 9.23 (a) Xanthelasma before treatment: yellow plaques on inner eyelids; (b) treatment of xanthelasma immediately after application of trichloracetic acid; (c) 7 days after treatment – crusts have formed; (d) 2 months after treatment there Is just a faint erythema

Non-erythematous lesions
Normal surface
Skin coloured, pink, yellow
Nodules

SKIN-COLOURED (PINK, YELLOW) NODULES

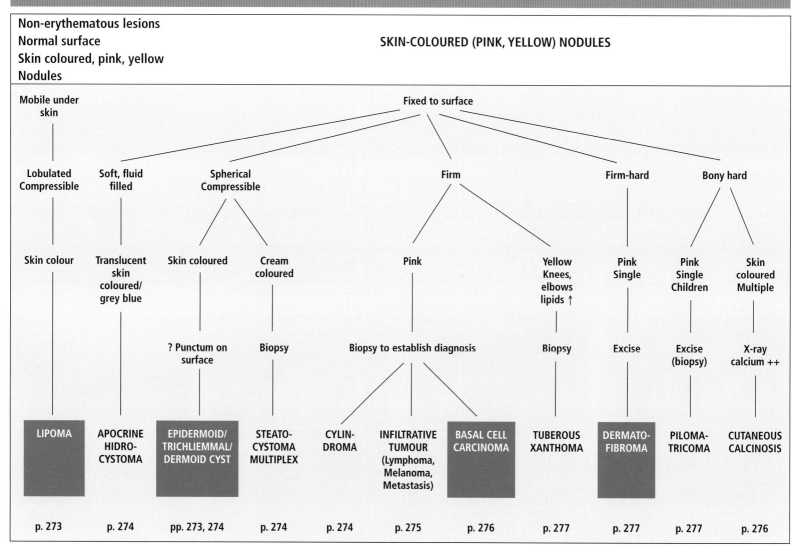

EPIDERMOID CYST

An epidermoid cyst (commonly misnamed a sebaceous cyst) is a well-circumscribed papule or nodule derived from the upper part of the external root sheath of a hair follicle or from a sweat duct. The lining of the cyst looks like normal epidermis. The cyst is situated in the dermis and there is usually a visible punctum on the surface. Through this punctum the cyst may become secondarily infected.

Epidermoid cysts are inherited as an autosomal dominant trait but do not appear until after puberty (usually 15–30 years). If they occur before puberty they may be associated with polyposis coli (Gardner's syndrome) or with the basal cell naevus syndrome. Similar cysts may occur in patients with acne after damage to hair follicles, or after penetrating injuries where bits of epidermis are implanted in the dermis.

DERMOID CYST

Dermoid cysts look like epidermoid cysts but they are present from birth or early childhood. They are due to the inclusion of epidermis and its appendages in the dermis at the time of embryonic skin closure. Most occur on the head and neck, either in the midline or at the lateral end of the eyebrow. They have an obvious punctum, which may have hairs protruding through it.

LIPOMA

This is a benign tumour of fat cells presenting as soft or firm subcutaneous nodules (you can move the skin over it), round or irregular in shape. They may be single or multiple and vary in size from 1 to 10 cm in diameter. The overlying skin is normal. Usually they are of no significance.

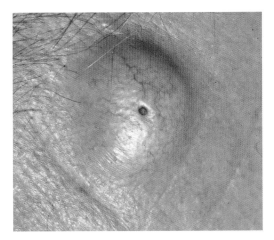

Fig. 9.24 Epidermoid cyst

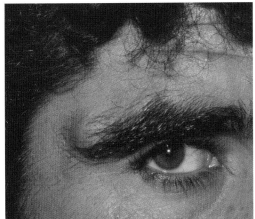

Fig. 9.25 Dermoid cyst

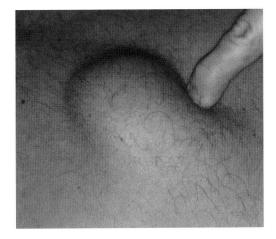

Fig. 9.26 Lipoma

TRICHILEMMAL (PILAR) CYST

These are derived from the external root sheath of a hair follicle between the opening of the sebaceous duct and the bulge (insertion of the erector pili muscle). Most occur on the scalp (*see* p. 95), although they can occur anywhere except the palms and soles. They do not have a punctum so they do not become infected. They are inherited as an autosomal dominant trait.

STEATOCYSTOMA MULTIPLEX

Multiple, symmetrical, small skin-coloured, white or yellowish papules or nodules occur on the skin of young adults. In females they are mainly in the axillae and between the breasts. In males they are mostly on the trunk in a diamond-shaped area between the xiphisternum and umbilicus or on the back. They are inherited as an autosomal dominant trait.

CYLINDROMA

Single or multiple, spherical or lobulated, red, smooth nodules occur on the scalp or face (*see* Fig. 9.29). They can grow to quite a large size. Sometimes they occur in association with multiple trichoepitheliomas (*see* p. 267). Alone or in combination they are inherited as an autosomal dominant trait. They are uncommon.

APOCRINE HIDROCYSTOMA

This is a solitary smooth, dome-shaped, cystic nodule, which may be skin coloured or blue grey in colour. It is found most commonly around the eyelids. It is usually misdiagnosed as a basal cell carcinoma.

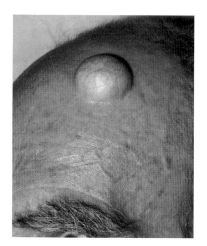

Fig. 9.27 Trichilemmal cyst on scalp

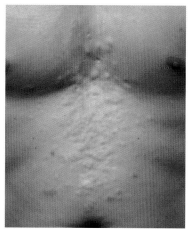

Fig. 9.28 Steatocystoma multiplex

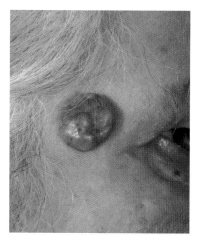

Fig. 9.29 Cylindroma: looks like a nodular basal cell carcinoma

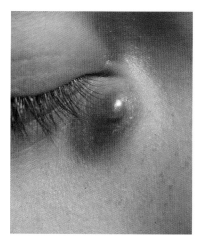

Fig. 9.30 Apocrine hidrocystoma

TREATMENT: LIPOMAS, CYSTS AND APPENDAGE TUMOURS

These can all be excised under local anaesthetic if they are large or a nuisance. **Lipomas** are removed by making an incision through the skin and shelling out an encapsulated tumour of fatty tissue. Pressing down around the lipoma often results in it popping out easily.

Appendage tumours (hidradenomas, cylindromas, pilomatricomas) can be excised together with the overlying skin.

When removing **cysts** first excise an ellipse of skin over the cyst so that the upper surface of the cyst is visible (*see* Fig. 3.44, p. 95). You will now be in the right plane to dissect out the cyst. The amount of skin you need to remove depends on how big the cyst is and how much redundant skin has been pushed up. The cyst is then dissected out using a pair of blunt curved scissors. If the resultant hole is large, close off the dead space with deep dissolving sutures before inserting ordinary interrupted sutures into the skin.

Epidermoid cysts are the most difficult to remove, since they are often stuck down to the surrounding connective tissue, particularly if they have ever been inflamed. **Trichilemmal** cysts shell out very easily once you are in the right plane, since they have a connective tissue sheath around them. If huge numbers of **steatocytoma multiplex** cysts are present, they can be incised with a no. 15 scalpel blade, the contents squeezed out and the cyst lining removed by pulling out with a pair of artery forceps. You have to pull quite hard to remove them. This will normally need to be done under a general anaesthetic.

Do not remove cysts while they are actively inflamed. It is important to remove all of the cyst wall during the procedure; if any of it is left behind, the cyst will recur.

TUMOURS

Many types of tumour (lymphoma, amelanotic melanoma, metastases, and so forth) present as skin-coloured or pink nodules growing within the dermis. They may be difficult to diagnose clinically, and urgent referral for a biopsy is usually necessary (*see* also p. 216).

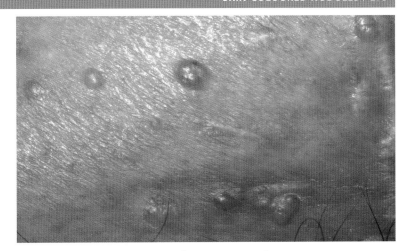

Fig. 9.31 Metastases on abdomen from carcinoma of ovary

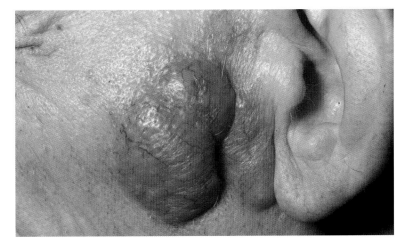

Fig. 9.32 B-cell lymphoma on cheek

BASAL CELL CARCINOMA

A nodular basal cell carcinoma can grow slowly without ulcerating to form a large nodule. It usually has a pearly translucent appearance with obvious telangiectasia on the surface (*see* p. 330).

CUTANEOUS CALCINOSIS

Bony hard papules and nodules due to the deposition of calcium within the dermis can occur in:

Localised lesions

- Various cysts (trichilemmal, pilomatricoma, *see* pp. 95 and 277)
- Pinneal (ear) calcification
- Venous disease on the lower legs (*see* pp. 391, 398)
- Cutaneous calculus (*see* p. 280)
- Scrotal calcinosis (*see* p. 364)

Generalised disease

- Chronic renal failure
- Dermatomyositis
- Hyperparathyroidism
- Sarcoidosis
- Systemic lupus erythematosus
- Systemic sclerosis (CREST syndrome)

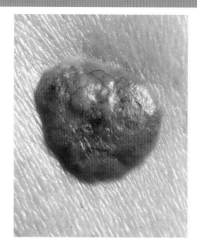

Fig. 9.33 Basal cell carcinoma: note the telangiectasia on the surface

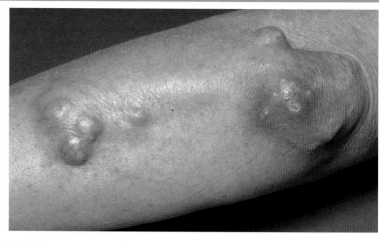

Fig. 9.34 Cutaneous calcinosis in a patient with CREST syndrome

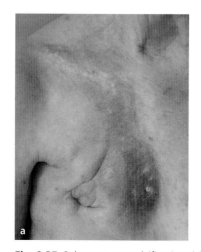
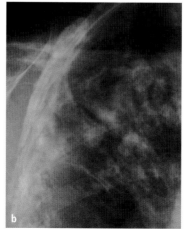
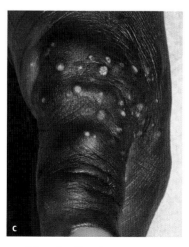

Fig. 9.35 Subcutaneous calcification: (a) in radiation-damaged skin; (b) X-ray of same; (c) on the thumb

PILOMATRICOMA

A pilomatricoma is a benign tumour of the hair follicle most commonly seen in children. It presents as a nodule resembling a cyst, which is usually pink red in colour. It is often calcified so is bony hard on palpation. It can be excised under local anaesthesia.

DERMATOFIBROMA

A slow-growing nodule that is firm but not bony hard growing within or out of the surface is likely to be a dermatofibroma. It can be shaved or excised under local anaesthetic.

TUBEROUS XANTHOMA

These are firm lobulated tumours appearing at sites of pressure, usually the extensor surface of the knees or elbows in patients with hypercholesterolaemia. The lesions will regress slowly once the hyperlipidaemia has been treated.

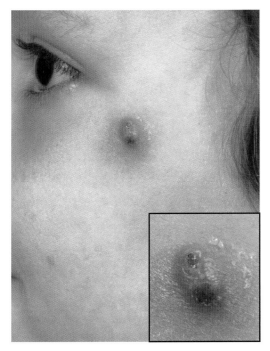

Fig. 9.36 Pilomatricoma on the cheek of a young boy (inset: close-up of lesion)

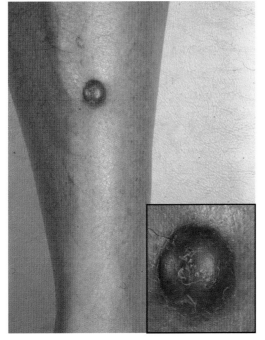

Fig. 9.37 Dermatofibroma on the leg (inset: close-up of lesion – hard on palpation)

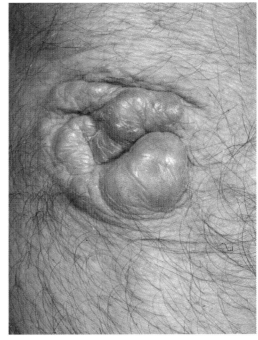

Fig. 9.38 Tuberous xanthoma on the elbow

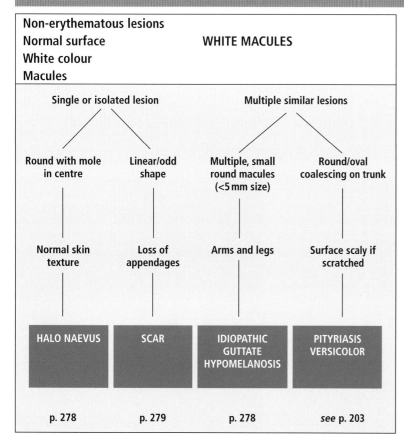

Non-erythematous lesions
Normal surface
White colour
Macules

WHITE MACULES

Single or isolated lesion

Round with mole in centre → Normal skin texture → **HALO NAEVUS** — p. 278

Linear/odd shape → Loss of appendages → **SCAR** — p. 279

Multiple similar lesions

Multiple, small round macules (<5 mm size) → Arms and legs → **IDIOPATHIC GUTTATE HYPOMELANOSIS** — p. 278

Round/oval coalescing on trunk → Surface scaly if scratched → **PITYRIASIS VERSICOLOR** — see p. 203

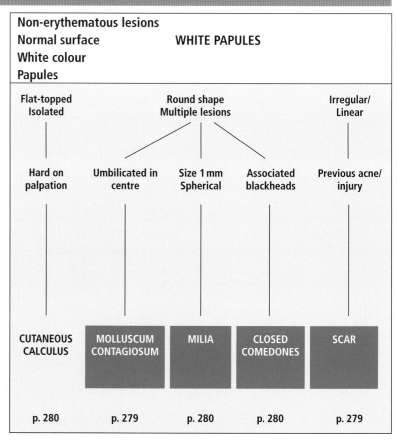

Non-erythematous lesions
Normal surface
White colour
Papules

WHITE PAPULES

Flat-topped Isolated → Hard on palpation → **CUTANEOUS CALCULUS** — p. 280

Round shape Multiple lesions

Umbilicated in centre → **MOLLUSCUM CONTAGIOSUM** — p. 279

Size 1 mm Spherical → **MILIA** — p. 280

Associated blackheads → **CLOSED COMEDONES** — p. 280

Irregular/Linear → Previous acne/injury → **SCAR** — p. 279

HALO NAEVUS

An immunological reaction against the melanocytes in a mole produces a halo of depigmentation around it. Eventually the mole disappears. This reaction is common in children, quite benign and does not indicate that the mole has undergone malignant change.

IDIOPATHIC GUTTATE HYPOMELANOSIS

Numerous symmetrical, small (1–5 mm), white macules on the arms or legs are extremely common, especially in individuals with black or pigmented skin. Individual lesions have well-defined borders and normal skin markings within them. Reassurance that they are harmless is all that is required.

SCARRING

Scars with triangular or rectangular shapes
may be due to self-inflicted damage; those
that are crescent-shaped or star-shaped
may be due to tearing of the skin after
minor trauma in elderly patients or those
on oral steroids or using potent topical
steroids. Acne can leave white, round,
papular scars on the back

MOLLUSCUM CONTAGIOSUM

This is a poxvirus infection of the skin usually affecting children. Small 1–5 mm white or
pink umbilicated papules (*see* Fig. 9.42) are found anywhere on the skin and there may
be few or many. They can become inflamed and red in colour. They last 6–24 months and
then disappear spontaneously. In children with atopic eczema, they may be extensive
particularly at the sites of the eczema. Isolated lesions in adults can be confused with a
basal cell carcinoma.

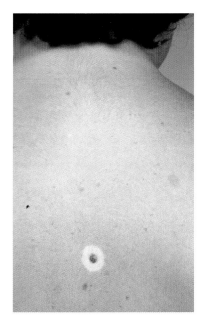

Fig. 9.39 Halo naevus

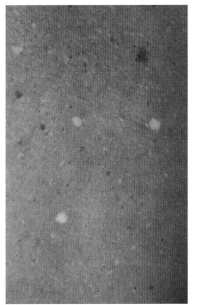

Fig. 9.40 Idiopathic guttate
hypomelanosis

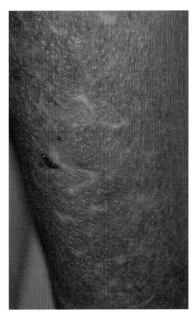

Fig. 9.41 Scars on the forearms due
to steroids

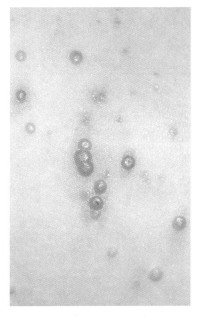

Fig. 9.42 Molluscum contagiosum

TREATMENT: MOLLUSCUM CONTAGIOSUM

Trauma to individual lesions results in their resolution. 5% potassium hydroxide solution (MolluDab) can be applied twice a day for 3–5 days (until an inflammatory reaction is seen). This is an effective treatment that is not painful and can be applied by the child's parents.

CUTANEOUS CALCULUS

A single white, round, flat-topped papule on the face of a child that feels firm to hard on palpation is likely to be a cutaneous calculus. It is due to calcium deposited in the upper dermis and is quite harmless.

MILIA

These are very small superficial epidermoid cysts. They are small (1–2 mm diameter only) white spherical papules protruding above the surface on the cheeks and eyelids. They can occur spontaneously or follow any acute sub-epidermal blister, e.g. after burns or other blistering diseases. To remove, open the skin over each cyst with a sharp needle; press on either side and it will pop out.

CLOSED COMEDO

A closed comedo (whitehead) is a single blocked pilosebaceous follicle in which the follicular opening is not visible (*see* acne, p. 116).

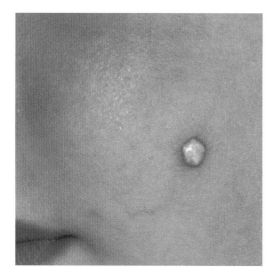

Fig. 9.43 Cutaneous calculus on child's face

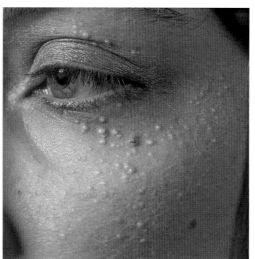

Fig. 9.44 Milia

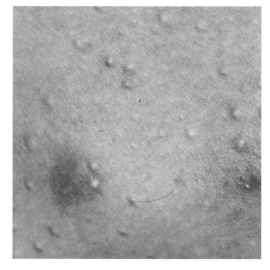

Fig. 9.45 Closed comedones on the back

Non-erythematous lesions
Normal surface
White colour
Patches and plaques

WHITE PATCHES AND PLAQUES

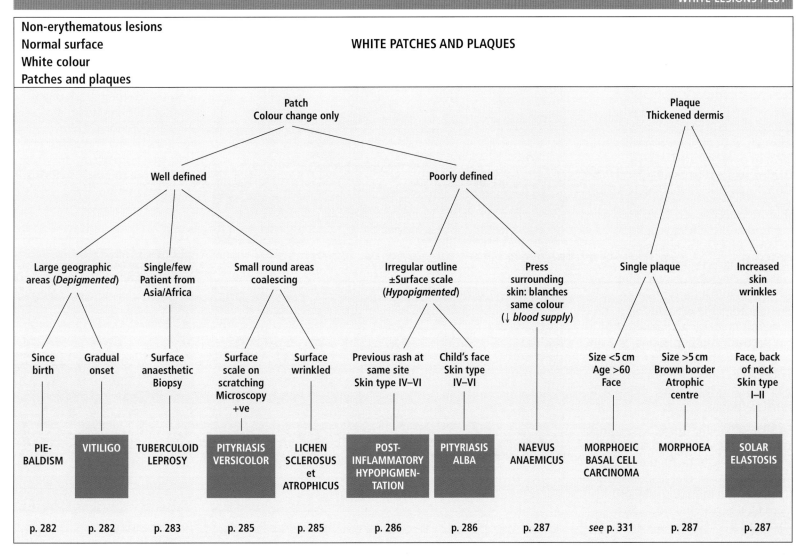

VITILIGO

Vitiligo is thought to be an autoimmune disease in which the melanocytes disappear from the epidermis. The patient presents with symmetrical white patches on any part of the skin. The skin is depigmented rather than hypopigmented, which distinguishes it from all other white skin lesions (other than piebaldism).

It is often confused with pityriasis versicolor, but vitiligo consists of large patches with no surface scale. Vitiligo on visible skin can be very unsightly, especially in dark-skinned individuals. Sometimes there is a band of hyperpigmentation at the edge of the patches, and in patients who are very fair skinned this may be more noticeable than the depigmented areas. On exposed sites vitiligo will burn in the sun.

In 30% of patients there is a positive family history of vitiligo, and it may also be associated with the organ-specific autoimmune diseases such as hypo- and hyperthyroidism, pernicious anaemia, Addison's disease and diabetes mellitus.

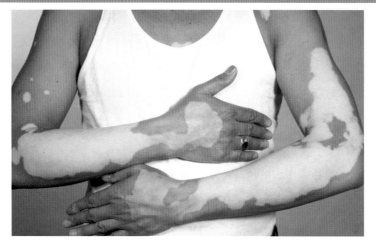

Fig. 9.46 Vitiligo: symmetrical areas of depigmentation

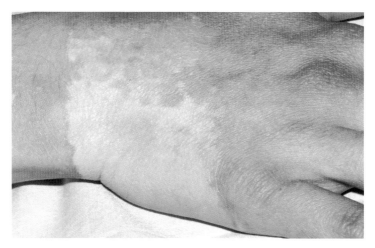

Fig. 9.47 Vitiligo on dorsum of hand: note burning in depigmented areas and hyperpigmentation at the edge of the patches

PIEBALDISM

This is an inherited condition (autosomal dominant) where white patches are present at birth and remain unchanged throughout life. It may be associated with a white forelock of hair if the skin in that area is affected. The white patches are identical to those of vitiligo.

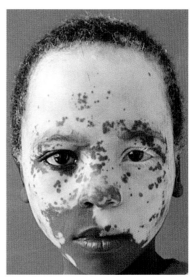

Fig. 9.48 Vitiligo on face of African girl

TREATMENT: VITILIGO

In white-skinned individuals the best advice is probably to keep out of the sun and to apply a high-factor sunblock all over to prevent the normal skin from tanning and the depigmented skin from burning.

If it is spreading very rapidly you can to switch it off with systemic steroids. In adults, give three doses of triamcinolone 40 mg intramuscularly at monthly intervals. In children, give prednisolone 5–10 mg/day for 2–3 weeks. Systemic steroids have no effect on stable vitiligo.

Repigmentation can be attempted by any of the following treatments.

- Apply a potent[UK]/group 2–3[USA] topical steroid cream to the white areas in the morning followed by half an hour of sun exposure a day (or narrowband UVB at your local hospital in the winter). After this period of sun exposure, the patient should use a high-protective-factor sunscreen on any exposed sites to prevent burning. Topical steroids should not be used for more than 3 months if used daily (6 months if used on alternate days).
- Topical 0.1% tacrolimus ointment may be used instead of a potent topical steroid, especially on the face. Both of these treatments can be used in children.
- Narrowband UVB (311 nm) two to three times a week to whole body if more than 15%–20% of the body's surface involved.
- Localised areas on the face can be treated with the excimer laser at 308 nm.
- PUVA therapy twice weekly (*see* p. 61). It may need to be given for 12–24 months for maximum effect.

When the vitiligo repigments, it does so initially from the hair follicles, so you will see small brown macules in the white patches.

The cosmetic appearance can be improved using cosmetic camouflage:
- fake tan applied every 3–5 days
- cover creams available on prescription after consultation with the Red Cross (*see* p. 39).

In very extensive vitiligo, depigmentation of the remaining normal skin can be attempted by using the monobenzyl ether of hydroquinone twice a day for several weeks. This depigmentation will be permanent.

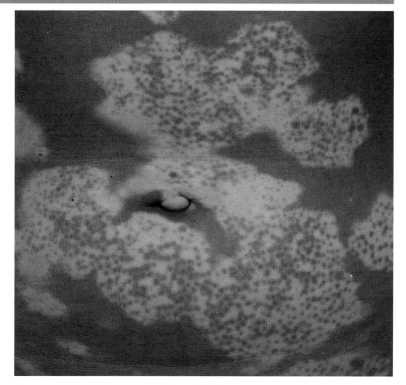

Fig. 9.49 Repigmenation around hair follicles in a patient with vitiligo

LEPROSY

Leprosy is a chronic bacterial infection due to *Mycobacterium leprae*. It is spread by droplet infection and has a long incubation period (anything from 2 months to 40 years). It principally affects peripheral nerves and the skin. The clinical features are very variable depending on the patient's cell-mediated immunity to the leprosy bacillus.

In **tuberculoid (TT) leprosy** (where patients have good cell-mediated immunity) few/no bacteria are found in the skin (paucibacillary leprosy). There are one to five hypopigmented anaesthetic patches with a raised red-copper-coloured border. Often this is associated with a single enlarged cutaneous nerve nearby.

At the other end of the spectrum, in **lepromatous (LL) leprosy**, the patient has no cell-mediated immunity and consequently there are numerous organisms in the skin (multibacillary leprosy). Clinically there are multiple papules, nodules and plaques that are not anaesthetic, and a 'glove and stocking' peripheral neuropathy due to widespread nerve damage.

In between are various forms of **borderline leprosy** (BT, borderline tuberculoid; BB, mid borderline; BL, borderline lepromatous) with clinical features gradually changing from tuberculoid to lepromatous.

The diagnosis is made by recognising the typical clinical features, doing slit-skin smears looking for organisms or by doing a skin biopsy.

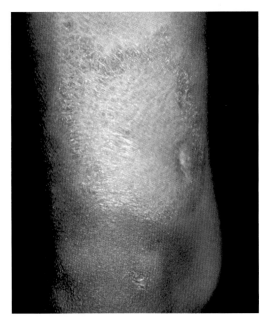

Fig. 9.50 Tuberculoid leprosy: single anaesthetic hypopigmented plaque on arm with a raised border

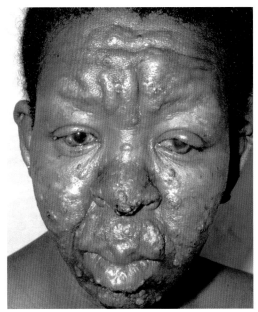

Fig. 9.51 Lepromatous leprosy: nodules on the face

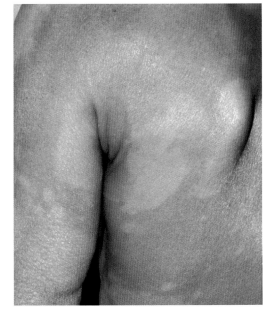

Fig. 9.52 Borderline leprosy: multiple asymmetrical hypopigmented patches

TREATMENT: LEPROSY

Patients suspected of having leprosy should be referred to a leprologist, since management requires careful monitoring of the skin and nerve lesions and regular supervision. All patients must have multidrug therapy.

	TT and BT *Paucibacillary*	BB, BL and LL *Multibacillary*
Duration of Rx	6 months	24 months
Rifampicin	600 mg monthly	600 mg monthly
Dapsone	100 mg daily	100 mg daily
Clofazimine		300 mg monthly and 50 mg daily

PITYRIASIS VERSICOLOR

White round or oval macules coalesce to form large hypopigmented patches on the upper trunk and proximal limbs in young adults with tanned or pigmented skin. The surface is always slightly scaly when scratched (*see* p. 203).

LICHEN SCLEROSUS ET ATROPHICUS

This condition usually presents with genital itching and is seen as white atrophic plaques in the perineum (*see* p. 368). Rarely the trunk and limbs may also be involved. Small flat white atrophic macules and papules with a shiny wrinkled surface occur, most commonly on the upper trunk. Fortunately they are usually asymptomatic. Trunk lesions tend to be unresponsive to treatment.

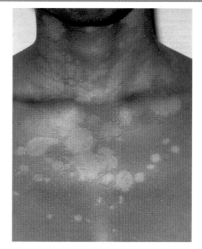

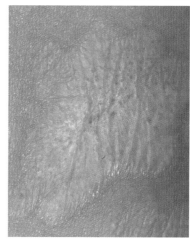

Fig. 9.53 Pityriasis versicolor: hypopigmented patches occurring on black skin

Fig. 9.54 Lichen sclerosus et atrophicus: close-up of lesions showing surface atrophy and wrinkled surface

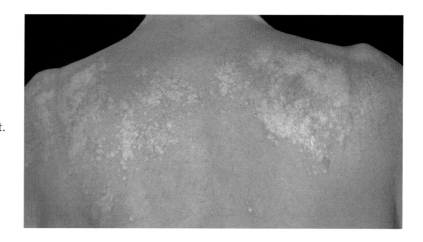

Fig. 9.55 (right) Lichen sclerosus et atrophicus: white macules, patches and plaques on upper back

PITYRIASIS ALBA

Multiple poorly defined hypopigmented, slightly scaly patches can occur on the face of children. In Caucasians they may only be visible in the summer when the normal skin tans. In dark-skinned individuals it is relatively common. It is considered to be a form of post-inflammatory hypopigmentation following mild eczema.

POST-INFLAMMATORY HYPOPIGMENTATION

Partial loss of pigment may follow any inflammatory skin condition affecting the epidermis, e.g. eczema or psoriasis, just as some individuals develop hyperpigmentation in response to the same stimulus. It is distinguished from pityriasis versicolor in being more ill-defined and irregular in outline, and producing little or no scale on scratching the surface, and from vitiligo by being hypopigmented rather than depigmented. Treat the underlying disease if it is still active, but reassure the patient that the pigmentation will return to normal in due course.

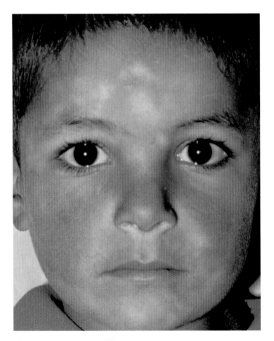

Fig. 9.56 Pityriasis alba

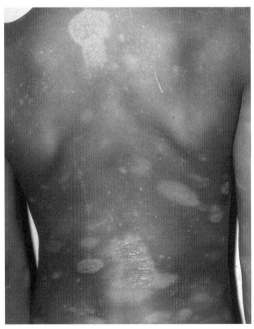

Fig. 9.57 Post-inflammatory pigmentation following atopic eczema in black skin

Fig. 9.58 Post-inflammatory hypopigmentation following eczema: poorly defined macules

NAEVUS ANAEMICUS

There is no structural abnormality in the skin. This is a pharmacological naevus with the blood vessels overreacting to adrenaline[UK]/epinephine[USA] and noradrenaline[UK]/norepinephrine[USA]. Pressure through the edge of the lesion will make the naevus disappear as the surrounding blood vessels are compressed. It is completely harmless.

SOLAR ELASTOSIS

This is a yellowish discolouration of the skin with more obvious skin creases and follicular openings on the face and neck due to chronic sun damage. This is the first sign of chronic sun damage and will always be seen in patients with basal cell carcinomas and squamous cell carcinomas. Both open and closed comedones can be found within solar elastosis (Favre–Racouchot syndrome, *see* Fig. 1.38, p. 10).

MORPHOEA

This is a localised thickening of the dermis due to excess collagen with loss of appendages (sweat glands and hair follicles). It occurs at any age (peak incidence from 20 to 40) and is more common in females. The lesions are firm oval plaques with a shiny smooth surface. The edge is often purple or brown, while the centre is white or yellow. It feels thickened compared with the surrounding skin. Rarely it may be linear, going down an arm or leg, or on the forehead (*see* p. 80).

In rare instances, morphoea can be extensive, and when involving large areas of the chest wall breathing, may be impeded. It is not related to systemic sclerosis, which is a widespread multi-system disease. There is a rare and mutilating form of linear morphoea in children in which the underlying muscle and bone are involved as well as the skin, causing problems with growth and permanent deformity.

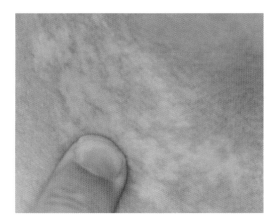

Fig. 9.59 Naevus anaemicus: white patch due to localised vasoconstriction

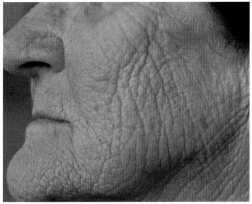

Fig. 9.60 Solar elastosis on side of face and neck: chronic sun damage in a patient with skin type I

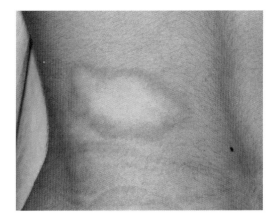

Fig. 9.61 Morphoea: purple border with white atrophic centre

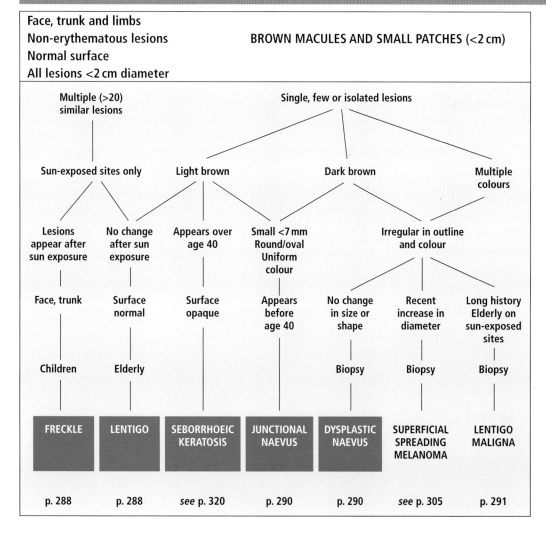

Face, trunk and limbs
Non-erythematous lesions
Normal surface
All lesions <2 cm diameter

BROWN MACULES AND SMALL PATCHES (<2 cm)

Multiple (>20) similar lesions — Single, few or isolated lesions

Sun-exposed sites only — Light brown — Dark brown — Multiple colours

Lesions appear after sun exposure — No change after sun exposure

Face, trunk — Surface normal

Children — Elderly

Appears over age 40 — Surface opaque

Small <7 mm Round/oval Uniform colour — Appears before age 40

Irregular in outline and colour

No change in size or shape — Recent increase in diameter — Long history Elderly on sun-exposed sites

Biopsy — Biopsy — Biopsy

FRECKLE	LENTIGO	SEBORRHOEIC KERATOSIS	JUNCTIONAL NAEVUS	DYSPLASTIC NAEVUS	SUPERFICIAL SPREADING MELANOMA	LENTIGO MALIGNA
p. 288	p. 288	see p. 320	p. 290	p. 290	see p. 305	p. 291

FRECKLES (EPHELIDES)

These well-demarcated, small (1–5 mm in diameter) orange-brown macules occur on sun-exposed sites (face, dorsum of hands and forearms). They appear after sun exposure in summer and disappear in winter. They occur in red-haired, blue-eyed individuals who burn rather than tan in the sun. Histologically they contain normal numbers of melanocytes but increased melanin pigment. They do not usually present a diagnostic problem or need any treatment.

LENTIGO

Lentigines are larger and darker than freckles and may have irregular edges. They occur mainly on the sun-exposed skin of middle-aged and elderly people and are present all the year round. They are caused by chronic sun exposure and if seen on the trunk in younger people (age <40) are evidence of too much sun exposure as a child. They are due to increased numbers of melanocytes in the basal cell layer of the epidermis.

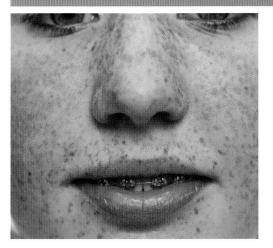

Fig. 9.62 Freckles

Skin-lightening creams do not work. Reassure the patient that lentigines are part of the normal ageing process. Individual lesions can be frozen with liquid nitrogen or treated with the NdYAG laser at 532 nm.

SEBORRHOEIC KERATOSIS

These lesions are usually raised; an early seborrhoeic keratosis may be flat and light brown, but under close inspection it will have an uneven surface.

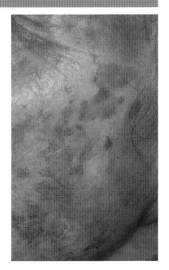

Fig. 9.65 (right) Lentigines on face of elderly lady with skin type I

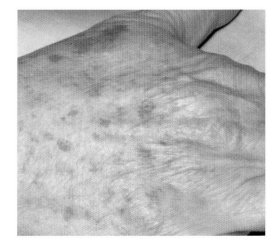

Fig. 9.63 Lentigines on dorsum of hand

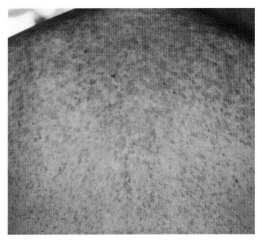

Fig. 9.64 Multiple lentigines over back in an individual who spent his or her childhood in Africa

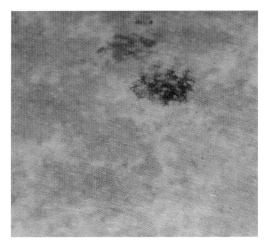

Fig. 9.66 Dark star-shaped lentigines – these are benign

JUNCTIONAL NAEVUS

A flat dark-brown mole that is round or oval in shape is a junctional naevus. Most are smaller than 7 mm in diameter. They can occur anywhere on the skin including the palms, soles and nail matrix (*see* Fig. 14.15, p. 440). They appear at any age but usually before the age of 35. Histologically groups of melanocytes are found in contact with the basal layer, hence the term junctional naevus (*see* Fig. 9.102a).

DYSPLASTIC (ATYPICAL) NAEVUS

A dysplastic (atypical) naevus is a flat or slightly raised mole, often >7 mm in diameter, that looks like a junctional naevus but which has an irregular edge and different shades of brown within it.

The atypical mole (dysplastic naevus) syndrome

There are a small number of families where some members have large numbers of moles (often >100), most of which are dysplastic, and a family history of malignant melanoma. Such individuals have an increased risk of developing multiple malignant melanomas.

TREATMENT: JUNCTIONAL AND DYSPLASTIC NAEVI

Junctional naevi do not need to be removed unless there is doubt over the diagnosis. Indeed, if lesions on the trunk are excised in young adults, the subsequent scarring can be unsightly. If the lesion has changed or developed any irregularity in colour, shape or border it should be excised and sent for histology to exclude a malignant melanoma. In patients with multiple dysplastic naevi, professional medical photographs taken of the whole body and given to the patient will help him or her identify any new or changing naevi.

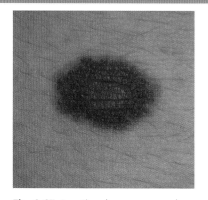

Fig. 9.67 Junctional naevus: round, symmetrical evenly pigmented
ABCDDEEE score (*see* p. 307) = 0 (not dark)

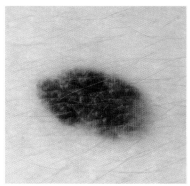

Fig. 9.68 Dysplastic naevus: irregular shape and pigmentation
Border irregular, colour variable, dark: score = 3

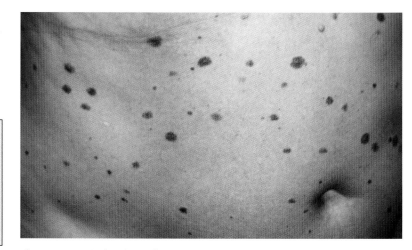

Fig. 9.69 Atypical mole syndrome: multiple large and irregular naevi on the trunk

LENTIGO MALIGNA

This looks very similar to an ordinary lentigo but is larger (usually >20 mm), has irregular margins and variation in pigment colour. It occurs only on sun-damaged skin, most commonly on the cheeks of the elderly. It may be difficult to distinguish from a benign lentigo, but slow extension over several years is characteristic. The diagnosis should be confirmed by a skin biopsy, which shows a malignant melanoma confined to the epidermis (melanoma in situ), *see* p. 304. These can sometimes progress to become an invasive malignant melanoma.

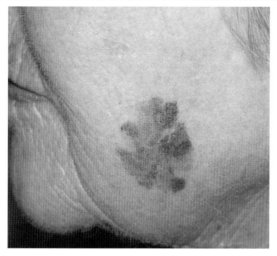

Fig. 9.70 Lentigo maligna on cheek

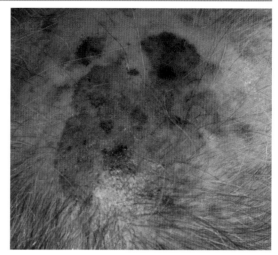

Fig. 9.71 Lentigo maligna melanoma arising in lentigo maligna on scalp

TREATMENT: LENTIGO MALIGNA

Excision is the treatment of choice, although for very large lesions on the face this may be impractable. Slow Mohs surgery using routine histopathology (*see* p. 332) can be used to control margins.

Alternatives include:

- topical 5% imiquimod (Aldara) cream applied three times a week for 12 weeks; this causes marked inflammation (*see* Fig. 9.72b) and the patient should be warned about this
- cryotherapy.

Recurrence can occur, so follow-up is essential.

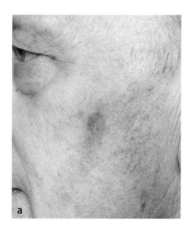
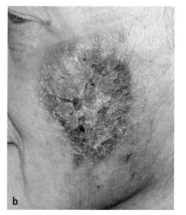
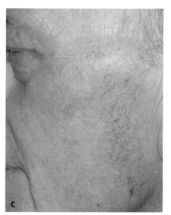

Fig. 9.72 (a) Lentigo maligna before imiquimod treatment; (b) treatment with imiquimod has produced an intense inflammatory reaction; (c) 4 weeks after completion of imiquimod treatment

Non-erythematous lesions
Normal surface
Brown, blue or grey   BROWN LESIONS (>2 cm) before AGE 10
Large patches and plaques (>2 cm)
Present from birth or before age 10

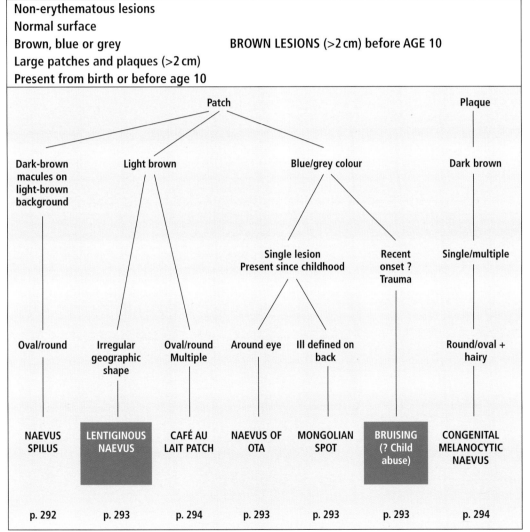

NAEVUS SPILUS

This is a birthmark where dark, speckled macules or papules occur in a larger pale-brown pigmented patch.

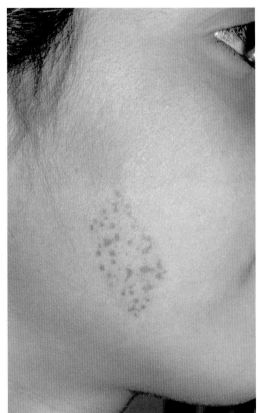

Fig. 9.73 Naevus spilus

NAEVUS OF OTA

This is blue-grey patch of pigmentation around the eye and on the sclera on one side only. It is a type of blue naevus with the melanocytes situated deep within the dermis. It is common among the Japanese and is present from birth or early childhood. It remains present throughout life. A similar lesion on the shoulder is called a **naevus of Ito**.

MONGOLIAN SPOT

A large blue-grey patch on the back of an oriental baby is extremely common. It disappears spontaneously by the end of the first year of life. It can occur in any race.

BRUISING (? CHILD ABUSE)

Bruising (*see* Fig. 9.77) can appear as blue-grey discolouration as it settles. In children the possibility of abuse always needs to be considered.

LENTIGINOUS NAEVUS

This is a flat, pigmented birthmark, light or medium brown in colour and oval or geographic in outline. There is no surface abnormality (*see* Fig. 9.79).

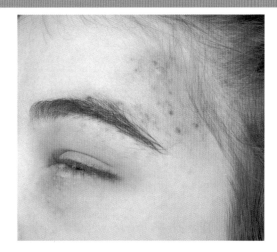

Fig. 9.74 Naevus of Ota

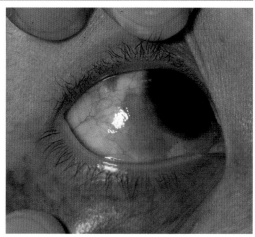

Fig. 9.75 Neavus of Ota on the sclera

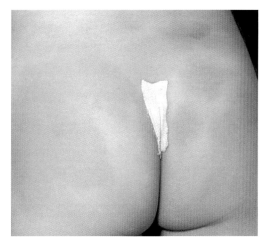

Fig. 9.76 Mongolian spot on buttocks and lower back

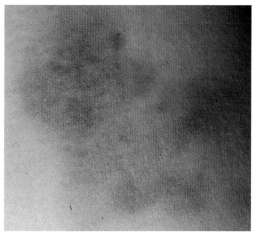

Fig. 9.77 Bruising

CAFÉ AU LAIT PATCH

These are light-brown patches, round or oval in shape, and often large (2–10 cm diameter). They are present at birth or appear in early childhood. If more than six are found, or the patient also has freckles in the axillae and multiple neurofibromas in the skin or peripheral nerves, the diagnosis of neurofibromatosis (von Recklinghausen's disease) can be made (*see* p. 266).

CONGENITAL MELANOCYTIC NAEVUS

Congenital melanocytic naevi are moles that are present at birth. They are normally >2 cm in diameter. At birth they may be red, rather than brown, but within a few months are obviously pigmented. They may be flat or raised, hairy or warty. They may sometimes be very large, covering up to half the body surface. For the very large naevi there is a 9% lifetime risk (greatest before puberty) of developing one or more malignant melanomas within the naevus.

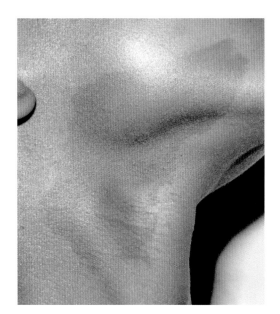

Fig. 9.78 Lentiginous naevus

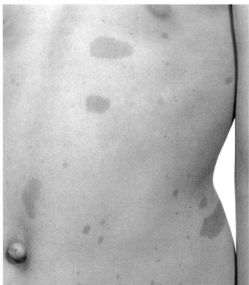

Fig. 9.79 Multiple café au lait patches

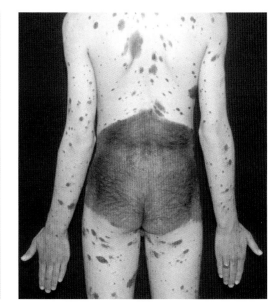

Fig. 9.80 Congenital melanocytic naevus: large 'bathing trunk' naevus with multiple smaller ones

Non-erythematous lesions
Normal surface
Brown, blue or grey
Large patches and plaques (>2 cm)
Appear after age 10 years

BROWN LESIONS (>2 cm) after AGE 10

Poorly defined borders

Well-defined border

Side of neck only	Female Face only	Site of previous rash	Lower legs ? Previous purpura	Recent oral medication, or skin application	Upper trunk/upper arms		Slowly enlarging	Round/oval Recurrent same site

Mottled Red-brown	?Contraceptive pill/pregnant	Brown colour	Orange-brown	Brown/orange/ blue-grey *See list*	Unilateral Geographic outline	Bilateral Small lesions coalescing	? Skin thickened	Previous blister/ erythema

POIKILODERMA OF CIVATTE	MELASMA/ CHLOASMA	POST-INFLAMMATORY HYPERPIGMENTATION	HAEMOSIDERIN PIGMENTATION LICHEN AUREUS	DRUG-INDUCED PIGMENTATION	BECKER'S NAEVUS	PITYRIASIS VERSICOLOR	MORPHOEA	FIXED DRUG ERUPTION
p. 296	p. 296	p. 297	pp. 279, 299	p. 298	p. 299	*see p. 203*	p. 299	p. 297

POIKILODERMA OF CIVATTE

Poikiloderma is identified by the combination of pigment, atrophy and telangiectasia. Poikiloderma of Civatte is the commonest type and occurs in middle-aged and older patients on the sides of the neck. The skin becomes a mottled red-brown colour with atrophic areas. The area immediately under the chin and ears is spared. It is thought to be due to UV exposure, possibly associated with cosmetics acting as photosensitisers. It is very common and patients rarely bring it to the attention of their doctors. No treatment is available other than using a sunblock.

MELASMA (CHLOASMA)

Unsightly symmetrical pigmented patches occur in women on the forehead, cheeks and moustache area that darken after sun exposure. They occur most commonly during pregnancy or on taking the contraceptive pill. The pigmentation usually fades after delivery or on stopping the pill, but it may be permanent. Identical pigmentation is sometimes seen in men, and in women who are not pregnant or on the pill.

TREATMENT: MELASMA

If on the contraceptive pill, stop taking it. A mixture of 0.05% tretinoin, 4% hydroquinone and 0.01% fluocinolone acetonide in a hydrophilic cream base (Pigmanorm[UK], Triluma[USA] – *available over the internet with private prescription*) applied twice a day for 8 weeks works well. Once the pigment has gone, the patient must keep out of the sun and/or use a high factor (15+) sunscreen or it will reoccur.

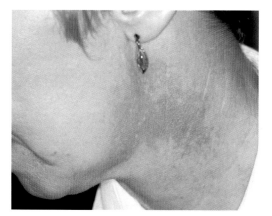

Fig. 9.81 Poikiloderma of Civatte

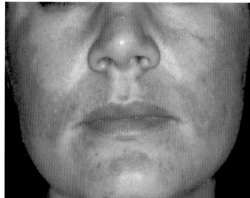

Fig. 9.82 Melasma

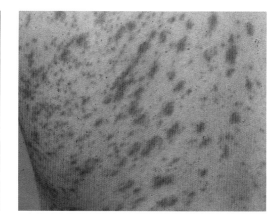

Fig. 9.83 Post-inflammatory pigmentation following lichen planus

POST-INFLAMMATORY HYPERPIGMENTATION

Brown patches on the skin may occur after any inflammatory process in the epidermis (e.g. eczema, psoriasis, lichen planus). It is commoner in darker-skinned individuals. There is usually a history of a rash before the pigment change. No treatment is available but it usually improves with time. The inflammatory phase of a **fixed drug eruption** (*see* p. 181) can also be followed by a dark-brown patch that remains for several months.

HAEMOSIDERIN PIGMENTATION

This is seen following purpura where haemoglobin is broken down to haemosiderin. The haemosiderin pigment looks similar to melanin except that it is a more rust-brown colour. It is usually seen on the lower legs (*see* p. 400). In cases of varicose eczema the pigmentation may be a mixture of melanin and haemosiderin.

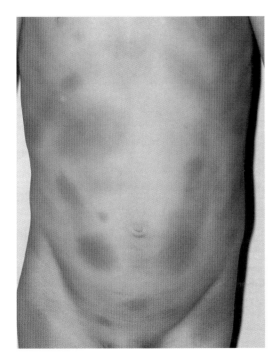

Fig. 9.84 Post-inflammatory pigmentation following a fixed drug reaction

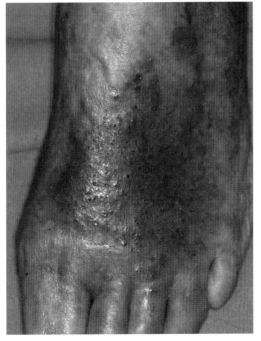

Fig. 9.85 Post-inflammatory pigmentation following foot eczema

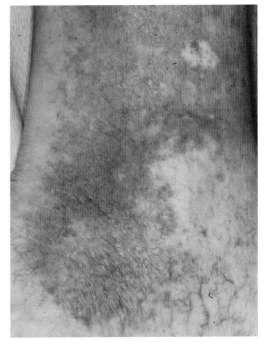

Fig. 9.86 Haemosiderin pigmentation: the colour is a rust-brown rather than dark brown

PIGMENTATION DUE TO DRUGS

The following drugs can cause pigmentation in the skin:

- amiodarone, chloroquine, minocycline, chlorpromazine (and other phenothiazines), dapsone, gold: blue-grey pigmentation in sun-exposed sites
- phenytoin and oral contraceptive pill: pigmentation similar to melasma (*see* Fig. 9.82)
- clofazimine (red pink)
- β-carotene (orange)
- mepacrine (yellow),
- bleomycin: flagellate brown or purple (linear streaks usually on back)

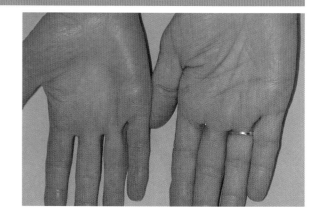

Fig. 9.87 (right) Carotenemia on right, compared with normal on left

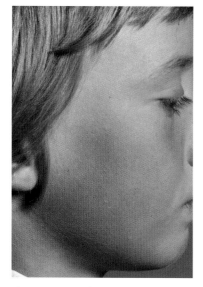

Fig. 9.88 Amiodarone pigmentation

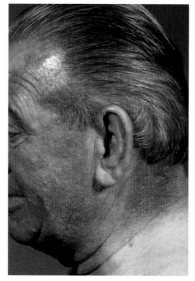

Fig. 9.89 Minocycline pigmentation.

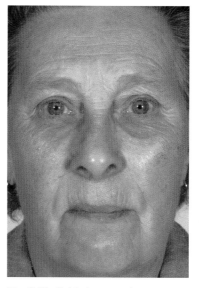

Fig. 9.90 Gold pigmentation (chrysiasis)

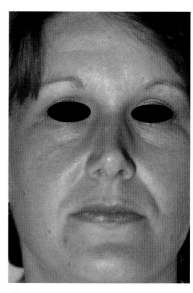

Fig. 9.91 Mepacrine pigmentation

BECKER'S NAEVUS

This is a congenital hamartoma of the skin that is androgen-sensitive so appears in the mid to late teens and then persists for life. It is an irregularly shaped patch of hyperpigmentation containing more hairs than is normal. It most commonly occurs over the shoulder region but can occur anywhere. No treatment is available, although the hair can be removed with a laser (Alexandrite, *see* p. 67); this can make the hyperpigmentation worse.

LICHEN AUREUS

A localised form of capilaritis where blood leaks from superficial vessels and the residual haemosiderin is seen as an orange/golden-coloured patch.

MORPHOEA

Morphoea can present as a brown patch or plaque with a purple-brown border (*see* also p. 287).

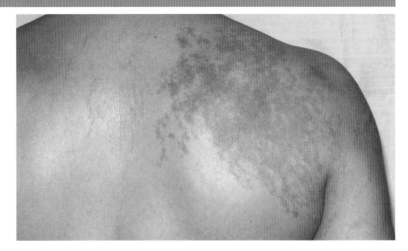

Fig. 9.92 Becker's naevus

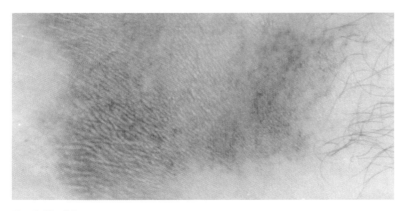

Fig. 9.93 Lichen aureus

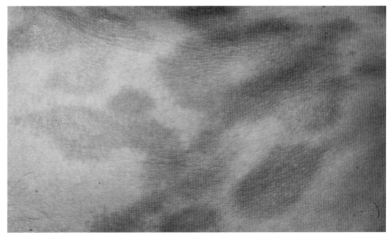

9.94 Brown patches of morphoea

Face, trunk and limbs
Non-erythematous lesions
Normal surface
Papules, plaques, nodules

BROWN – raised lesions

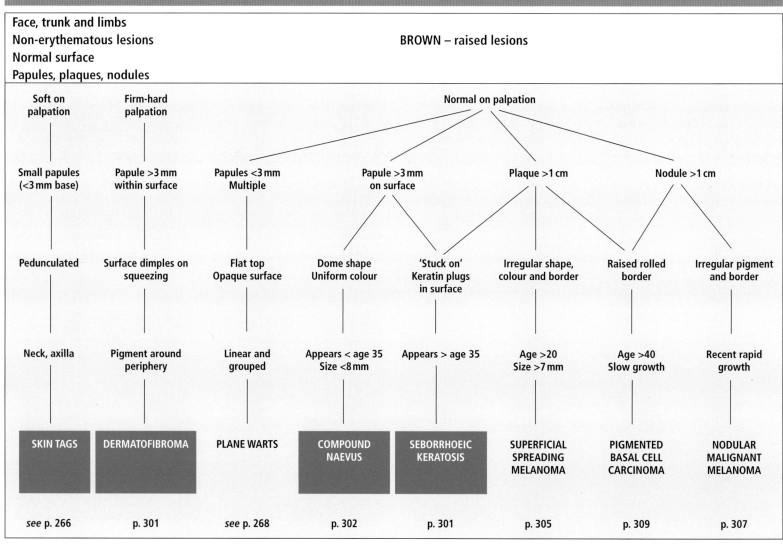

Soft on palpation	Firm-hard palpation			Normal on palpation			
Small papules (<3 mm base)	Papule >3 mm within surface	Papules <3 mm Multiple	Papule >3 mm on surface		Plaque >1 cm	Nodule >1 cm	
Pedunculated	Surface dimples on squeezing	Flat top Opaque surface	Dome shape Uniform colour	'Stuck on' Keratin plugs in surface	Irregular shape, colour and border	Raised rolled border	Irregular pigment and border
Neck, axilla	Pigment around periphery	Linear and grouped	Appears < age 35 Size <8 mm	Appears > age 35	Age >20 Size >7 mm	Age >40 Slow growth	Recent rapid growth
SKIN TAGS	**DERMATOFIBROMA**	PLANE WARTS	**COMPOUND NAEVUS**	**SEBORRHOEIC KERATOSIS**	SUPERFICIAL SPREADING MELANOMA	PIGMENTED BASAL CELL CARCINOMA	NODULAR MALIGNANT MELANOMA
see p. 266	p. 301	*see* p. 268	p. 302	p. 301	p. 305	p. 309	p. 307

DERMATOFIBROMA (HISTIOCYTOMA)

This is a firm-hard papule situated in the dermis and occurs anywhere on the body. It often follows an insect bite, so is most commonly found on the legs. It is usually small (<5 mm), attached to the skin and mobile over deeper structures. Squeezing the lesion from the sides results in puckering of the skin since dermatofibromas are situated very high in the dermis. The colour ranges from skin coloured, to pink to brown, often with a darker ring at the edge. The surface may be smooth or slightly scaly. It looks like a compound naevus but is distinguished by being much firmer on palpation.

SEBORRHOEIC KERATOSIS/WART

Seborrhoeic keratoses usually have a warty or keratotic surface (*see* p. 320). Occasionally they have a smooth surface and can be confused with compound naevi or even malignant melanomas if very heavily pigmented. If you look carefully at the surface you may see small keratin plugs, which are specific to seborrhoeic keratoses. In addition the lesion will tend to be sitting on top of the skin and have no deep component at all.

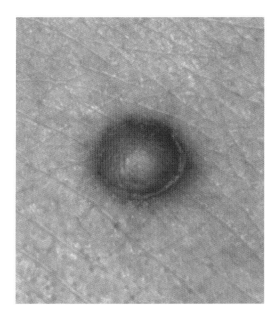

Fig. 9.95 Dermatofibroma showing halo of pigmentation around edge

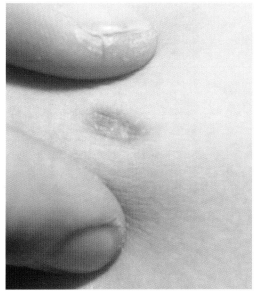

Fig. 9.96 Puckering of the skin over a dermatofibroma when squeezed

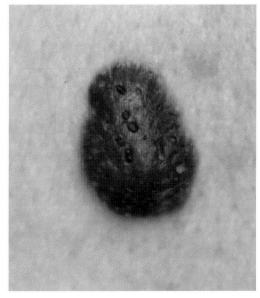

Fig. 9.97 Seborrhoeic keratosis: note tiny keratin plugs in surface

COMPOUND NAEVUS

These are melanocytic naevi that are raised and pigmented, and may be hairy. On histology the melanocytes are both at the dermo-epidermal junction and within the dermis (hence compound). The melanocytes at the dermo-epidermal junction give moles their brown colour while the intradermal melanocytes result in elevation. The natural history of moles is a maturation from junctional naevi (flat and dark brown) to compound naevi (brown and dome-shaped or papillomatous) to intradermal naevi (skin-coloured papules) *see* Fig. 9.102, p. 303.

Established benign moles change (*see* previous paragraph) and new moles occur or get bigger around puberty, during pregnancy and after sun exposure. Assuming that all moles that change are malignant is misleading. It is the type of change that is important.

If a benign mole becomes more *elevated* and at the same time *lightens* in colour, this is the normal change from junctional to intradermal naevus. Sometimes moles can look irregular if part of the periphery of the mole is flat and brown (junctional) and the centre raised and lighter in colour (intradermal) (*see* Fig. 9.101). Malignant change should be thought of if there is lateral spread of pigment (*see* Fig. 9.103b).

TREATMENT: COMPOUND NAEVUS AND DERMATOFIBROMA

Only remove if they are very unsightly or get caught on clothing. For compound naevi removal by shave biopsy will generally leave an acceptable scar, which is flat and no bigger than the original lesion, although recurrence of pigment may occur. Dermatofibromas need to be excised but in young people this can leave ugly scars. Always send the lesion off for histology.

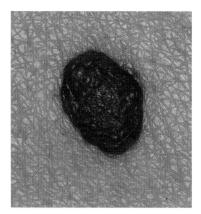

Fig. 9.98 Compound naevus: dark-brown, elevated mole
ABCDDEEE score (*see* p. 307) dark, elevated: score = 2

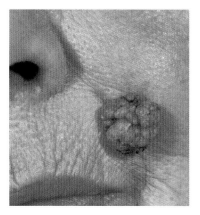

Fig. 9.99 Compound naevus with a papillomatous surface
ABCDDEEE score not applicable: warty surface

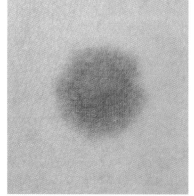

Fig. 9.100 Compound naevus in patient with type I skin
colour variable, elevated: score = 2

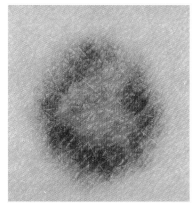

Fig. 9.101 Compound naevus with peripheral junctional area
colour variable, diameter >1 cm: score = 2

a. Junctional naevus (p. 290)

Histological features:

Naevus cells at dermo-epidermal junction.

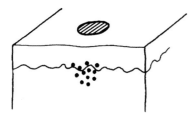

Clinical features:

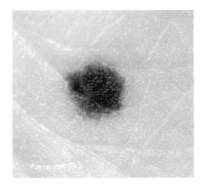

Flat and dark brown.
(ABCDDEEE score, *see* p. 307)
dark: score = 1

b. Compound naevus (p. 302)

Naevus cells at dermo-epidermal junction and within the dermis.

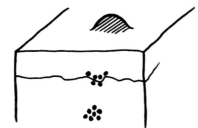

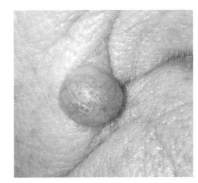

Raised (dome shaped or papillomatous) and brown.
dark, elevated: score = 2

c. Intradermal naevus (p. 264)

Naevus cells only within dermis.

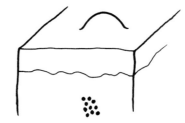

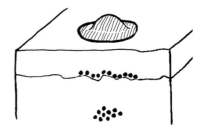

Raised (dome shaped or papillomatous) and skin coloured.
elevated: score = 1

d. Combined junctional and compound naevus

Junctional cells throughout lesion, intradermal naevus cells centrally only.

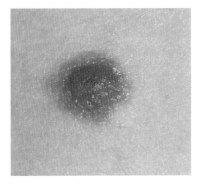

Periphery flat and brown, centre raised and brown.
colours multiple, elevated: score = 2

Fig. 9.102 Clinicopathological correlation of melanocytic naevi (moles)

a. Lentigo maligna (p. 291)

Histological features:

*Malignant melanocytes restricted to epidermis only. Has an **excellent prognosis.***

b. Superficial spreading malignant melanoma (p. 305)

*Malignant melanocytes migrating laterally along dermo-epidermal junction. Has a **good prognosis.***

c. Superficial spreading melanoma with nodule (p. 306)

*Malignant melanocytes growing downwards as well as laterally. Has a **worse prognosis.***

d. Nodular malignant melanoma (p. 306)

*Malignant melanocytes migrating vertically downwards only. Has a **poor prognosis.***

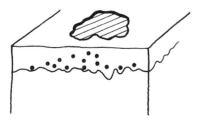 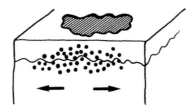 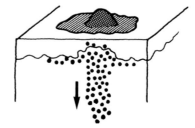 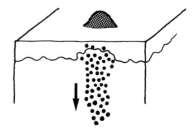

Clinical features:

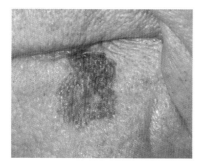 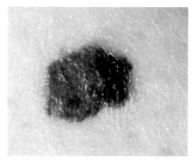 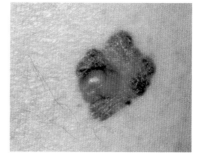 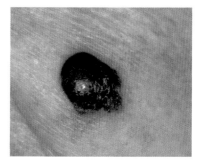

Large irregular patch on sun-exposed skin in the elderly – long history.
ABCDDEEE scoring (see p. 307)
Asymmetry, border irregegular, colour variable, diameter >10 mm: score = 4

Flat plaque with irregular shape and pigment, recent increase in diameter.
Asymmetry, border irregular, colour variable, diameter >10 mm, dark: score = 4

Black irregular plaque out of which is growing a brown nodule.
Asymmetry, border irregular, colour variable, diameter >10 mm, dark, elevated: score = 6

Black bleeding nodule. No surrounding pigmentation.
Border irregular, diameter >10 mm, dark, elevated: score = 4

Fig. 9.103 Clinicopathological correlation of malignant melanoma

MALIGNANT MELANOMA

A malignant melanoma is malignant tumour of melanocytes. Two-thirds arise from normal skin and one-third from a pre-existing mole. There are four clinical patterns of malignant melanoma.

1. **Lentigo maligna**. A large (1–3 cm size) brown patch on sun-exposed skin in an elderly patient. The tumour cells are confined to the epidermis (*see* p. 304). Later an invasive melanoma can develop with a lentigo maligna as a papule or nodule within the original patch (*see* Fig. 9.71, p. 291).

2a. **Superficial spreading malignant melanoma (SSMM)**. The initial growth phase of malignant melanocytes is along the dermo-epidermal junction (*radial growth phase*). This change is seen clinically as a flat brown patch enlarging in diameter. Because the radial growth is usually uneven, there will be variation in the degree of pigmentation and an irregular border, often with scalloped edges. There may also be evidence of inflammation, erythema and sometimes an altered sensation. Tumour cells remain high in the dermis and are unlikely to invade blood vessels or lymphatics. As a result superficial spreading melanomas generally carry a good prognosis. If however regression has occurred, then the depth of invasion may have been greater previously than it is at removal, raising the possibility that the prognosis based on thickness may be false.

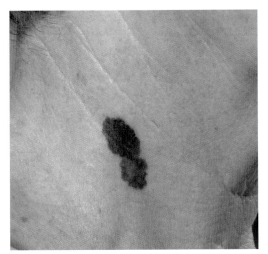

Fig. 9.104 Superficial spreading melanoma: note size, irregular border and pigment.
(Scores 5 points on ABCDDEEE, *see* p. 307)

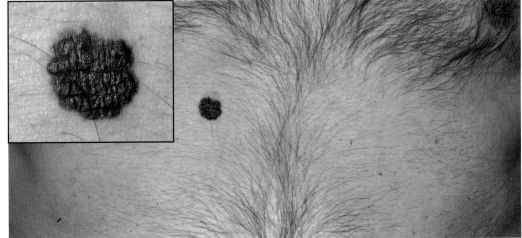

Fig. 9.105 Small early superficial spreading melanoma on chest: close-up (above left).
(Scores 4 points on ABCDDEEE, *see* p. 307; border irregular, diameter >10 mm, dark, elevated)

2b. Superficial spreading melanoma with nodular component. Eventually the malignant melanocytes grow downwards (*vertical growth phase*). A papule or nodule will appear within the flat irregular brown patch (*see* Figs 9.103c and 9.106). Once this happens the prognosis becomes worse because tumour cells are more likely to have entered dermal blood vessels and lymphatics leading to metastases.

3. Nodular malignant melanoma. This type needs to be distinguished from the superficial spreading melanoma. Here there is no radial growth and the malignant melanocytes grow down vertically from the start. The lesion is a nodule without any surrounding irregular pigmentation. A typical nodular melanoma is a black, dome-shaped nodule. The surface of the lesion will eventually break down to bleed, ooze and crust over. Sometimes nodules may be red (amelanotic – *see* also Fig. 8.47, p. 216) rather than brown-black. The diagnosis can be delayed as there is no superficial spread to alert the patient, and prognosis is often poor as the lesion will be relatively thick before it has been diagnosed and removed. The ABCDDEE list may not help with nodular melanomas. Black or red nodules should be referred for biopsy.

4. Acral lentiginous melanomas occur on the palms, soles or under the nails (*see* p. 440).

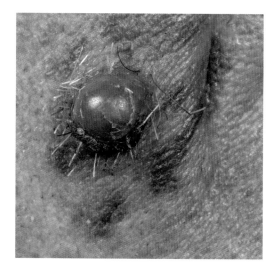

Fig. 9.106 Nodule arising in a lentigo maligna (scores 6 points with ABCDDEEE – asymmetry, border irregular, colour variable, diameter >10 mm, darkness, elevation)

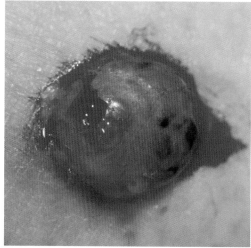

Fig. 9.107 Nodular melanoma with no horizontal growth phase (scores 6 points on ABCDDEEE – colour variable, diameter >10 mm, darkness, erythema, elevation, exudate)

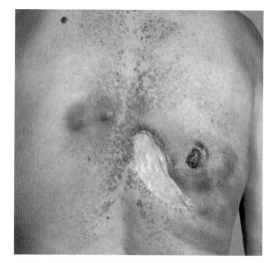

Fig. 9.108 Recurrence of melanoma around a large skin graft on the back

Diagnosis of melanoma

It is important to diagnose malignant melanomas while they are thin so that removal results in cure. In practice this means distinguishing them from lentigines, junctional and compound naevi. Remember that benign moles can change (*see* Fig. 9.102). Malignant lesions tend to be larger, darker, palpable, and may ooze or bleed.

To identify melanomas this checklist (**ABCDDEEE**) may be helpful. If four or more are present, a melanoma is possible. Biopsy if three are present. *Only apply this check list if the surface is smooth* (i.e. not warty, papillomatous, scale, keratin or crust). Dermoscopy will also be useful in distinguishing the benign from malignant (*see* p. 18).

- **Asymmetry**: there will not be an axis of symmetry in any direction
- **Border** irregular: the border should be definite but irregular with notches; fade-out of border does not count (*see* Fig. 9.109)
- **Colour** variable: definite areas of light and dark brown, or black
- **Diameter** >10 mm
- **Darkness** of colour (dark brown or black)
- **Erythema**
- **Elevation**
- **Exudate**: any evidence of serum or blood on the surface

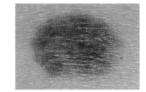

Fig. 9.109 Benign naevus with border fade-out

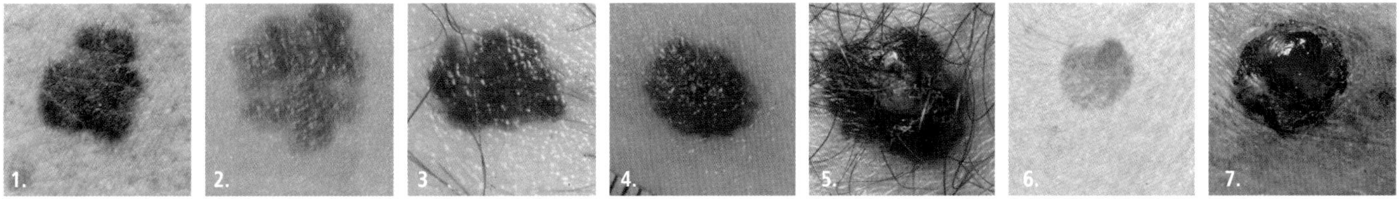

	1.	2.	3.	4.	5.	6.	7.
Asymmetry	yes	yes	yes	no	yes	no	no
Border irregular	yes	yes	yes	no	yes	no	no
Colour variable	no	yes	no	no	no	yes	no
Diameter >10 mm	yes	yes	no	no	yes	yes	yes
Darkness	yes	no	yes	yes	yes	no	yes
Erythema	no	yes	no	no	no	no	yes
Elevation	no	no	no	no	yes	no	yes
Exudate	no	no	no	no	no	no	yes
SCORE	4	5	3	1	5	2	5
Diagnosis:	SSMM	SSMM	Dysplastic naevus	Junctional naevus	Nodular MM	Lentigo (cheek)	Ulcerated nodular MM

Fig. 9.110 Using the ABCDDEEE checklist in diagnosing melanomas

Aetiology of malignant melanoma

Malignant melanoma is more likely to occur in:

- those with fair or red hair who burn rather than tan in the sun (skin types I and II)
- those who have been badly sun burnt on more than one occasion in *childhood (< age 18)*, but not as an adult

- those who have a large number of moles (>50); duration of sun exposure in childhood is linked to number of moles
- those with a past or family history of malignant melanoma
- those with atypical mole syndrome (*see* p. 290)
- giant congential melanocytic naevus, p. 294
- the use of tanning beds before age 35.

Prognosis of malignant melanoma (*See* Table 9.01.)

The following have been found to accurately predict prognosis.

- **Breslow's thickness** (*see* Fig. 9.111): measure in millimeters the depth from the top of the granular cell layer of the epidermis to the deepest point of invasion. This is by far the most important prognostic indicator.
- **Ulceration**: for any given thickness this worsens the prognosis.
- **Involvement of regional lymph nodes** or satellite/in-transit metastases makes the prognosis worse (stage III). The more nodes involved (>3) and if the metastases are clinically apparent, the worse the prognosis.
- **Distant metastases** and elevated levels of lactic dehydrogenase in the blood imply a very poor prognosis (stage IV).

Table 9.01 Prognosis of malignant melanoma showing % survival rates at 1–15 years

Prognosis of malignant melanoma (% survival rates 1–15 years)							
No lymph node involvement or distant metastasis							
Stage	Thickness	Ulceration	1 year	2 years	5 years	10 years	15 years
IA	<1 mm	No	99.7	99.0	95	88	85
IB	<1 mm	Yes	99.8	98.7	91	83	72
	1–2 mm	No	99.5	97.3	89	79	72
IIA	1–2 mm	Yes	98.2	93	77	64	57
	2–4 mm	No	98.7	94	79	64	57
IIB	2–4 mm	Yes	95.1	85	63	51	44
	>4 mm	No	95	89	67	54	44
IIC	>4 mm	Yes	90	71	45	32	29
With lymph node involvement or distant metastasis – any thickness							
Stage	Nodes	Ulceration	1 year	2 years	5 years	10 years	15 years
IIIA	1–3 micro	No	95	86	67	60	59
IIIB	1–3 micro	Yes	88	75	53	38	31
	1–3 macro	No	88	75	53	38	31
IIIC	1–3 macro	Yes	71	49	27	19	17
	>4 or in-transit	Yes/No	71	49	27	19	17
IV	Distant metastases		50	25	10	7	5

Note: from Balch CM, Gershenwald JE, Soong SJ, *et al.* Final version of 2009 AJCC melanoma staging and classification. *J Clin Oncol.* 2009; **27**(36): 6199–206.

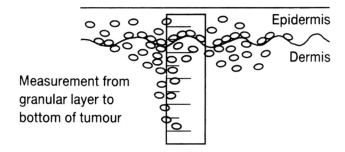

Fig. 9.111 Breslow's thickness: measure in millimeters the depth of invasion from the granular layer to the deepest tumour cells

TREATMENT: MALIGNANT MELANOMA

All suspicious lesions should be excised with a 2 mm margin of normal skin and sent for histology. Having confirmed the diagnosis histologically, wider excision is carried out as follows (UK and Australian guidelines):

- confined to the epidermis – excise with 0.5 cm margin
- tumours <1 mm thick – excise with 1 cm margin
- tumours 1–2 mm thick – excise with 1–2 cm margin
- tumours >2 mm thick – excise with 2 cm margin.

SENTINEL NODE BIOPSY AND ADVANCED DISEASE

Removal of the nearest lymph node (the sentinel node) to which the lymphatics at the site of the tumour drain may help predict the prognosis. It is found by injecting a radioactive tracer and a blue dye. If this node does not contain tumour, the *prognosis* is obviously better than if it does. Block dissection of the nodes is usually done if the sentinel node is positive. Otherwise lymph nodes are not removed unless clinically involved.

There is *no evidence* that sentinel node biopsy or removal of lymph nodes improves the prognosis. It should only be performed to give the patient or physician a better idea of prognosis (usually in clinical trials).

Metastatic melanoma can be treated with immunotherapy: ipilimumab (blocks CTLA-4) plus vemurafenib (blocks BRAF), *see* p. 57.

PREVENTION OF MELANOMAS

Almost all melanomas are induced by sun exposure, particularly short, sharp bursts leading to sunburn. Everyone should protect themselves from sunburn and in particular parents should protect their children from sunburn by using a waterproof high-protective-factor sunscreen (SPF 30+) on all exposed skin and covering as much skin as possible.

There is no evidence that having a melanoma during pregnancy affects the prognosis; likewise, taking the contraceptive pill or hormone replacement therapy do not alter the natural history of melanoma.

PIGMENTED BASAL CELL CARCINOMA

Occasionally basal cell carcinomas are heavily pigmented and they may then be confused with a nodular malignant melanoma. The typical rolled edge should suggest the diagnosis (*see* p. 330).

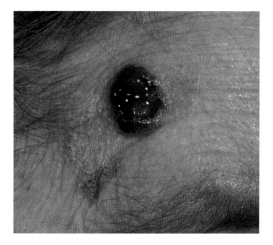

Fig. 9.112 Pigmented basal cell carcinoma: note pigment in the rolled edge

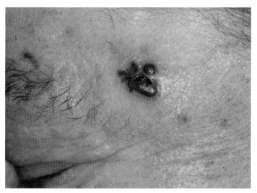

Fig. 9.113 Pigmented basal cell carcinoma: clinically it is not possible to distinguish this lesion from a melanoma except by histology (scores 7 points with ABCDDEEE list, *see* p. 307)

Face, trunk and limbs
Non-erythematous lesions
Normal surface
Macules, papules and nodules

BLACK, BLUE, PURPLE or GREY LESIONS

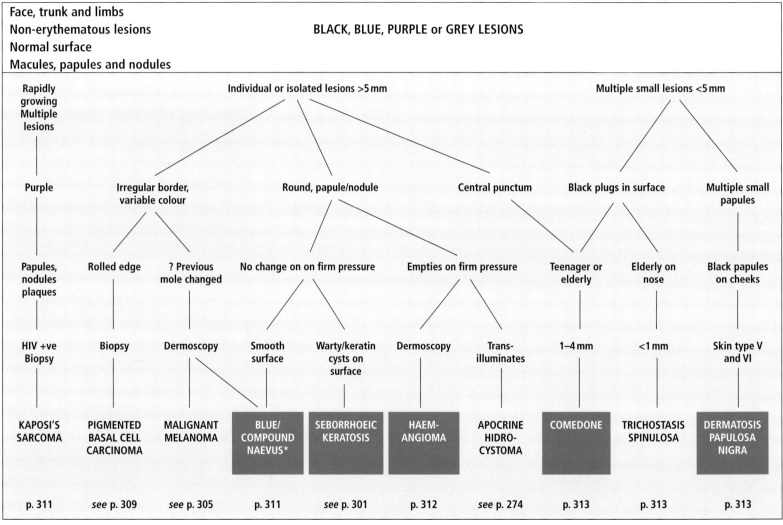

KAPOSI'S SARCOMA	PIGMENTED BASAL CELL CARCINOMA	MALIGNANT MELANOMA	BLUE/ COMPOUND NAEVUS*	SEBORRHOEIC KERATOSIS	HAEM- ANGIOMA	APOCRINE HIDRO- CYSTOMA	COMEDONE	TRICHOSTASIS SPINULOSA	DERMATOSIS PAPULOSA NIGRA
p. 311	*see* p. 309	*see* p. 305	p. 311	*see* p. 301	p. 312	*see* p. 274	p. 313	p. 313	p. 313

*Seen in heavily pigmented skin

KAPOSI'S SARCOMA

This is a malignant growth of blood vessels caused by human herpes virus 8. It is seen mainly in patients with HIV/AIDS. The lesions begin as small reddish-purple, reddish-brown or purple macules or papules that grow to form nodules and plaques. Screening for HIV and a biopsy will confirm the diagnosis.

TREATMENT: KAPOSI'S SARCOMA

In patients with AIDS, the appearance of Kaposi's sarcoma would be a reason to introduce HAART (highly active antiretrovirus treatment) even with a normal CD_4 count.

For the Kaposi's sarcoma itself, no treatment is needed unless the lesions are unsightly or painful. Small lesions can be excised. Lesions localised to a limb can be treated with radiotherapy. Chemotherapy using vinblastine, doxorubicin, and bleomycin give good palliation for a while.

BLUE NAEVUS

This looks like a compound naevus except that it is blue or blue-black rather than brown in colour. It is dome shaped, usually less than 10 mm in diameter. Blue naevi appear during childhood and then remain fixed, a feature that will distinguish them from a malignant melanoma. In **pigmented skin**, ordinary **compound naevi** may be black in colour rather than brown. No treatment is needed, as this is a benign lesion.

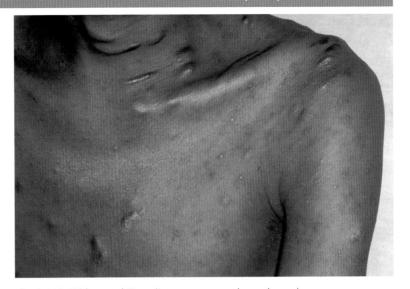

Fig. 9.114 Widespread Kaposi's sarcoma: macules and papules

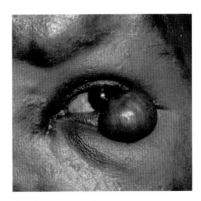

Fig. 9.115 Nodule of Kaposi's sarcoma

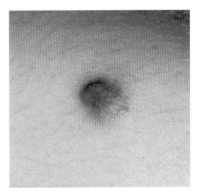

Fig. 9.116 Blue naevus

HAEMANGIOMA AND ANGIOKERATOMA

The terms angioma and haemangioma are interchangeable. Red or purple papules and plaques that have been present since childhood are due to a localised overgrowth of blood vessels. The stagnant blood within the lesion may be compressed partially, but the colour will never fade completely.

Those occurring in adult life may be very dark in colour and mimic an early melanoma. If you look carefully you will see a lobulated vascular pattern; this is easily seen using a dermatoscope (*see* Fig. 1.91, p. 18).

Angiokeratomas are similar but have a scaly surface. They may be almost black in colour.

TREATMENT: ANGIOMA AND HAEMANGIOMA

Small lesions can be excised or cauterised. Larger lesions are best left alone as the vascular malformation in the deeper tissue may be extensive.

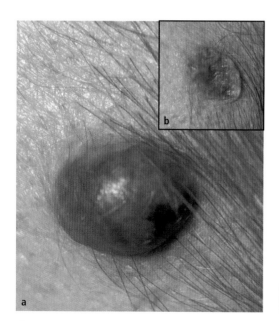

Fig. 9.117 Haemangioma: (a) compressible nodule on left temple; (b) same lesion after compression

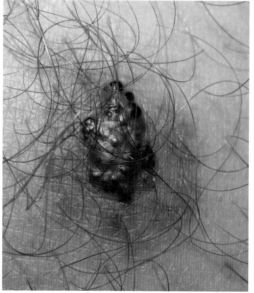

Fig. 9.118 Black coloured angioma: diagnosis made by dermoscopy (*see* p. 18)

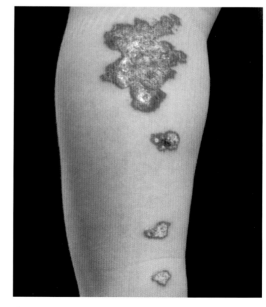

Fig. 9.119 Angiokeratoma on a child's leg: differs from an ordinary angioma in having a scaly surface

TRICHOSTASIS SPINULOSA

Small blackheads on the nose in elderly patients are very common. They are due to the failure of shedding of vellus hairs in the hair follicles of the nose.

If the patient complains about the problem and wants treatment, 0.05% isotretinoin (Isotrex) gel or lotion applied at night for 6–8 weeks will give a fairly dramatic improvement. It can be kept clear by using it twice a week.

GIANT COMEDONE

Single large comedones can occur on the trunk and face in the elderly. They are much larger than the blackheads associated with acne in teenagers, but the aetiology is basically the same, i.e. a single follicle with a keratin plug at its mouth, filling up with keratin and sebum behind it. Clinically it is a white/cream papule with a central black punctum.

DERMATOSIS PAPULOSA NIGRA

Multiple small black or brown papules occur on the cheeks particularly in black skin. Histologically the lesions are seborrhoeic keratoses. They are inherited as an autosomal dominant trait. They are harmless and best left alone.

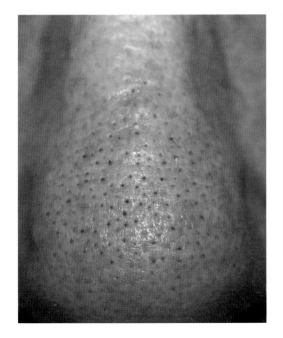

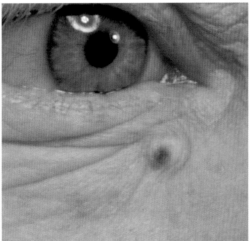

Fig. 9.121 Giant comedo

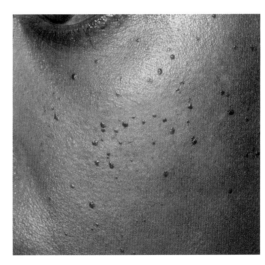

Fig. 9.122 Dermatosis papulosa nigra: tiny seborrhoeic keratoses on cheek in black skin

Fig. 9.120 (left) Trichostasis spinulosa on the nose

Non-erythematous lesions
Normal surface
Red, orange colour   **RED or ORANGE LESIONS**
Macules, papules, plaques
(Nodules *see* p. 213)

```
        Macule              Papule              Plaque


        Red/purple colour       Orange colour    Red/straw
                                                 coloured
                                                 Fluid filled


Middle age/elderly   Bleeds easily   Children      Lobulated


   CHERRY          PYOGENIC       SPITZ        LYMPHANGIOMA
   ANGIOMA         GRANULOMA      NAEVUS       CIRCUMSCRIPTUM
   (Cambell de
   Morgan spot)

   see p. 315      see p. 334     p. 314          p. 315
```

SPITZ NAEVUS

These look like moles but they are red/orange in colour.
They mainly occur in children. In adults they can be confused
histologically with malignant melanoma. Reassurance that they
are benign is all that is necessary.

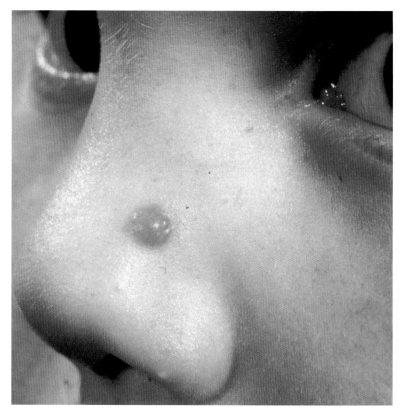

Fig. 9.123 Spitz naevus

CHERRY ANGIOMA (CAMPBELL DE MORGAN SPOT)

These small (1–4 mm) bright-red or purple papules appear on the trunk and proximal limbs in patients over the age of 35. Usually there are multiple lesions. They are a normal finding and do not need to be removed. Viewed through the dermatoscope (*see* p. 18), you can see that they are vascular.

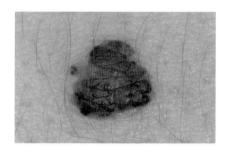

Fig. 9.124 (right) Angioma showing lobulated pattern

LYMPHANGIOMA CIRCUMSCRIPTUM

This is an uncommon malformation of lymphatics. Grouped straw-coloured papules that look like frogspawn are present in the skin. Usually there is some communication between lymphatics and blood vessels so some of the lesions can be red or black. The lesions may remain static or gradually increase in extent over the years.

TREATMENT: LYMPHANGIOMA CIRCUMSCRIPTUM

As well as the visible surface component, there is a deep component (muscular cistern) in the subcutaneous fat. If treatment is required, surgical excision is the treatment of choice but the deep component will have to be removed to prevent recurrence.

If surgical removal is not possible and the lesions get traumatised and leak, then the best thing is to produce a superficial scar over the surface to seal them using a carbon dioxide or Erbium-YAG laser.

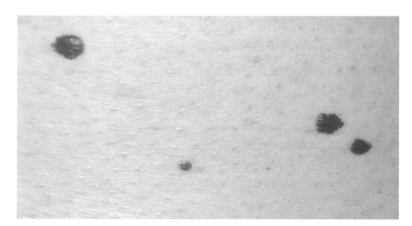

Fig. 9.125 Multiple cherry angiomas

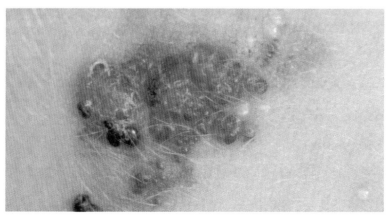

Fig. 9.126 Lymphangioma circumscriptum: close-up of a lesion on the neck

Non-erythematous lesions
Surface warty/papillomatous
Brown, skin coloured
Papules, plaques

WARTY or PAPILLOMATOUS LESIONS

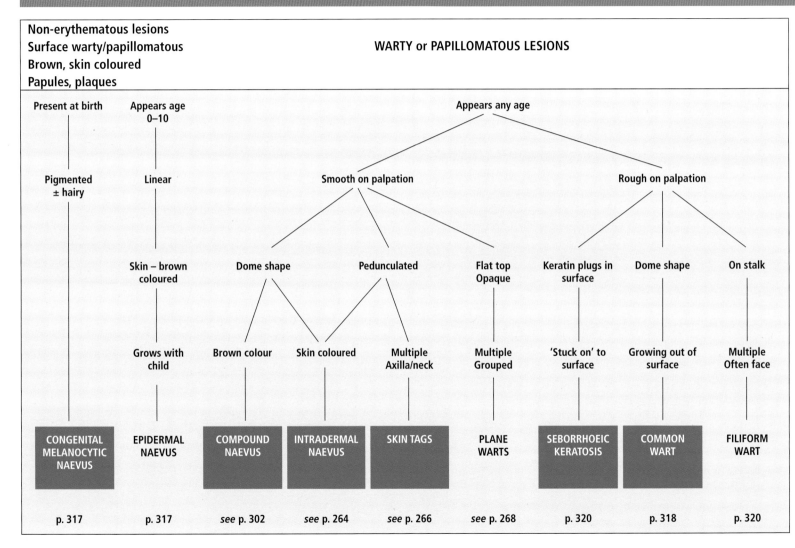

EPIDERMAL NAEVUS

An epidermal naevus is a developmental defect that presents as a skin-coloured or brown linear warty plaque. It often looks like a line of viral warts, but it is present from birth or early childhood. It may be quite small (1–2 cm long) or go down the length of an arm or leg, or in a line around one side of the trunk.

CONGENITAL MELANOCYTIC NAEVUS

Congenital melanocytic naevi, unlike acquired moles, are present at birth. They are usually >2 cm in diameter and are brown with a warty and sometimes hairy surface (*see* also Fig. 9.80, p. 294). Malignant melanoma may arise in congenital naevi, and any growing nodules will need to be biopsied.

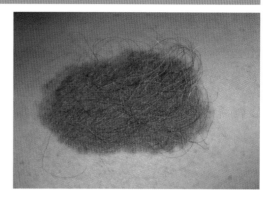

Fig. 9.129 Congenital melanocytic naevus: present from birth and grows with age

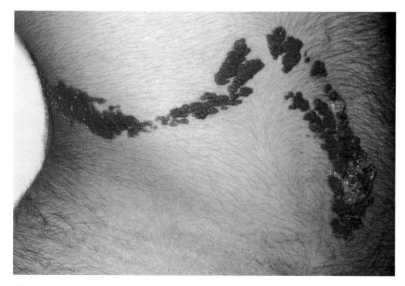

Fig. 9.127 Warty epidermal naevus on side of the trunk

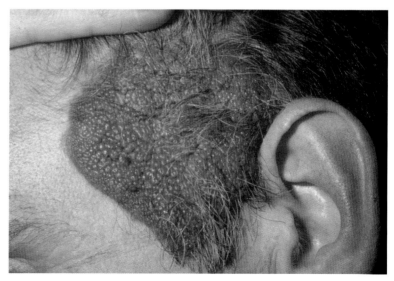

Fig. 9.128 Congenital melanocytic naevus with a papillomatous surface

TREATMENT: CONGENITAL AND EPIDERMAL NAEVI

Small naevi can be excised, although scarring is more prominent in children's skin. Giant naevi are too large to remove surgically. Treatment with a pigment laser may reduce the colour but is unlikely to produce a good cosmetic result, and does not reduce the risk of melanoma.

Surgical removal of epidermal naevi is difficult, especially if the lesion is large. A compromise is to shave and cauterise the superficial component. There is a tendency for the warty papules to regrow but this may take several years.

COMMON WARTS

Warts are an infection of the epidermis with one of the numerous human papilloma viruses. They are transmitted from one individual to another through broken skin (cuts, grazes, and so forth). They disappear spontaneously without scarring after weeks to years (average about 2 years) when the body has built up enough cell-mediated immunity. Unfortunately immunity to one type of wart virus does not confer immunity to any of the others, i.e. having had an infection with the common wart virus does not prevent infection with the plantar wart or plane wart virus.

Common warts are easily recognised as firm, rough, skin-coloured or brown papules with black pinpoint dots on the surface.

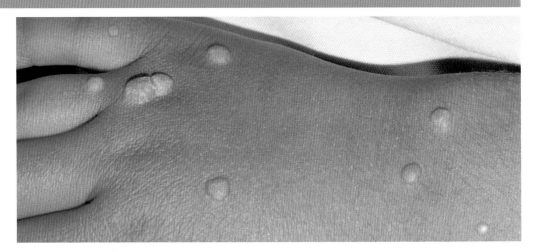

Fig. 9.130 Multiple common warts on the hand

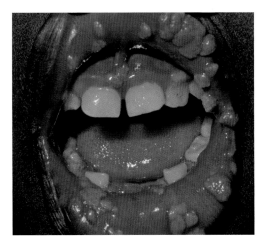

Fig. 9.131 Multiple warts in and around mouth in patient with HIV infection

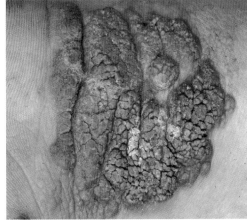

Fig. 9.132 Warts on wrist

TREATMENT: COMMON WARTS

Treatment of warts depends on the age of the patient and how many are present.

In **young children** the best treatment is to leave alone. You will need to explain to parents that they are a viral infection that will resolve spontaneously.

For **older children** and **adults**, if there is a *single wart or only a few warts* the options are as follows.

- Cryotherapy. First pare down any hyperkeratosis on the surface and then freeze with liquid nitrogen until the wart and a halo of normal skin goes white (10–30 seconds). The patient should get a blister at the site within 48 hours as the epidermis that contains the wart lifts off. It is important that the treatment is repeated every 2–3 weeks until the wart goes. Do not use several freeze–thaw cycles, as you may get necrosis of the underlying skin. Large warts (>5 mm) diameter *do not* respond well to cryotherapy.
- Curettage and cautery under local anaesthetic is very effective and should result in clearance immediately. This is a very good treatment for single warts on the face and elsewhere.

For *multiple warts* the options are:
- leave alone and await natural resolution
- a keratolytic agent (salicyclic + lactic acid) – apply at night before going to bed; pare down any excess keratin before the agent is applied, and cover with a plaster unless it contains a collodian gel that sets; this should be carried out for several weeks to months; you should remind the patient that keratolytic agents do not cure warts themselves; any effect is probably secondary as an adjunct to the development of natural immunity
- 20% podophylline applied at night – this is brown and unsightly
- 5% imiquimod cream applied three times a week for 12 weeks – use a keratolytic agent first to reduce surface keratin to allow better penetration of the imiquimod
- pulsed dye laser – this results in coagulation of the blood vessels within the wart; a single shot of 8 joules/cm is given to each wart; treatment is expensive but in many cases two or three treatments will be effective.

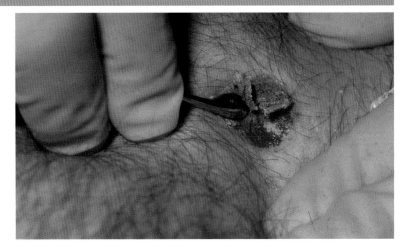

Fig. 9.133 Curettage of a wart using a Volkmann spoon, which allows blunt dissection of the wart off the skin: the base is cauterised and curetted twice

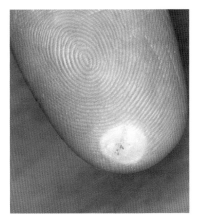

Fig. 9.134 Wart treated with liquid nitrogen showing halo of frozen normal skin

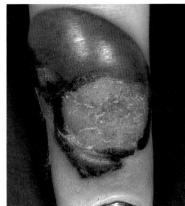

Fig. 9.135 Blister after treatment with liquid nitrogen

FILIFORM WARTS

These are warts with long finger-like protrusions. They occur around the eyelids, on the nose, lips and beard area.

TREATMENT: FILIFORM WARTS

For single or few lesions curettage and cautery under local anaesthetic is the treatment of choice. Cryotherapy is also effective. For multiple warts in the beard area, frizzle them up with a hyfrecator.

SEBORRHOEIC KERATOSIS/WART (BASAL CELL PAPILLOMA)

These very common lesions have a flat but warty surface, and typically look as if they are 'stuck on' to the skin. Sometimes small keratin cysts can be seen in the surface (*see* Fig. 9.97, p. 301). These can be black or white in colour and easily visualised through a dermatoscope (*see* Fig. 1.95, p. 18). Initially seborrhoeic keratoses are skin coloured and not very noticeable, but gradually become more prominent and deepen in colour from light brown to jet black. They are usually multiple and occur most commonly on the face and trunk of middle-aged or elderly people. They are usually easy to diagnose but their appearance late in life, the black or brown colour and the increase in size are all features that cause alarm to the patient. Occasionally they may become inflamed, particularly if they have been caught in clothing and partly torn off (*see* Fig. 9.165).

They need to be distinguished from moles, solar keratoses, and occasionally from pigmented basal cell carcinomas and malignant melanomas. Moles (melanocytic naevi) are more dome shaped and do not have the 'stuck on' appearance, while solar keratoses are rough to palpation, being felt more easily than seen. Basal cell carcinoma has a more shiny surface and a rolled edge with telangiectasia running over it, while a malignant melanoma has an irregular edge, colour variation and does not look as if it is 'stuck on' to the surface.

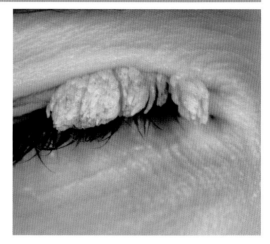

Fig. 9.136 Filiform warts on eyelid

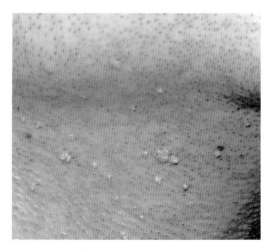

Fig. 9.137 Filiform warts on the beard area

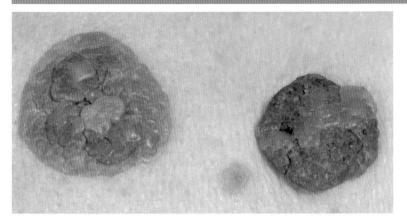

Fig. 9.138 Seborrhoeic keratoses: note the variation in colour (left lesion) and small keratin cysts within the lesion on the right

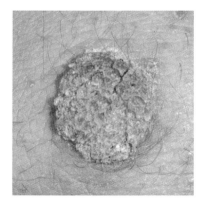

Fig. 9.139 Seborrhoeic keratosis: non-pigmented lesion with papillomatous surface

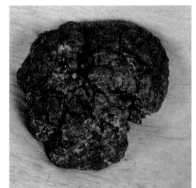

Fig. 9.140 Seborrhoeic keratosis: deeply pigmented lesion – might be confused with a malignant melanoma, but 'stuck on' to surface and with papillomatous surface

TREATMENT: SEBORRHOEIC KERATOSIS

Most lesions require no treatment. Unsightly lesions on the face and trunk can be removed by curettage and cautery under local anaesthesia or by freezing with liquid nitrogen.

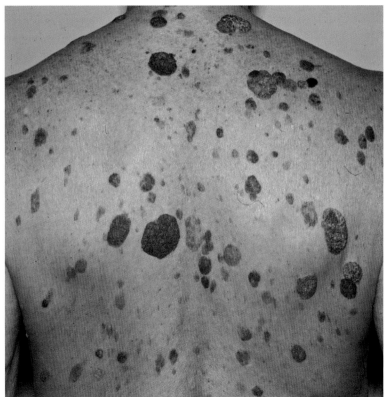

Fig. 9.141 Multiple seborrhoeic keratoses on the back

Non-erythematous lesions
Surface scaly or keratin
Papules, patches, plaques
Multiple (more than five) lesions/rash

SCALE or KERATIN: MULTIPLE LESIONS or DRY SKIN

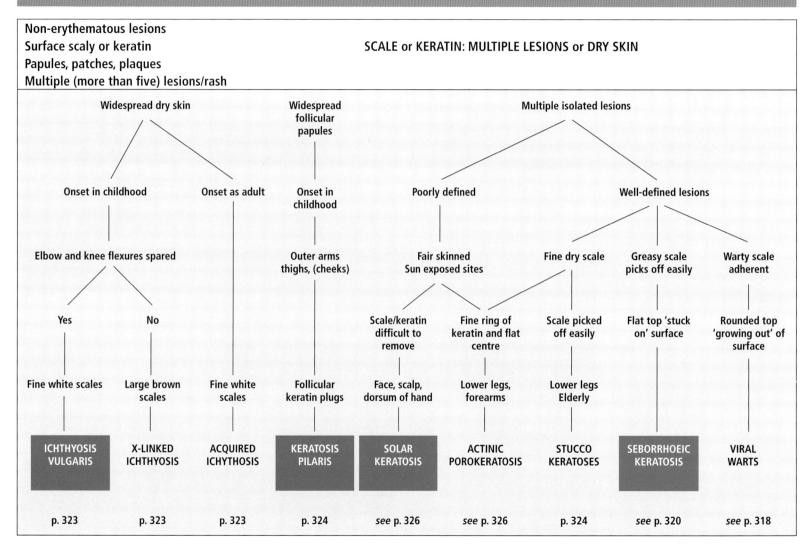

Widespread dry skin

- Onset in childhood
  - Elbow and knee flexures spared
    - Yes
      - Fine white scales
        - **ICHTHYOSIS VULGARIS** — p. 323
    - No
      - Large brown scales
        - **X-LINKED ICHTHYOSIS** — p. 323
- Onset as adult
  - Fine white scales
    - **ACQUIRED ICHYTHOSIS** — p. 323

Widespread follicular papules

- Onset in childhood
  - Outer arms thighs, (cheeks)
    - Follicular keratin plugs
      - **KERATOSIS PILARIS** — p. 324

Multiple isolated lesions

- Poorly defined
  - Fair skinned Sun exposed sites
    - Scale/keratin difficult to remove
      - Face, scalp, dorsum of hand
        - **SOLAR KERATOSIS** — see p. 326
    - Fine ring of keratin and flat centre
      - Lower legs, forearms
        - **ACTINIC POROKERATOSIS** — see p. 326
- Well-defined lesions
  - Fine dry scale
    - Scale picked off easily
      - Lower legs Elderly
        - **STUCCO KERATOSES** — p. 324
  - Greasy scale picks off easily
    - Flat top 'stuck on' surface
      - **SEBORRHOEIC KERATOSIS** — see p. 320
  - Warty scale adherent
    - Rounded top 'growing out' of surface
      - **VIRAL WARTS** — see p. 318

ICHTHYOSIS VULGARIS

This is a genetic disorder transmitted as an autosomal dominant trait. It is first noticed at or soon after birth. The skin is dry with small fine white scales, affecting the whole of the skin except the antecubital and popliteal fossae. There are increased skin markings on the palms and soles (*see* Fig. 8.85, p. 237), and some individuals will also have keratosis pilaris and atopic eczema. The patient will complain of the appearance and the associated itching. It often improves in the sun and with increasing age.

Acquired ichthyosis is clinically similar to ichthyosis vulgaris but occurs later in life. It may be idiopathic or due to an underlying lymphoma.

X-LINKED ICHTHYOSIS

This is transmitted by an X-linked recessive gene, so appears in boys but is transmitted though females. It is much less common than ichthyosis vulgaris, from which is distinguished by the fact that the scales are large and dirty brown in colour and the flexures are involved. Sunshine does not help and it does not usually improve with age.

TREATMENT: ICHTHYOSIS

Since central heating tends to dry out the skin, this should be kept to a minimum and if the weather is cold and the humidity low, then this needs to be increased with a humidifier.

Add a capful of one of the proprietary dispersible bath oils to the bath water (*see* Table 2.01b, p. 27) and stay in the bath for 15 minutes a day. Wash with Dermol 500[UK] or Epaderm[UK] ointment instead of soap, because soap removes the natural grease and makes the skin even drier.

After getting out of the bath, while the skin is moist and warm, apply a greasy moisturiser. There is a wide range available. Some contain keratolytic agents such as urea (Aquadrate[UK], Calmurid[UK], Calmol[USA]), salicylic or lactic acid, which also help remove the excess keratin (*see* Table 2.01a, pp. 26).

Severe cases may be improved by systemic retinoids such as acitretin 10–25 mg/day (*see* p. 49). These are available only from a dermatologist.

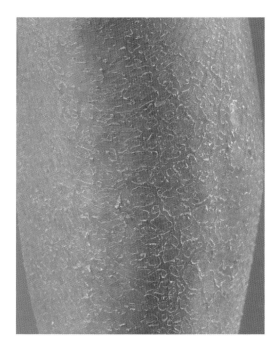

Fig. 9.142 Ichthyosis vulgaris: fine white scale

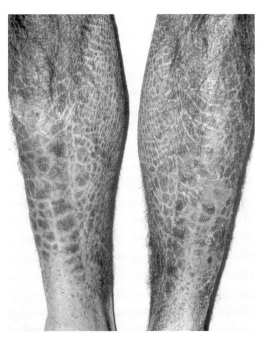

Fig. 9.143 X-linked ichthyosis: large dark scales

KERATOSIS PILARIS

This is such a common condition in childhood and adolescence that it can be regarded as one end of the normal spectrum of skin changes. Many patients will not notice it or complain about it. It often improves spontaneously in the summer. Skin-coloured follicular papules develop on the cheeks, the upper arms and thighs. Sometimes the papules are red rather than skin coloured. It may be associated with ichthyosis vulgaris or atopic eczema, and is often familial (*see* also p. 115).

TREATMENT: KERATOSIS PILARIS

If treatment is required, a topical keratolytic agent can be applied: 10% urea cream (Calmurid) or 2% salicylic acid ointment put on once or twice a day will not cure it but will remove the rough surface temporarily and make it feel more comfortable.

STUCCO KERATOSES

This is a term used to describe multiple fine scaly papules scattered over the lower legs in some elderly people. The lesions are seborrhoeic keratoses. They may improve by applying a urea or lactic acid based moisturiser such as Calmurid cream.

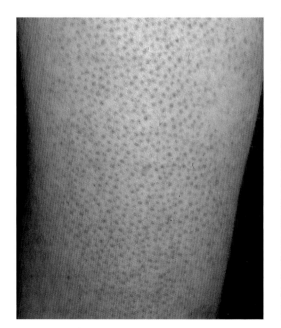

Fig. 9.144 Keratosis pilaris on upper arm: rough follicular pink papules on upper arm of young girl

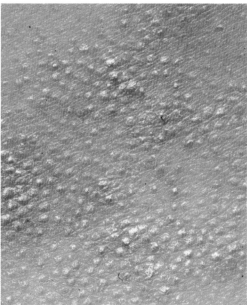

Fig. 9.145 Keratosis pilaris: close-up of follicular plugs

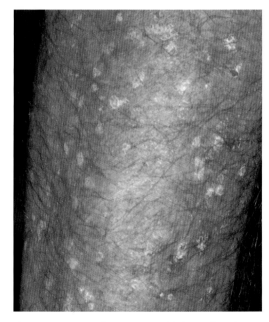

Fig. 9.146 Stucco keratoses: multiple small scaly papules on lower legs

Face, trunk and limbs
Non-erythematous lesions
Scale, keratin surface
Papules and nodules
Single/few (<5) lesions

SCALE/KERATIN – single/few lesions

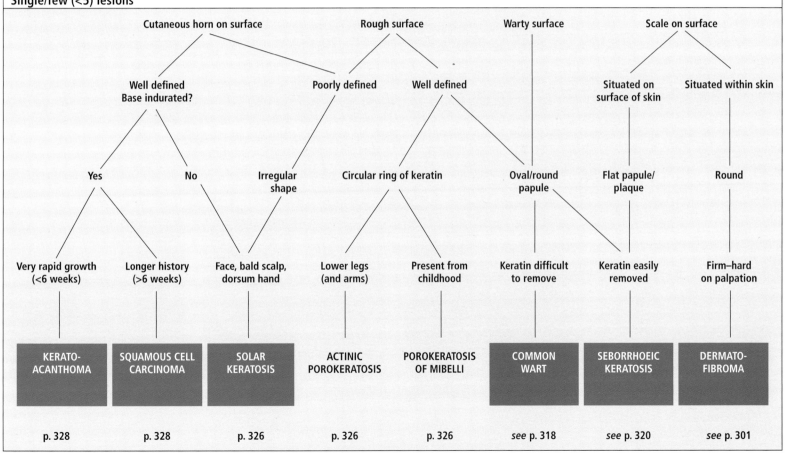

ACTINIC POROKERATOSIS

This is problem on the lower legs and forearms mainly in women. Numerous small (5 mm), round, slightly scaly macules are seen. All have a raised edge like a thread of cotton stretched around, which can be more easily seen if illuminated from the side. The lesions are caused by chronic sun exposure. Usually the patient only notices the lesions when they itch or become erythematous in the sun. Similar but larger lesions called **porokeratosis of Mibelli** can occur in childhood.

TREATMENT: ACTINIC POROKERATOSIS

If they are symptomless it is best to leave them alone, although the patient should be encouraged to wear long-sleeved shirts and trousers to prevent further sun exposure. Treatment options include cryotherapy, 5-FU cream, retinoic acid cream or a vitamin D_3 analogue, but none are particularly effective.

SOLAR (ACTINIC) KERATOSES

A **cutaneous horn** is a keratotic outgrowth from the skin (*see* Fig. 9.150). At its base will be a solar keratosis, Bowen's disease or squamous cell carcinoma.

Solar keratoses are rough, scaly papules on chronically sun-exposed skin. They are most commonly seen on the bald scalp, face and dorsum of the hands and forearms in patients over the age of 50 who have fair skin and other evidence of sun damage (*see* p. 287). Generally they are more easily felt than seen due to the roughness of the abnormal keratin. The surrounding skin may be normal or pink/red. Sometimes scaling is not present and the lesion is just a fixed pink macule (*see* p. 112). Seborrhoeic warts may look similar but are not so rough to the touch, and are generally more easily seen than felt.

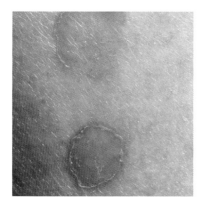

Fig. 9.147 Porokeratosis: close-up of lesions, note collar of scale

Fig. 9.148 Solar keratoses: these are more easily felt than seen

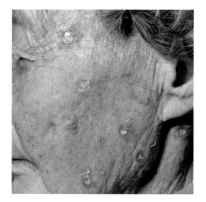

Fig. 9.149 Multiple solar keratoses: more obvious lesions than in Fig. 9.148.

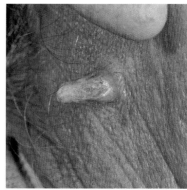

Fig. 9.150 Cutaneous horn below the earlobe

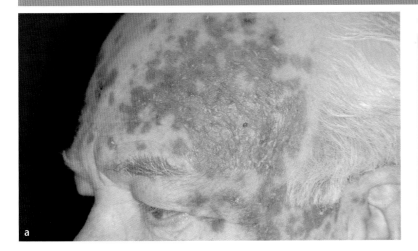

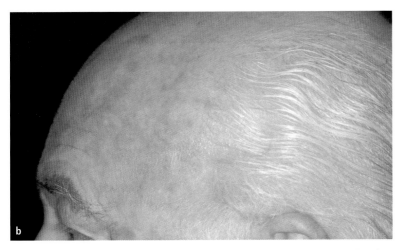

Fig. 9.151 (a) Solar keratoses treated with 5-fluorouracil cream for 4 weeks: this is the reaction to expect at the end of the treatment; (b) same patient 1 month later, after the inflammation has settled down

TREATMENT: SOLAR KERATOSIS

A **single or a few lesions** can be treated with the following.
- The treatment of choice is cryotherapy. You should freeze them just enough to cause a blister at the dermo-epidermal junction. This is done by freezing the lesion until a 2 mm halo of normal skin goes white around it (5–10 seconds). Warn the patient that he or she will develop a blister and that it will crust and drop off after 7–10 days.
- 0.5% 5-fluorouracil (5-FU) and 10% salicylic acid solution (Actikerall) painted on daily for up to 12 weeks is a useful alternative if cryotherapy is not available.
- If there is any doubt over the diagnosis or you suspect a squamous cell carcinoma, remove the lesion by excision and send for histology.

Large numbers of solar keratoses can be treated with the following.
- 5% 5-fluorouracil (Efudix) cream: this is applied twice a day for 4 weeks. You can treat just local areas or the whole of the bald scalp and/or face. Not a lot will be seen for the first 2 weeks, but over the second 2 weeks the area will become inflamed and sore. At the end of 4 weeks all the solar keratoses (even ones not clinically apparent) will be red and eroded (*see* Fig. 9.151a). 1% hydrocortisone cream can then be applied for a further week to settle the inflammatory reaction down (*see* Fig. 9.151b). The effectiveness of 5-FU therapy may be increased by using 0.05% isotretinoin gel for the first 1–2 weeks as well as the 5-FU. Patients who cannot cope with the severe reaction to 5-FU can use it twice a day on 2 days/week for 2 months instead (2,2,2 regimen). This produces less inflammation but is probably less effective.
- Photodynamic therapy: 5% methyl aminolaevulinic ester (Metvix) is applied to affected skin and irradiated 3 hours later with a red light source for 12 minutes. The Metvix is preferentially taken up by solar keratoses. Treatment is repeated after 1 week (*see* p. 63).
- 5% imiquimod (Aldara) cream applied three times a week for 12 weeks: the skin will look inflamed but does not hurt as it does after 5-FU cream (*see* Fig. 9.72b, p. 291).
- 3% diclofenac (Solaraze) gel applied twice a day: this results in less of a reaction than 5FU but is also less effective. It needs to be applied for 2–3 months.
- Chemical peels using glycolic or trichloroacetic acid: a single application of 35% trichloroacetic acid (Jessner's solution) produces a severe reaction like 5-FU.
- Carbon dioxide or Erbium-YAG laser (two to three passes) will remove the epidermis and allow regeneration from the residual follicles.

KERATOACANTHOMA

A rapidly growing benign tumour occurring on sun exposed skin. It grows fast for about 3 months, reaching a size of up to 3 cm in diameter. It then regresses spontaneously and should have disappeared within 6 months. It has a symmetrical configuration with an erythematous or translucent circumference and a horny volcano-like centre. It looks a bit like a basal cell carcinoma but it grows too quickly, and a basal cell carcinoma has crust rather than keratin in the centre. A well-differentiated squamous cell carcinoma tends to be more irregular in shape, slower growing and does not regress spontaneously.

TREATMENT: KERATOACANTHOMA

If the patient is prepared to wait, the lesion will resolve spontaneously. In most instances it is best removed either by excision or curettage and cautery, as it is not always possible to be certain that it is not a squamous cell carcinoma.

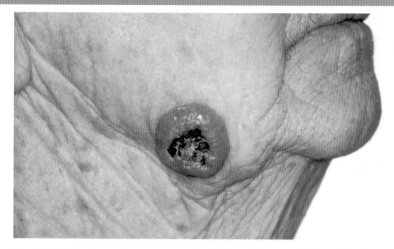

Fig. 9.152 Keratoacanthoma: symmetrical lesion with central plug of keratin

SQUAMOUS CELL CARCINOMA (WELL DIFFERENTIATED)

A squamous cell carcinoma is a tumour of keratin producing cells. Well differentiated tumours produce keratin on the surface like a solar keratosis, but as they are invasive into the dermis they have a thickened or indurated base. Basal cells do not produce keratin, so a basal cell carcinoma will not have a hyperkeratotic surface. Squamous cell carcinomas grow more rapidly than basal cell carcinomas, but both will tend to ulcerate as they get bigger. Tumours on the scalp, ears and lower lip are squamous cell carcinomas until proved otherwise. Squamous cell carcinomas are differentiated from a solar keratosis by being indurated (thickened) at the base, or becoming ulcerated or tender on palpation. Any of these signs are an indication for a biopsy or removal (*see* p. 332).

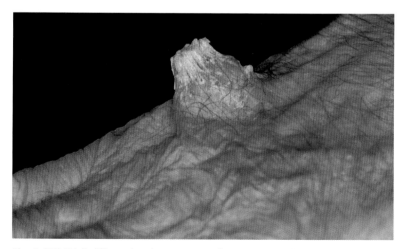

Fig. 9.153 Well-differentiated squamous cell carcinoma with keratotic surface and thickened base

Face, trunk and limbs
Non-erythematous lesions
Papules, plaques, nodules
Single/few (<5) fixed lesions
(Multiple [>5] lesions/rash variable in site and time, *see* p. 245)

CRUST / ULCERATED / BLEEDING SURFACE

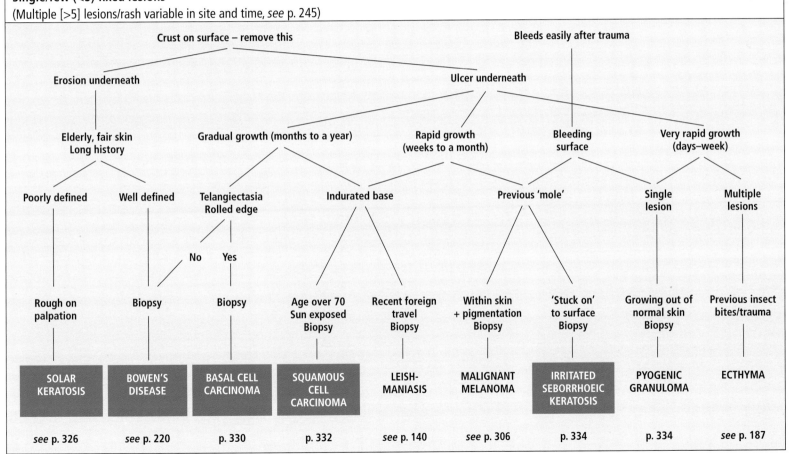

SOLAR KERATOSIS	BOWEN'S DISEASE	BASAL CELL CARCINOMA	SQUAMOUS CELL CARCINOMA	LEISH-MANIASIS	MALIGNANT MELANOMA	IRRITATED SEBORRHOEIC KERATOSIS	PYOGENIC GRANULOMA	ECTHYMA
see p. 326	*see* p. 220	p. 330	p. 332	*see* p. 140	*see* p. 306	p. 334	p. 334	*see* p. 187

BASAL CELL CARCINOMA (RODENT ULCER)

This is the commonest malignant tumour of the skin. It usually occurs in middle-aged or elderly fair-skinned individuals who have worked at out of doors all their lives, or who have spent a lot of time gardening, fishing, sailing, and so forth. Although due to sun damage, they do not occur at the sites of maximum sun exposure, i.e. rarely on the bald scalp, lower lip or dorsum of the hands. Most occur on the face, some on the trunk and limbs.

There are three growth patterns. A **nodular** basal cell carcinoma starts as a small translucent (pearly) papule with obvious telangiectasia over the surface. It gradually increases in size either to form a nodule or sideways to produce the classic rolled edge. The centre may then ulcerate and form surface crust. Growth is very slow – some may reach a diameter of 1 cm only after 5 years. If there is any doubt over the diagnosis, stretch the skin and you will see the raised rolled edge, like a piece of string around the edge.

In a **superficial** basal cell carcinoma the growth is along the base of the epidermis, and

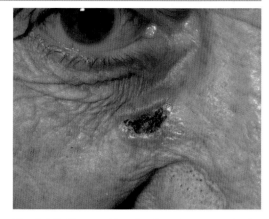

Fig. 9.156 Ulcerated basal cell carcinoma on cheek with typical rolled edge

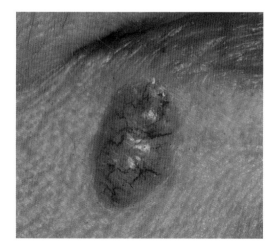

Fig. 9.154 Typical nodular basal cell carcinoma with telangiectasia over the edge

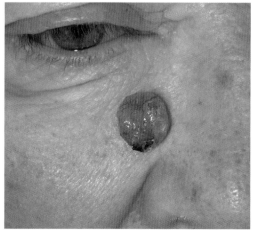

Fig. 9.155 Ulcerated nodular basal call carcinoma with telangiectasia over the edge

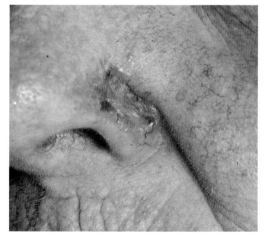

Fig. 9.157 Basal cell carcinoma in nasolabial fold, a common site – will need Mohs surgery

presents more as a scaly plaque (*see* p. 220). It may become quite large (>1–2 cm diameter).

A **morphoeic** or infiltrating basal cell carcinoma has fine strands of tumour cells infiltrating into the dermis. These may be difficult to diagnose early because they present like a scar with an indistinct border. Sometimes the lesion may be quite extensive without obvious surface features. Resection by Mohs surgery where the margins can be assessed histologically is recommended.

Pigmented basal cell carcinomas are the same as nodular basal cell carcinomas except for the increased melanin pigment (*see* Fig. 9.112) which makes differentiation from a malignant melanoma difficult (*see* p. 309). If you look carefully and put the skin on the stretch, the typical rolled edge is usually present.

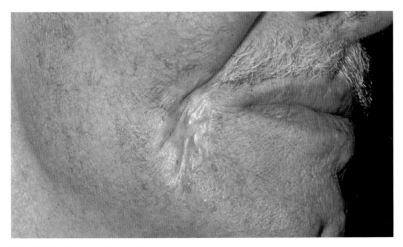

Fig. 9.158 Morphoeic basal cell carcinoma at angle of jaw – will need Mohs surgery

TREATMENT: BASAL CELL CARCINOMA

1. Local excision with a 2–4 mm margin is the treatment of choice. If the lesion is completely excised recurrence is unlikely (<5%).
2. Mohs micrographic surgery (*see* Fig. 9.159): removal of the lesion and assessment of the peripheral and deep margins by frozen section results in recurrence rates of less than 1%. Since this process is time consuming and requires the assistance of a pathology technician, Mohs surgery should be restricted to:
   - central facial lesions in those requiring a skin flap or graft
   - recurrent lesions (especially after radiotherapy) on the face
   - lesions with indistinct margins
   - morphoeic (infiltrating) basal cell carcinoma.
3. Curettage and cautery has a higher recurrence rate than excision but is useful in elderly patients with multiple tumours or when there are multiple lesions on the trunk. The lesion is curetted out and the margin cauterised for 1 mm around. This is repeated three times to give a 3 mm margin. The subsequent wound will heal by secondary intention over a period of 2–4 weeks. This should be cleaned daily with damp cotton wool and a topical antibiotic ointment applied.
4. Radiotherapy is only indicated when surgery is inappropriate, e.g. large lesions in the elderly. Ten daily fractions of 3.75Gy are given. If the patient is very frail, the time between fractions can be increased, e.g. 10 fractions are given over 10 weeks. This will cause virtually no local reaction and will be much more pleasant for the patient.
5. Topical imiquimod (Aldara) cream works for superficial basal cell carcinomas on the trunk and limbs. The cream is applied to lesions three times a week for 12 weeks (*see* pp. 34 and 291).
6. Photodynamic therapy is useful if the patient has numerous tumours. A photosensitiser is applied and this is irradiated with a red light source (*see* p. 63).
7. Cryotherapy is not recommended, since the recurrence rate is unacceptably high.
8. Vismodegib, an orally active small molecule inhibitor of the 'hedgehog pathway' can sometimes be used to reduce tumour bulk in inoperable basal cell carcinomas (*see* p. 57).

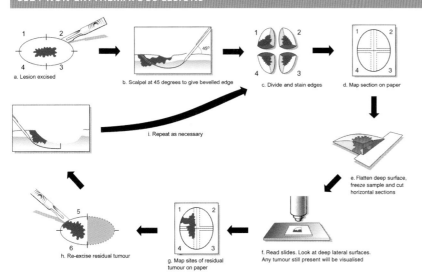

a. The tumour is debulked using a curette or Volkmann spoon.

b. The debulked tumour is completely removed by bevelling the angle of the scalpel at 45°.

c. The removed tissue is divided into half or quarter sections and the edges stained.

d. The sections are numbered and colour of edges recorded on a map.

e. The sections are flattened, inverted and mounted on a cryostat chuck, and sections cut.

f. These sections are read.

g. The presence of any tumour is marked on the map. This indicates the exact site of any residual tumour.

h. The residual tumour is resected and steps c–g repeated.

i. When the final reading shows no tumour in the sections, then full clearance of the basal cell carcinoma has been achieved, and the defect can be repaired.

Fig. 9.159 How Mohs surgery is carried out (adapted with permission from Rook A. *et al. Textbook of Dermatology*, Blackwell Science)

SQUAMOUS CELL CARCINOMA

Squamous cell carcinoma arises from previously normal (sun-damaged) skin or from a pre-existing lesion such as a solar keratosis or Bowen's disease. A well-differentiated squamous cell carcinoma can be distinguished from a basal cell carcinoma by the production of keratin (*see* Fig. 9.153) and its faster growth (it may grow to 1–2 cm in diameter over a few months). They occur at sites of maximum sun exposure, on a bald head, the lower lip, cheeks, nose, top of earlobes and dorsum of hands and in the elderly (usually over 70). There is always other evidence of sun damage such as solar elastosis (*see* p. 287) and solar keratoses (*see* p. 326). Poorly differentiated squamous cell carcinomas tend to ulcerate (*see* Fig. 9.160), and be may be covered with crust. The edge of the ulcer is craggy and indurated, while the base bleeds easily. On the scalp the crust may become matted down with hair, which will hide a pus-filled ulcer (*see* Fig. 9.162).

Squamous cell carcinomas can also occur on non-sun-exposed skin – at sites of previous radiotherapy, or in chronic scars such as in old burn scars, osteomyelitis, lupus vulgaris or leg ulcers.

The prognosis of squamous cell carcinoma depends on several factors:
- size of lesion >2 cm diameter
- depth of invasion >4 mm or Clark level IV (reticular dermis)
- poorly differentiated cell type
- immunosuppression
- perineural invasion
- site: lip, ear, non-sun exposed
- recurrent lesions.

The presence of two or more of these factors indicate a high-risk tumour. None of these factors suggest low risk.

TREATMENT: SQUAMOUS CELL CARCINOMA

- **Low-risk** lesions: excise the lesion with a 4 mm margin of normal skin around it.
- **High-risk** lesions: these require a 6 mm margin. Lesions in patients under 70 years age around the central face should have their margins checked by frozen section (Mohs surgery, *see* p. 332).

Most cutaneous lesions do not spread so the prognosis is excellent, but always check the regional lymph nodes.

Radiotherapy is a possibility for primary lesions in the very elderly who cannot tolerate surgery, or when the lesion is too large to remove surgically. Ten daily fractions of 3.75Gy work well. Electrons rather than superficial X-rays are useful on the ear and nose, as they are less likely to damage the cartilage.

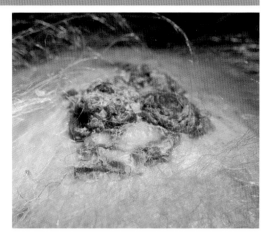

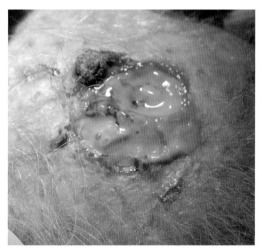

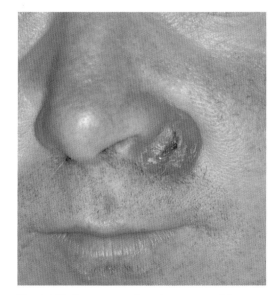

Fig. 9.160 Squamous cell carcinoma: a rapidly growing nodule in 40-year-old patient that needed Mohs surgery to remove

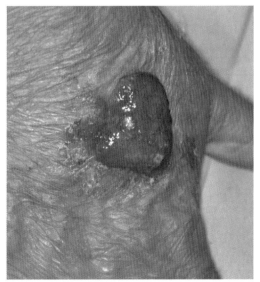

Fig. 9.161 Squamous cell carcinoma: typical ulcerated nodule on dorsum of hand of elderly patient

Fig. 9.162 Crusting on scalp of elderly patient (top): always remove the crust to see what is underneath; in this case an ulcer was present (below) which on biopsy showed a squamous cell carcinoma

PYOGENIC GRANULOMA

This is due to a localised overgrowth of blood vessels in response to trauma, often a graze or a prick. There is very rapid growth over a few weeks, and usually a history of the lesion having bled spontaneously at some stage. The lesion is round in shape, bright red or purple in colour, and the surrounding skin will be quite normal. In contrast an amelanotic malignant melanoma is usually irregular in shape, has some surrounding pigmentation and grows over a period of months rather than days or weeks.

Kaposi's sarcoma can also ulcerate but there will be other lesions elsewhere.

TREATMENT: PYOGENIC GRANULOMA

The best treatment is curettage and cautery under local anaesthetic. Sometimes there is quite a large blood vessel at the base but cautery will eventually seal this. **Always send the lesion for histology.**

IRRITATED SEBORRHOEIC KERATOSIS

A seborrhoeic keratosis (*see* p. 320) may be caught in clothing, half torn off and become red and inflamed. It may then be easily mistaken for a melanoma. The lesion usually has the 'stuck on' appearance of the original lesion, but will have surrounding erythema rather than pigmentation. If the diagnosis is in doubt, it should be removed for histological examination

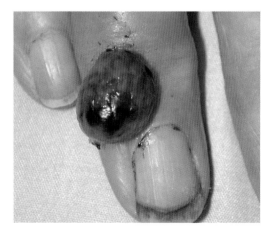

Fig. 9.163 Pyogenic granuloma: rapidly growing red papule that bleeds after trauma; normal surrounding skin

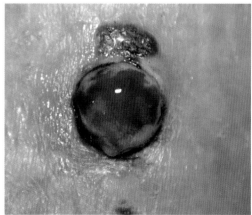

Fig. 9.164 Nodular malignant melanoma: note pigment at edge of the lesion

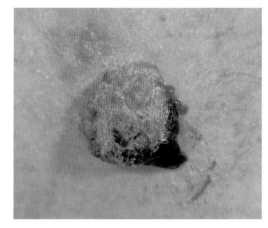

Fig. 9.165 Irritated seborrhoeic keratosis: it has been caught in clothing and partially torn off, hence the bleeding; lesion sits on surface, normal skin around

Flexures

Axilla, groin, natal cleft, sub-mammary folds

10

Flexures
Erythematous lesions
Papules, patches and plaques

ERYTHEMATOUS RASH

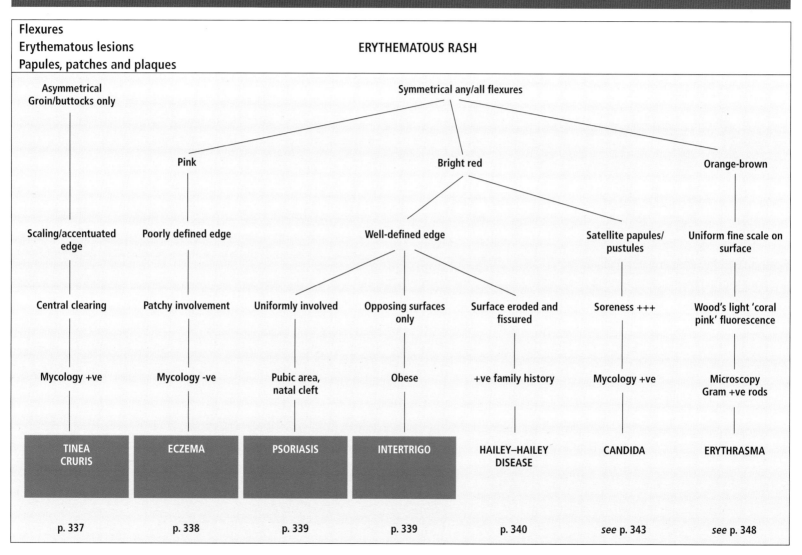

Asymmetrical Groin/buttocks only		Symmetrical any/all flexures		

Pink — Bright red — Orange-brown

Scaling/accentuated edge — Poorly defined edge — Well-defined edge — Satellite papules/ pustules — Uniform fine scale on surface

Central clearing — Patchy involvement — Uniformly involved — Opposing surfaces only — Surface eroded and fissured — Soreness +++ — Wood's light 'coral pink' fluorescence

Mycology +ve — Mycology -ve — Pubic area, natal cleft — Obese — +ve family history — Mycology +ve — Microscopy Gram +ve rods

TINEA CRURIS — **ECZEMA** — **PSORIASIS** — **INTERTRIGO** — HAILEY–HAILEY DISEASE — CANDIDA — ERYTHRASMA

p. 337 — p. 338 — p. 339 — p. 339 — p. 340 — *see* p. 343 — *see* p. 348

TINEA CRURIS

Flexural tinea only occurs in the groin; it does not involve the axillae or sub-mammary folds. It is caused by the same organisms that cause tinea pedis, i.e. *Trichophyton mentagrophytes*, *Trichophyton rubrum* or *Epidermophyton floccosum*.

Infection is nearly always from the patient's own feet, and men are affected more often than women. The rash starts in the fold of the groin and gradually spreads outwards and down the thigh. The leading edge is scaly unless treated with topical steroids, when the whole area may become red (tinea incognito). The rash is usually asymmetrical, one side being more involved than the other.

The infection may also involve the buttocks and back of thighs. The genitalia, including the scrotum, are never involved. It may be difficult to differentiate between eczema and tinea of the groin,

especially if partially treated. Eczema is usually symmetrical and tinea is usually unilateral or asymmetrical (unless treated with topical steroids or in someone who is immunocompromised, *see* Fig. 10.02). Always check the mycology if in doubt (*see* p. 20).

TREATMENT: TINEA CRURIS

An imidazole (clotrimazole, econazole, ketoconazole, miconazole or oxiconazole[USA]) cream should be applied to the affected area of the groin (and buttock) and to the toe webs twice a day for 2–3 weeks or until it is clear. Alternatively, use terbinafine (Lamisil) cream for 7–10 days. Almost all groin infections have been acquired from the patient's own feet, so the feet must always be examined and treated at the same time if they are involved.

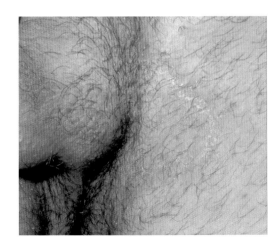

Fig. 10.01 Tinea cruris: rash in one groin only, with obvious scaly edge

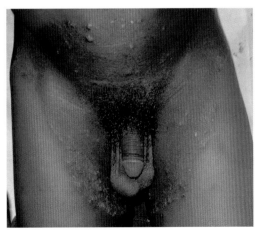

Fig. 10.02 Tinea cruris: note extensive symmetrical rash in a patient with HIV infection

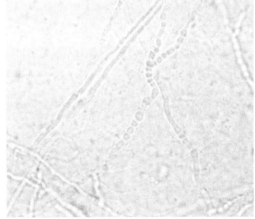

Fig. 10.03 Dermatophyte fungal hyphae on direct microscopy

FLEXURAL ECZEMA

Eczema in the flexures looks like eczema elsewhere – a poorly defined pink (scaly) rash that is usually symmetrical. The eczema may be localised to only the flexures or it may be part of seborrhoeic eczema elsewhere. Contact dermatitis in the **axillae** may be due to irritants (depilatories, deodorants) or allergens. Deodorants cause a rash in the centre of the axilla; dyes and resins in clothing cause a rash around the edge of the axilla but spare the vault. Patch testing will distinguish between these, *see* p. 21. Eczema in the groin often also involves the genitalia, which distinguishes it from tinea. Tinea does not occur in other flexures, it is usually unilateral and it does not involve the scrotum. If in doubt, take skin scrapings for mycology, *see* p. 20.

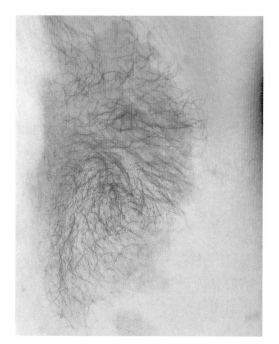

Fig. 10.04 Seborrhoeic eczema in axilla

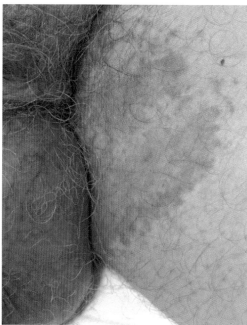

Fig. 10.05 Eczema in groin and on scrotum: this cannot be tinea because of involvement of the scrotum

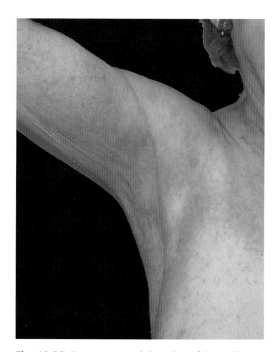

Fig. 10.06 Eczema around the edge of the axilla due to allergic contact dermatitis from resins in clothes

INTERTRIGO

The word 'intertrigo' comes from the Latin word *intertrerere*, meaning to rub together. Intertrigo therefore describes painful, red skin due to two moist surfaces rubbing together. It occurs in the summer months in the flexures of individuals who are too fat, usually in the sub-mammary, lower abdominal and groin folds. Only the areas of skin that are touching are involved. In the summer it is impossible to prevent intertrigo from developing in patients who are overweight, because the sweaty skin surfaces will rub together.

TREATMENT: FLEXURAL ECZEMA AND INTERTRIGO

Use a moderately potent[UK]/group 4–5[USA] topical steroid initially daily, such as 0.05% clobetasone butyrate (Eumovate) or 0.1% hydrocortisone 17-butyrate (Locoid) cream or ointment. For maintenance, use only two to three times a week. The occlusion that naturally occurs in the flexures will increase the potency of the steroid, so avoid strong steroids, as they are likely to cause atrophy and striae. Loss of weight is the only real answer for persistent intertrigo.

PSORIASIS

Psoriasis of the flexures (any flexure) is distinguished from all other rashes by its bright-red colour and well-defined edge. Silvery scaling will not be seen on the moist skin of the flexure, but it may be seen at the very edge of the plaque. Often psoriasis is present elsewhere to confirm the diagnosis. Characteristically the pubic area and natal cleft are involved.

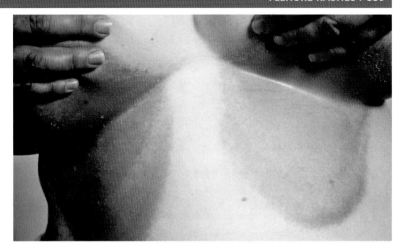

Fig. 10.07 Intertrigo: only skin folds affected

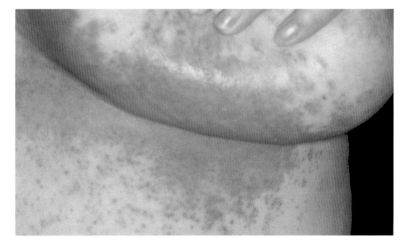

Fig. 10.08 Intertrigo in a patient who also has eczema

TREATMENT: FLEXURAL PSORIASIS

Tar, dithranol and retinoids are likely to make the skin sore in the flexures and on the genitalia, so they should not be used. The vitamin D₃ analogues calcitriol (Silkis) and tacalcitol (Curatoderm) are non-irritant and can be used in flexures twice daily and should be tried first. If they do not help, then you can use a topical steroid. The weakest possible steroid to clear the skin is required, but 1% hydrocortisone is ineffective and not worth trying. Use a moderate^{UK}/group 4–5^{USA} topical steroid such as 0.05% clobetasone butyrate (Eumovate) or 0.1% hydrocortisone 17-butyrate (Locoid) cream or ointment applied twice a day. Do not use topical steroids in the flexures for long periods of time, as steroid atrophy and striae are likely.

HAILEY–HAILEY DISEASE

Also termed chronic benign familial pemphigus, this rare condition is inherited as an autosomal dominant trait. The patient complains of soreness in any of the flexures, and on examination the surface is red and finely fissured (*see* Fig. 10.11). As in pemphigus vulgaris (*see* p. 257), there is an abnormality of cohesion of epidermal cells. This disease typically remits and relapses. It is exacerbated by friction, heat, secondary infection with *Staphylococcus aureus*, *Candida albicans*, or herpes simplex, and by stress. The patient complains of itching, pain and smell. There may be long periods when the patient is entirely asymptomatic, especially in the winter.

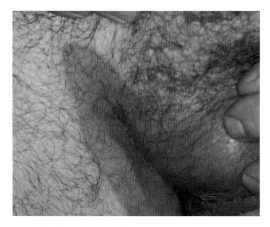

Fig. 10.09 Psoriasis in the groin and on scrotum (*see* also Figs 11.13 and 11.14, p. 360)

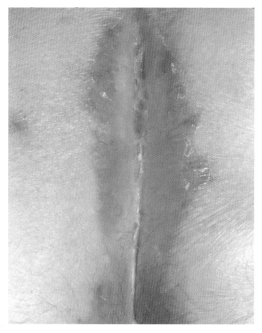

Fig. 10.10 Psoriasis of perianal skin and natal cleft

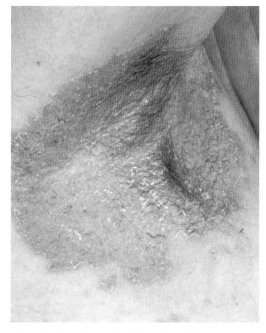

Fig. 10.11 Hailey–Hailey disease in axilla: note erosions, crusting and fine fissures

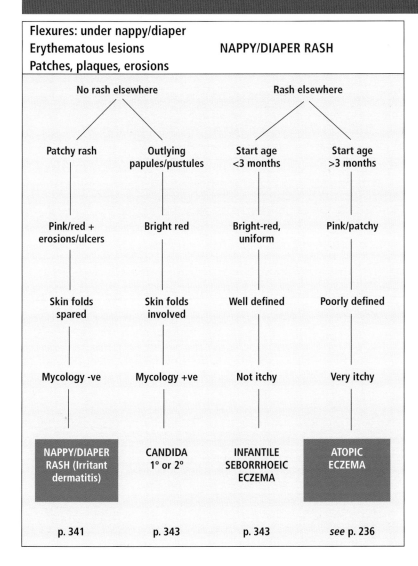

Flexures: under nappy/diaper
Erythematous lesions   NAPPY/DIAPER RASH
Patches, plaques, erosions

TREATMENT: HAILEY–HAILEY DISEASE

If the skin is weeping, wet dressings of aluminium acetate (Burow's solution) or dilute potassium permanganate solution (*see* p. 30) can be applied to the affected areas once or several times a day. Topical steroids are often helpful. Use the weakest possible steroid that is effective so as to reduce the risk of skin atrophy in the flexures. Start with a moderate[UK]/group 4-5[USA] topical steroid bid, and increase the strength when required. Secondary infection should be treated early. Rarely patients may need systemic steroids, methotrexate or superficial X-ray treatment.

NAPPY/DIAPER RASH (CONTACT IRRITANT DERMATITIS)

The common type of nappy/diaper rash is an irritant reaction to urine and faeces held next to the skin under occlusion. Bacteria in the faeces break down urea in urine into ammonia, which is very irritant to the skin. Clinically the rash is patchy and tends to involve the convex skin in contact with the nappy (buttocks, genitalia, thighs) rather than the skin in the folds (*see* Fig. 10.12). In mild cases there is just erythema, but when severe, erosions or even ulcers can develop. The affected area is sore and cleaning or bathing the area produces a lot of discomfort.

TREATMENT: NAPPY/DIAPER RASH

Nappies/diapers should be changed as soon as they are wet or soiled and the skin cleaned and dried. A moisturiser such as zinc and castor oil cream is then applied to the area that is covered by the nappy. If the rash is very bad and does not improve after taking these simple measures, a weak[UK]/group 7[USA] topical steroid such as 1% hydrocortisone ointment can be applied twice daily for a few days to speed things up.

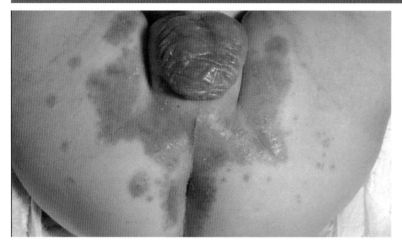

Fig. 10.12 Contact irritant nappy/diaper rash

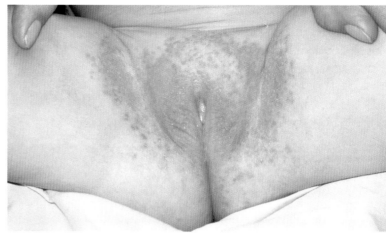

Fig. 10.14 Candidiasis: note bright-red colour with outlying satellite lesions

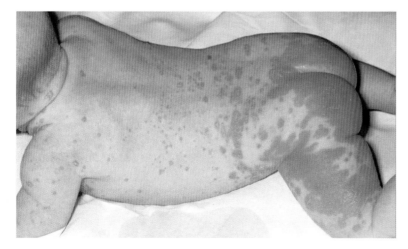

Fig. 10.13 Infantile seborrhoeic dermatitis

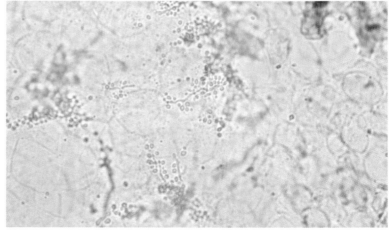

Fig. 10.15 Direct microscopy of *Candida albicans* (spores and short hyphae)

CANDIDIASIS

Candida affecting the skin most often occurs in patients at the extremes of life – babies and old people – but it can occur at any age. There is always a reason for the presence of the pathogenic form of *Candida* and this should be looked for and treated. The commonest causes are:

- broad-spectrum antibiotics
- contraceptive pill
- diabetes
- iron deficiency
- obesity
- pregnancy
- immunosuppression – AIDS, systemic steroids, cytotoxic drugs, cancer.

It affects **all the flexures** (axillae, groins, sub-mammary area, toe webs) and is usually symmetrical. The rash is bright red, and the key feature is that outlying papules or pustules occur around the main rash (*see* Fig. 10.14). In addition, the skin is sore rather than itchy, a feature that may help distinguish it from psoriasis or tinea cruris.

Scrapings taken from the edge of the lesions can be examined under the microscope (*see* Fig. 10.15) for spores and hyphae, or cultured to prove the diagnosis. It is important to do this, because flexural rashes are often assumed to be 'fungal' without any evidence.

TREATMENT: CANDIDIASIS

Take scrapings for mycology before treatment, as treatment 'failure' may be due to the misdiagnosis of eczema or intertrigo as candida. Look for predisposing factors and treat these.

An imidazole cream twice daily is most convenient for the patient. In women, if the pubic area or groin is involved also treat the vagina with a single clotrimazole 500 mg pessary, or a single oral dose of fluconazole 150 mg. Involvement of the perianal skin will necessitate oral treatment with nystatin tablets (100 000 units) qid for 5 days to clear the gut. Oral nystatin is not absorbed from the gut, so is not useful for *Candida* infection elsewhere.

Alternative oral treatments are itraconazole 200 mg for 7 days or fluconazole 50 mg daily for 2 weeks.

INFANTILE SEBORRHOEIC DERMATITIS (NAPKIN PSORIASIS)

Infants under 3 months of age may develop an eruption that starts in the nappy/diaper area but later spreads to involve the scalp, face and trunk. It looks like psoriasis, consisting of well-demarcated bright-red plaques. In the nappy/diaper area involvement extends into the flexures (unlike the usual nappy/diaper rash). There is no itching and the infant remains unaffected by the rash. The condition goes away by itself after a few months. This rash is distinct from adult seborrhoeic eczema and has nothing to do with atopic eczema or psoriasis; is a type of nappy rash secondarily infected with *C. albicans*. Once it disappears it does not recur; it is good to reassure the parents.

TREATMENT: INFANTILE SEBORRHOEIC DERMATITIS

Parents are usually very distressed because infantile seborrhoeic dermatitis looks unsightly. The application of 1% hydrocortisone ointment to the affected areas two or three times a day will clear it up fairly speedily. Usually there is secondary infection with *Candida* or bacteria, so use a cream containing both hydrocortisone and an imidazole, nystatin, or clioquinol (e.g. Daktacort, Vioform HC or Nystaform). This is one of the rare instances where combined steroid/antifungal preparations can be recommended.

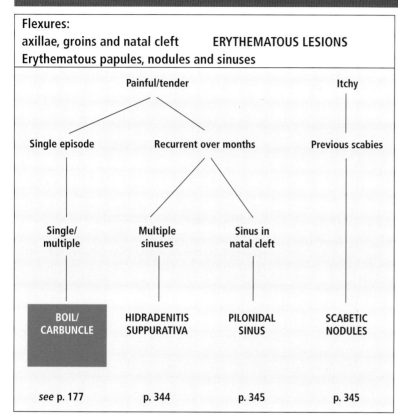

Flexures:
axillae, groins and natal cleft   ERYTHEMATOUS LESIONS
Erythematous papules, nodules and sinuses

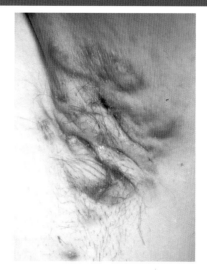

Fig. 10.16 Hidradenitis suppurativa in the axilla

Fig. 10.17 Hidradenitis suppurativa in the perineum

HIDRADENITIS SUPPURATIVA

This is a disease of the apocrine sweat glands that are found in the axillae and perineum. Tender papules, nodules and discharging sinuses occur in the axillae, groins, perianal area and very occasionally on the breasts. They heal leaving scars. It is thought to be due to an infection with *Streptococcus milleri*, but it does not always respond to antibiotics.

TREATMENT: HIDRADENITIS SUPPURATIVA

Minor degrees of hidradenitis can be controlled by long-term, low-dose antibiotics as for acne. Erythromycin or clindamycin 250 mg bid, or one to two co-trimoxazole tablets twice a day, given over a period of years will keep some patients free of disease. If they do not work, a combination of rifampicin 600 mg/day plus doxycycline 100 mg/day may work better. Systemic retinoids such as acitretin 10–50 mg daily may also be of benefit, and in severe cases they can be combined with antibiotics (clindamycin) and steroids (prednisolone). Surgery is really the last resort. All the apocrine glands in the affected area need to be removed. Excision of the abnormal skin together with the underlying sinuses and abscesses is a major undertaking. In the axillae it is often possible to excise the affected area and close the defect as a primary procedure. In the perineum that is not usually possible, so the patient will be left with a large, open wound that is left to granulate up on its own. This may take many months.

PILONIDAL SINUS

A tender papule or nodule in the midline of the natal cleft may be due to a pilonidal sinus, where hairs become buried within the skin. Usually the patient has hairy skin and a sedentary occupation. The sinus needs to be opened up, laid open and allowed to granulate up from the base. This is best done by a surgeon and under a general anaesthetic.

SCABETIC NODULES

A few patients with scabies develop persistent itchy papules, especially around the axillae. These may last for weeks or months after the patient has been successfully treated for scabies. Their presence does not mean that the scabies is active, so further treatment for scabies is unnecessary. Treat these lesions with a topical steroid.

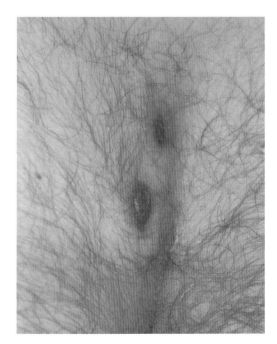

Fig. 10.18 Pilonidal sinuses above the natal cleft

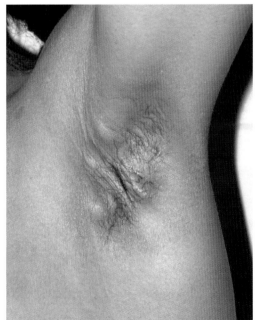

Fig. 10.19 Multiple tender boils in axilla due to infection with *Staphylococcus aureus*: treat with flucloxacillin

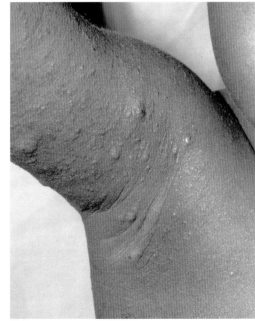

Fig. 10.20 Scabetic nodules

Flexures
Non-erythematous lesions
Macules, patches, papules, plaques, nodules
Skin coloured, brown

NON-ERYTHEMATOUS LESIONS

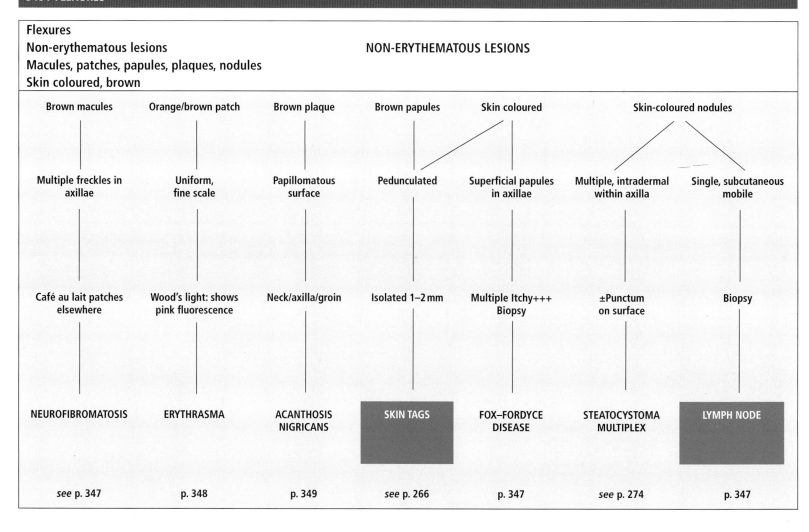

Brown macules	Orange/brown patch	Brown plaque	Brown papules	Skin coloured	Skin-coloured nodules	
Multiple freckles in axillae	Uniform, fine scale	Papillomatous surface	Pedunculated	Superficial papules in axillae	Multiple, intradermal within axilla	Single, subcutaneous mobile
Café au lait patches elsewhere	Wood's light: shows pink fluorescence	Neck/axilla/groin	Isolated 1–2 mm	Multiple Itchy+++ Biopsy	±Punctum on surface	Biopsy
NEUROFIBROMATOSIS	ERYTHRASMA	ACANTHOSIS NIGRICANS	SKIN TAGS	FOX–FORDYCE DISEASE	STEATOCYSTOMA MULTIPLEX	LYMPH NODE
see p. 347	p. 348	p. 349	*see* p. 266	p. 347	*see* p. 274	p. 347

FOX–FORDYCE DISEASE

Very itchy skin-coloured or yellowish papules occur in the axillae due to blockage of the apocrine ducts. The itching may be precipitated by the emotional stimuli that can cause axillary sweating. It mainly occurs in young women, and treatment is unsatisfactory.

NEUROFIBROMATOSIS

'Axillary freckles' or light-brown macules are pathognomonic of neurofibromatosis. In children this sign may predate the development of the neurofibromas (*see* p. 266), but there will be café au lait patches present on the trunk (*see* Fig. 9.79, p. 294).

LYMPH NODES

Lymph node enlargement may be reactive to a local infection, or due to malignancy, either a lymphoma or a secondary carcinoma. If in doubt, do a fine needle aspiration for cytology or refer to a surgeon for biopsy. Non-erythematous nodules in the axilla may also be due to steatocystoma multiplex (*see* p. 274).

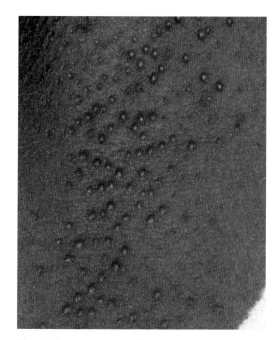

Fig. 10.21 Fox–Fordyce disease

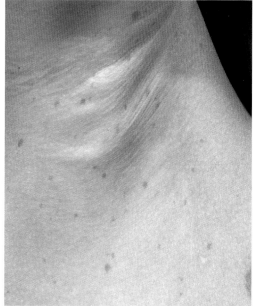

Fig. 10.22 Axillary freckling in neurofibromatosis

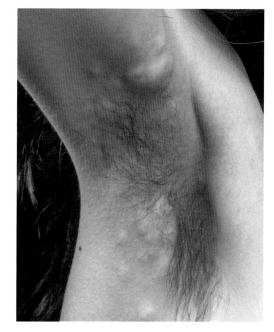

Fig. 10.23 Steatocystoma multiplex in axilla

ERYTHRASMA

Erythrasma is caused by an infection with *Corynebacterium minutissimum* in the flexures. Symmetrical, orange-brown, scaly plaques spread across the folds. Usually all flexures are involved – axillae, groins, sub-mammary areas and toe webs – although the natal cleft is spared. The condition may be confused with tinea cruris, but the colour is different, more orange-brown, the scale is not just at the edge, the axillae are involved and mycology will be negative. A Gram stain on the scales will reveal Gram-positive rods, and on Wood's light (UVA) examination there is bright-pink fluorescence (*see* Fig. 10.27).

TREATMENT: ERYTHRASMA

Erythromycin 250 mg orally qid for 14 days will clear erythrasma at any site. Nothing needs to be applied to the skin (topical imidazoles are ineffective).

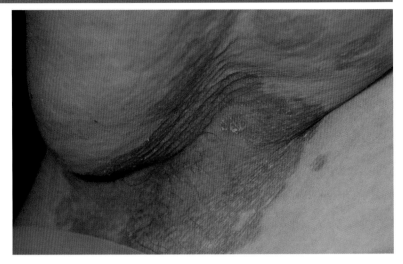

Fig. 10.25 Erythrasma in axilla

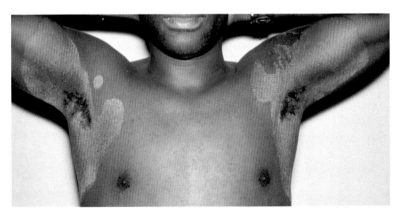

Fig. 10.24 Erythrasma in both axillae: in patients with black skin the scale is grey rather than brown

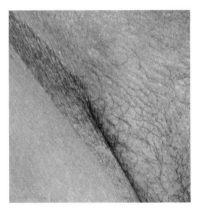

Fig. 10.26 Erythrasma in groin

Fig. 10.27 Coral-pink fluorescence of erythrasma under ultraviolet light

ACANTHOSIS NIGRICANS

This is a rare condition but it is important, because when it occurs in patients over the age of 40 you should look for an underlying malignancy – carcinoma of the lung, stomach or ovary. In younger patients it is usually associated with obesity and insulin resistance. It is then called **pseudoacanthosis nigricans**. The skin of the flexures becomes dark brown, dry and thickened, with a papillomatous velvety surface. In the malignant form the skin changes are often associated with marked itching, and there may be widespread lesions that look like viral warts. Treatment involves finding the cause and treating this. Weight loss is necessary for pseudoacanthosis nigricans.

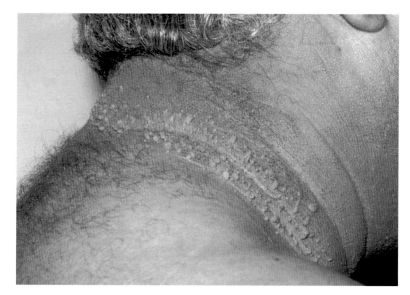

Fig. 10.28 Acanthosis nigricans

ABNORMALITIES OF SWEATING

PHYSIOLOGY OF SWEATING

Eccrine sweat glands are distributed all over the body surface, but they are most numerous on the palms of the hands, the soles of the feet and in the axillae. The secretary coil (sweat gland) is situated deep in the dermis and is linked to the skin surface by a straight duct. It produces an isotonic secretion that can be modified as it passes up the duct. Secretion of sweat is controlled by the sympathetic nervous system but the mediator is acetylcholine.

Generalised sweating is usually due to an underlying medical condition, i.e. thyrotoxicosis, diabetes, menopause, fever, infections such as tuberculosis and HIV, lymphoma, phaeochromocytoma and some drugs, e.g. tricyclic antidepressants and tamoxifen.

AXILLARY HYPERHIDROSIS

Hyperhidrosis is excessive production of sweat. In the axillae it causes embarrassment because of staining of clothes, the need to change clothes frequently and the rotting of clothes.

BROMHIDROSIS (BODY ODOUR)

Smelly armpits are not due to smelly apocrine sweat but to the breakdown of the sweat by bacteria on the skin. It can also be caused by secretion of smelly substances in the sweat such as garlic. Frequent washing of the axilla with soap and water is all that is needed. Control of excessive sweating does not help. Avoid spicy foods.

TREATMENT: AXILLARY HYPERHIDROSIS

The options available for treatment are as follows.

- 20% **aluminium chloride hexahydrate** in absolute (or 95%) alcohol: this is available commercially as Anhydrol Forte^{UK}, Drichlor^{UK}, Drysol^{USA}. It works by the aluminium ions migrating down the sweat ducts and blocking them. If applied to a sweaty axilla it will combine with the water in sweat to form hydrochloric acid, which will make the skin sore. It should be applied before going to bed, after washing and drying the axillae carefully. It can be applied every night for about a week to control the sweating, and thereafter applied only when the sweating reoccurs (usually every 7–21 days). Mild irritation of the axilla can be relieved by applying 1% hydrocortisone cream in the morning. Commercially available antiperspirants contain aluminium hypochlorite. These work well for normal individuals but are ineffective for excessive sweating.
- **Botulinum toxin**: up to 50 units of Azzalure, Botox, Xeomin or 125 units of Dysport dissolved in 2 mL saline is injected intradermally into each axilla. The hairy axillary vault is divided into 1 cm squares and about 0.05 mL injected into each square. This will abolish sweating for any time from a few weeks to a year. It is very effective and safe, but it is expensive and needs to be repeated when sweating reoccurs. It is the treatment of choice for severe, disabling hyperhidrosis.
- **Surgery**: removal of the axillary vault will remove most of the eccrine sweat glands and so stop sweating.

TREATMENT: GENERALISED SWEATING

Treat the underlying cause. If no cause is found it is worth trying propantheline 15 mg tid, but its anticholinergic side effects are often not tolerated (blurred vision, dry mouth, constipation, urinary retention, dizziness and palpitations). Glycopyrrolate (*Robinul*) 1–2 mg tid (named-patient prescription) and oxybutynin 2.5–5 mg bid are better tolerated. A β-blocker is an alternative, but do not use in patients with asthma or peripheral vascular disease.

CHROMHIDROSIS (COLOURED SWEAT)

Apocrine sweat may be coloured yellow, blue or green when it is secreted. More commonly, colourless apocrine sweat is broken down to different colours by bacteria on the skin surface or on axillary or pubic hair. The main problem is staining of the clothes.

TRICHOMYCOSIS AXILLARIS

This is a superficial infection of axillary or pubic hairs with a variety of corynebacteria. White or coloured concretions are fixed to the hair. Most people do not notice this but occasionally some complain of it. Treat by shaving off the axillary hair and wash the axilla with soap and water at least once a day.

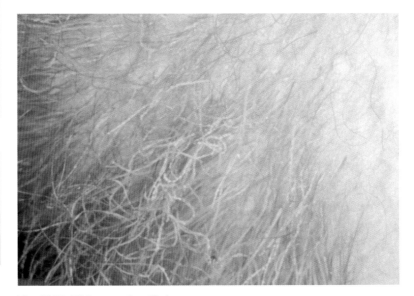

Fig. 10.29 Trichomycosis axillaris

Genitalia

Including pubic, perianal and perineal areas

11

Genitalia

ULCERS AND EROSIONS

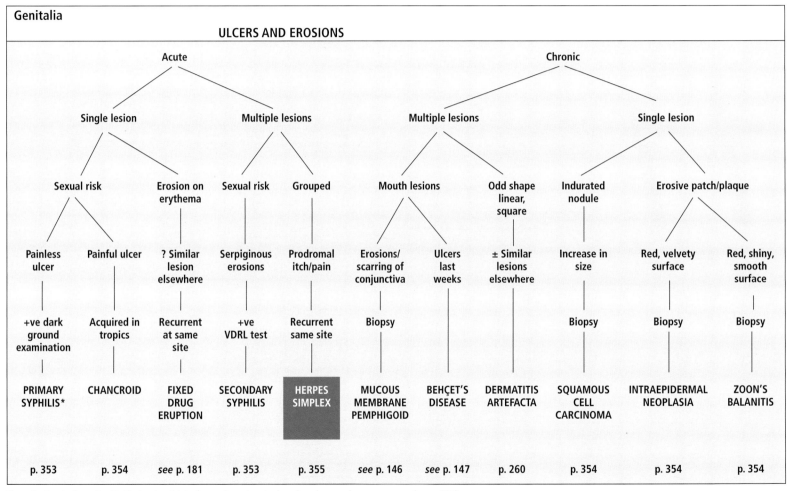

p. 353	p. 354	*see* p. 181	p. 353	p. 355	*see* p. 146	*see* p. 147	p. 260	p. 354	p. 354	p. 354

*In patients who have lived in the tropics, think of **granuloma inguinale** or **lymphogranuloma venereum** (*see* p. 354)

PRIMARY SYPHILIS

Primary syphilis presents as a round painless ulcer (1° chancre) with an indurated base about 3 weeks after infection (can be 10–90 days). The chancre is seen on the penis, scrotum, vulva, perianal skin or lip, but it may also be found on the cervix or within the anal canal. Suspect the diagnosis in any genital ulcer, and confirm by demonstrating *Treponema pallidum* on dark ground microscopy. Serology (EIA, TPHA, RPR) is helpful because it becomes positive within a week of the primary sore developing.

SECONDARY SYPHILIS

Irregular shallow serpiginous erosions on the penis, scrotum or vulva should suggest secondary syphilis. Similar lesions can occur on the buccal mucosa and tongue. These lesions are very infectious and the spirochaetes can be demonstrated in the exudate from such lesions by dark ground microscopy. Serology (VDRL) will always be positive. The patient will also have lymphadenopathy; general malaise; a widespread rash on the trunk (*see* p. 207), palms of the hands and soles of the feet; 'moth-eaten' alopecia; and flat warty papules and plaques on the genitalia and around the anus (condylomata lata).

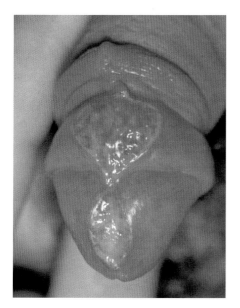

Fig. 11.01 Primary syphilis: two chancres where glans in contact with foreskin

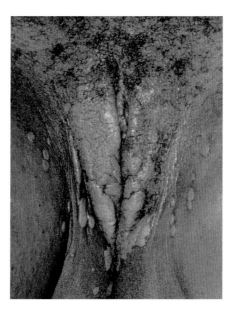

Fig. 11.02 Condylomata lata: these are much flatter than viral warts

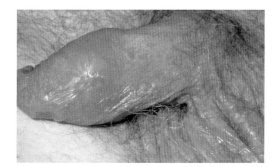

Fig. 11.03 (above) Secondary syphilis on shaft of penis and scrotum: serpiginous erosions

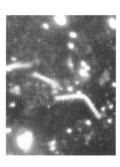

Fig. 11.04 (right) Dark ground microscopy showing spirochaetes of *Treponema pallidum* (×100)

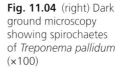

TREATMENT: SYPHILIS

All patients with syphilis should be seen in a department of genito-urinary medicine so that other sexually transmitted diseases can also be screened for and the patient's sexual contacts traced. **Early syphilis** (up to 1–2 years) is treated with a single dose of benzathine penicillin, 2.4 megaunits by intramuscular injection. To minimise the Jarisch–Herxheimer reaction, prednisolone 60 mg is given for 3 days, starting 24 hours before giving penicillin. If the patient is allergic to penicillin, the treatment is doxycycline 100 mg bid for 14 days. For **late syphilis** (over 2 years) 3 doses of benzathine penicillin, 2.4 megaunits is given by intramuscular injection at weekly intervals. If allergic to penicillin, doxycycline 100 mg bid is given for 28 days.

Contacts are treated with penicillin (if serology positive), or doxycyline (if negative).

OTHER SINGLE OR MULTIPLE GENITAL ULCERS

If the patient has multiple ulcers and has been to the tropics, consider **granuloma inguinale** (due to *Klebsiella granulomatis*), **lymphogranuloma venereum** (due to *Chlamydia trachomatis*) or **chancroid** (due to *Haemophilus ducreyi*). The latter two are usually associated with marked local lymphadenopathy. All such patients should be referred to a department of genito-urinary medicine, where the diagnosis can be confirmed.

Any indurated ulcer on the genitalia that is negative on dark ground microscopy should be biopsied to exclude a **squamous cell carcinoma** or **intraepithelial neoplasia**. Genito-urinary surgeons should manage these conditions. An ulcer that has an odd shape should make you think of **dermatitis artefacta** (*see* p. 260).

ZOON'S BALANITIS

Zoon's plasma cell balanitis is uncommon. It usually occurs as a single shiny, red plaque on the glans penis of a middle-aged or elderly man. Biopsy and histology is required to reach a correct diagnosis. Circumcision is usually curative.

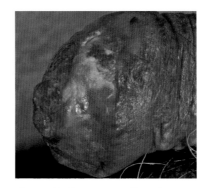

Fig. 11.05 Squamous cell carcinoma

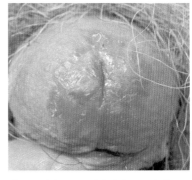

Fig. 11.06 Intraepithelial neoplasia

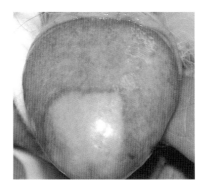

Fig. 11.07 Zoon's balanitis

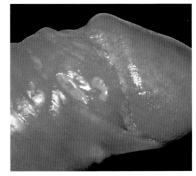

Fig. 11.08 Herpes simplex under foreskin

GENITAL HERPES SIMPLEX

Genital herpes simplex is by far the commonest cause of genital ulceration and is usually due to infection with herpes simplex type 2 (HSV-2). About 50% of **primary infections** with HSV-1 or 2 are asymptomatic. The rest present with localised burning, itching or soreness of the penis, vulva, anus or thighs, together with grouped vesicles that break down to form erosions/ulcers that heal in 7–10 days. Pain may be severe and there may be associated fever, malaise, headache and pain in the back and buttocks. In women there may be dysuria if there are ulcerated lesions on the vulva, and in patients of either sex there can be proctitis with anal infections.

Recurrent episodes of herpes simplex are common and can be precipitated by fever, stress and sexual trauma. Not all patients who have had a primary infection with HSV-2 will get recurrent episodes. For those who do, it is usually a lot less severe than the primary episode. It consists of painful grouped vesicles that break down to form erosions/ulcers. Ulcers in patients with HIV infection may last for months. Patients should be seen at the local genito-urinary medicine clinic. Here the diagnosis can be confirmed and the presence or absence of other sexually transmitted diseases checked for.

A primary infection with HSV-2 in the first 3 months of pregnancy can cause infection in the foetus and lead to spontaneous abortion. If there is active infection with HSV-2 at the time of birth, the child should be delivered by caesarean section to prevent encephalitis.

There is a considerable body of evidence to suggest that genital infection with HSV-2 is one of the causative factors in the development of carcinoma of the cervix. Other factors include early age of first coitus, multiple sexual partners and infection with genital warts.

TREATMENT: GENITAL HERPES SIMPLEX

PRIMARY INFECTION WITH HERPES SIMPLEX TYPE 1 OR 2

In both men and women, provided that they present within 48 hours of the appearance of the vesicles, treat with one of the following for 5–10 days:

- aciclovir 400 mg tid
- famciclovir 250 mg tid
- valaciclovir 500 mg bid.

This will relieve the pain and cut the attack short; it will also decrease the time that the virus is shed and therefore the time that the patient is infectious.

The following may be useful to bring symptomatic relief to patients of either sex:

- take aspirin or paracetamol for the pain
- apply lignocaine gel to the erosions/ulcers
- urinate in a warm bath if there is dysuria
- leave the affected area open if possible, to avoid clothes rubbing
- avoid sexual intercourse until the ulcers have healed.

RECURRENT INFECTION WITH HERPES SIMPLEX TYPE 1 OR 2

In some patients, recurrent episodes cause a lot of pain and this may ruin their sex life by causing dyspareunia, frigidity and impotence. Such patients should have a 2-day supply of oral aciclovir 800 mg tid (or alternatives, *see* first list in this box) at home to take at the first sign of recurrence. If they are getting frequent recurrences, long-term prophylaxis with oral aciclovir, 400 mg bid, can be used.

THE USE OF ACICLOVIR DURING PREGNANCY AND LACTATION

Aciclovir is not teratogenic or mutagenic in animals, so it is probably safe to give during pregnancy. Given during lactation, aciclovir will be present in the mother's breast milk; since it is not harmful to babies this probably does not matter.

Penis
Papules and plaques
(Note list is not exhaustive: see other chapters if necessary)

PENILE LESIONS AND RASH

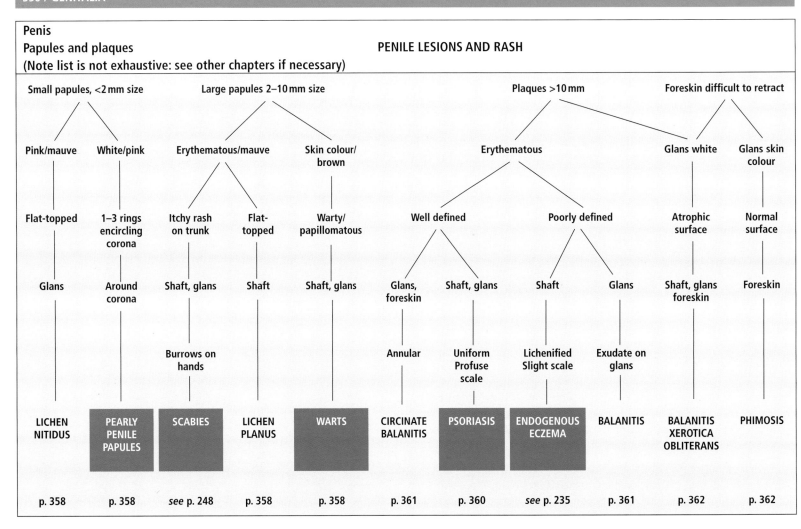

Small papules, <2 mm size		Large papules 2–10 mm size		Plaques >10 mm		Foreskin difficult to retract	
Pink/mauve	White/pink	Erythematous/mauve	Skin colour/brown	Erythematous		Glans white	Glans skin colour
Flat-topped	1–3 rings encircling corona	Itchy rash on trunk	Flat-topped	Well defined	Poorly defined	Atrophic surface	Normal surface
Glans	Around corona	Shaft, glans	Shaft	Warty/papillomatous			
		Burrows on hands		Shaft, glans → Glans, foreskin / Shaft, glans	Shaft / Glans	Shaft, glans foreskin	Foreskin
				Annular / Uniform Profuse scale	Lichenified Slight scale / Exudate on glans		
LICHEN NITIDUS	**PEARLY PENILE PAPULES**	**SCABIES**	**LICHEN PLANUS**	**WARTS** / **CIRCINATE BALANITIS** / **PSORIASIS**	**ENDOGENOUS ECZEMA** / **BALANITIS**	**BALANITIS XEROTICA OBLITERANS**	**PHIMOSIS**
p. 358	p. 358	*see* p. 248	p. 358	p. 358 / p. 361 / p. 360	*see* p. 235 / p. 361	p. 362	p. 362

Scrotum and pubic area
Papules, plaques and nodules   SCROTAL AND PUBIC LESIONS AND RASHES
(Note list is not exhaustive: *see* other chapters if necessary)

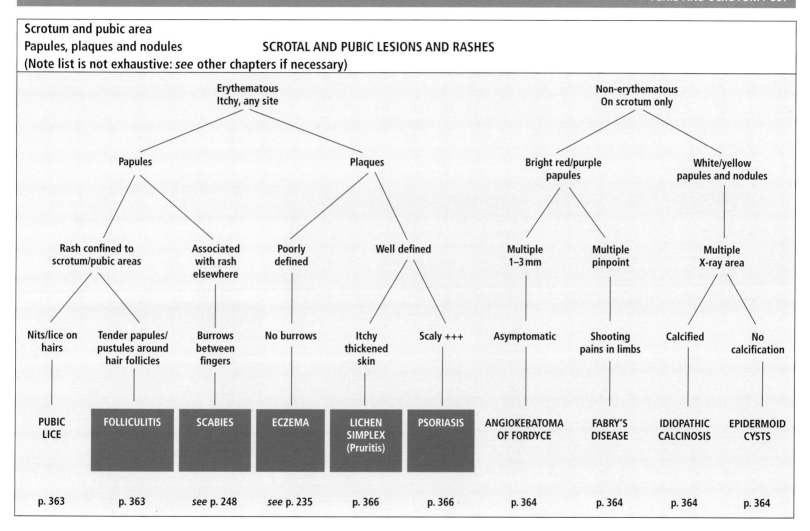

LICHEN NITIDUS / LICHEN PLANUS

Lichen planus nearly always affects the genital area. The lesions are identical to those elsewhere, i.e. flat-topped, shiny, mauve polygonal papules. If the papules are very small they are called lichen nitidus (*see* Fig. 8.04, p. 198). For treatment *see* p. 198.

PEARLY PENILE PAPULES

Small skin-coloured, pink or pearly papules 1–3 mm across occur around the corona in about 10% of males after puberty. Many young men go to their doctor when they first notice them, thinking that they are abnormal. Reassurance that they are normal is all that is needed.

WARTS

Warty lesions on the penis, scrotum, vulva or perianal skin may be due to the following.

- **Genital warts (condyloma acuminata):** these are due to one of the human papilloma viruses (HPV 6, 11, 16, 18) and are spread by sexual contact. These single or multiple, skin-coloured, pink or brown warty papules with a moist rather than rough surface can occur anywhere on the genitalia or perianal skin. The patient's sexual partner should also be checked and other sexually transmitted diseases looked for and excluded.

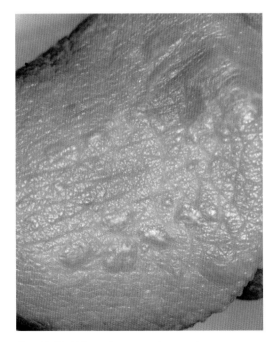

Fig. 11.09 Lichen planus on glans penis

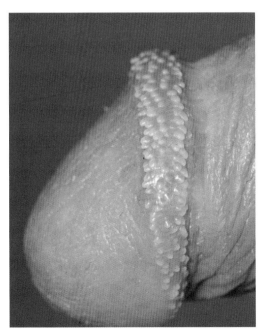

Fig. 11.10 Pearly penile papules around corona of the glans

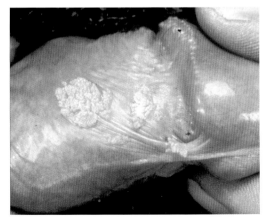

Fig. 11.11 Genital warts on shaft of penis and pearly penile papules on the corona

- **Common warts** (*see* p. 318)
- **Plane warts** (*see* p. 268)
- **Seborrhoeic warts** (*see* p. 320)
- **Condylomata lata**: lesions that look like flat viral warts (*see* Fig. 11.02) may occur in secondary syphilis. They are teeming with spirochaetes which can be demonstrated by dark ground microscopy (*see* Fig. 11.04). Think of this if the patient is unwell and check the VDRL.

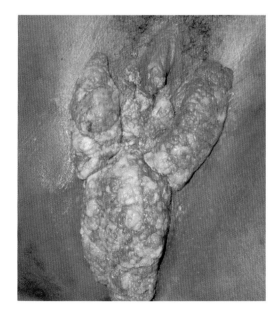

Fig. 11.12 Genital warts on vulva in a patient with HIV

TREATMENT: GENITAL AND PERIANAL WARTS

The most important part of the treatment for genital warts is to screen the patient for other sexually transmitted diseases, so referral to the local genito-urinary medicine department is required.

Modalities of treatment that are commonly used are as follows.

1. For non-keratinised genital warts: **0.5% podophyllotoxin** in an alcohol base or as a cream (Warticon) is applied to each wart twice a day for 3 consecutive days with a 4-day break weekly for 4 weeks. If warts still present, try points 2 and 3 below. It can be done by the patient himself but he needs to be able to see the warts so that it is applied carefully to the wart and not the surrounding skin, otherwise it can cause erythema, oedema and erosions.
2. For ano-genital and other keratinised warts: **imiquimod** (Aldara) **cream**. This has replaced podophyllotoxin as the treatment of choice. It is applied three times a week for up to 16 weeks (*see* p. 34). Each application is left on for 12 hours and then washed off with soap and water. It should be washed off before sexual intercourse, as it can produce a lot of irritation, inflammation and swelling.
3. **Freezing with liquid nitrogen** is a suitable treatment if there is a single wart or only a few warts present. It is the treatment of choice for meatal warts. The skin around the wart is put on the stretch so that the liquid nitrogen can be applied accurately to the wart and not to the adjacent normal skin. Treatment can be repeated every week until the wart has gone. Use with *extreme caution for warts on/near the clitoris or frenum* to avoid permanent scarring.
4. **Surgical removal** under a general anaesthetic is a useful treatment if there are very extensive warts, particularly if the anal canal is involved as well as the skin. Between 50 and 75 mL of 1:30 000 adrenaline in physiological saline is injected subcutaneously underneath the warts. This causes the skin to swell up like a balloon so that the warts are separated from one another and stick out like fingers. Taking hold of the warts with a pair of fine-toothed forceps, they are then snipped off with a pair of sharp-pointed scissors. The presence of adrenaline means that there will be very little bleeding; any persistent bleeding points can be diathermied.

PSORIASIS

The diagnosis of psoriasis on the glans or shaft of the penis is not usually difficult, since the bright-red colour is just like psoriasis elsewhere. On the glans, scaling may be absent, but on the shaft the plaques often have the typical silvery scaling. In boys between the ages of 5 and 15 years, psoriasis may first appear on the penis and cause considerable anxiety to the parents. In adults it often is a problem because of pain and embarrassment during sexual intercourse.

TREATMENT: PSORIASIS OF THE GENITALIA

Tar, dithranol and calcipotriol are likely to make the skin sore in the flexures and on the genitalia, so they should not be used. Calcitriol (Silkis) is the treatment of choice at these sites, since it produces less irritation than other vitamin D₃ analogues. Topical steroids can also be used to clear the skin, but 1% hydrocortisone is ineffective and is not worth trying. Start with a moderately potent[UK]/group 4–5[USA] topical steroid cream or ointment applied twice a day. Whether the patient will prefer a cream or ointment you will have to discover by trial and error.

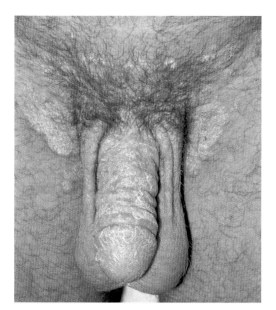

Fig. 11.13 Psoriasis on penis, pubic area and groins

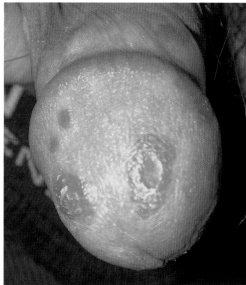

Fig. 11.14 Psoriasis on glans penis

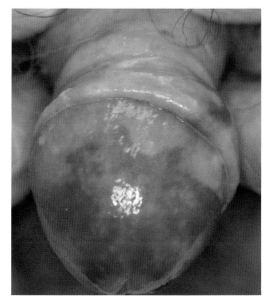

Fig. 11.15 Balanitis: you will need to biopsy this lesion to exclude Zoon's or neoplasia; histology showed it to be inflammatory and it responded to a weak steroid cream

BALANITIS

Balanitis means inflammation of the glans penis. It is uncommon in those who have been circumcised. It is usually an irritant dermatitis, which may be due to poor hygiene (particularly if the foreskin is tight and difficult to retract), urethral discharge or trauma. Always check for *Candida albicans*, which may not have the typical appearance with outlying pustules as in the groin, by taking a swab and sending it to the lab. If *Candida* is present, check a fasting blood sugar or HbA1c, since this may be a presenting sign of diabetes mellitus in middle or old age. If it occurs very acutely, consider an allergic contact dermatitis due to latex condoms, spermicidal foams or applied medicaments.

CIRCINATE BALANITIS

This occurs in some patients with **Reiter's syndrome** (arthritis [sacroiliitis ± polyarthritis], urethritis or dysentery, and conjunctivitis). A red scaly or eroded area occurs on the glans and spreads outwards in phases with a grey circinate edge. On the soles of the feet, tender keratotic papules or pustules can occur (keratoderma blennorrhagicum). Some or all of these symptoms usually occur 1–3 weeks after an infection of the genito-urinary tract (often with *Chlamydia*), or a bacterial gastro-intestinal infection causing diarrhoea. Predisposed individuals are usually HLA B27-positive young males. Patients should be screened for other sexually transmitted infections if at risk.

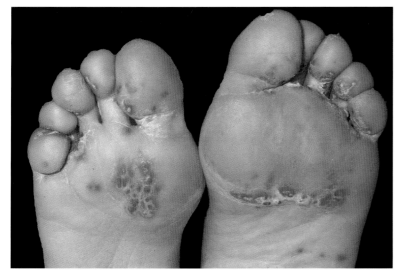

Fig. 11.16 Keratoderma blennorrhagicum: tender keratotic papules and pustules on the soles of feet in a patient with Reiter's syndrome

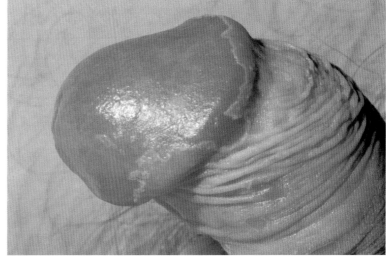

Fig. 11.17 Circinate balanitis in a patient with Reiter's syndrome

TREATMENT: BALANITIS

- If *Candida* is not present (check by taking a swab) and the patient is not diabetic, soaking the penis in normal saline (1 tablespoon of salt in one pint of water) for 10 minutes twice a day for a week will clear the problem in 80%–90% of patients. If it recurs this can be repeated.
- If the patient is diabetic or *Candida* is present, after soaking in saline, the patient should apply topical nystatin cream or ointment or one of the imidazole creams (e.g. miconazole cream) two or three times a day until it clears.
- If neither of these measures work, a urethral swab should be taken looking for anaerobes. If they are not found, the patient's sexual partner should also be examined. If anaerobes are found in the patient or his sexual partner, treatment is with oral metronidazole 400 mg tid for 10 days.
- If no infection is present, then 1% hydrocortisone cream is usually effective.
- If none of the above points work, then refer to a dermatologist for a biopsy.

BALANITIS XEROTICA OBLITERANS (BXO)

This is the same condition which in females is called **lichen sclerosus et atrophicus** (*see* p. 368). It most commonly affects young adults. It can present in a number of ways. The patient may notice white discolouration of the glans or prepuce, blistering or haemorrhage, difficulty in retracting the foreskin or the urine spraying out uncontrollably during micturition. On examination, ivory-white macules, papules or plaques are present on the glans with or without obvious atrophy. Blisters or haemorrhage may also be seen (*see* Fig. 11.18).

TREATMENT: BALANITIS XEROTICA OBLITERANS

If the man has not been circumcised, circumcision is probably the treatment of choice. If the problem is itching or soreness, a topical steroid in the form of 1% hydrocortisone cream applied twice daily is all that is needed. If that does not work, or if there is a problem with urethral stenosis, a very potent[UK]/group 1[USA] topical steroid cream will be required. It is applied twice a day to the affected area (and to the urethra if necessary) and produces a very rapid and dramatic improvement. This should not be continued for more than 2–3 weeks. Once the disease is under control, a weaker topical steroid usually works just as well.

PHIMOSIS

Difficulty in retracting the foreskin in a young adult without any clinical signs may be due to a congenitally tight foreskin, repeated trauma or underlying balanitis xerotica obliterans.

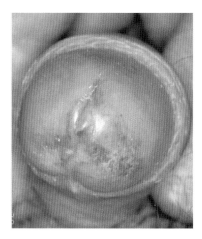

Fig. 11.18 Haemorrhagic erosions in balanitis xerotica obliterans

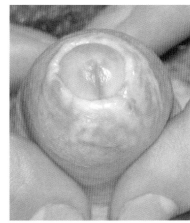

Fig. 11.19 Phimosis due to balanitis xerotica obliterans: note atrophic area on glans and foreskin

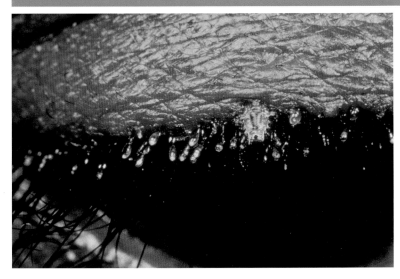

Fig. 11.20 Pubic (crab) louse and nits on eyelashes

PUBIC LICE

Pubic lice (crab lice) like other lice live on human blood. They grip the pubic hair and feed on blood through the pubic skin. The eggs are laid on the pubic hair. These look identical to the nits that are found in the scalp: oval, white, shiny capsules 1–2 mm long and firmly attached to the pubic hairs. In Negros the nits are sometimes very dark in colour but are otherwise the same. If no nits are present, look for other evidence of eczema or scabies to confirm the diagnosis of these. In individuals who are very hairy, pubic lice can also be found in the axillae, on the body hair and in the eyelashes (*see* Fig. 11.20).

FOLLICULITIS/BOIL

Small, red papules around a hair follicle, some of which have pus in the centre, are due to folliculitis. Larger nodules are boils. Both are caused by infection with *Staphylococcus aureus* (*see* pp. 177, 185 and 187). With both there may be painful lymphadenopathy in the groin. Bacteriology culture will confirm the diagnosis.

TREATMENT: PHIMOSIS

If there is no obvious infection present the patient will need to be circumcised; he should be referred to a surgeon.

If a urethritis is present (urethral discharge), the commonest causes are non-specific urethritis and gonorrhoea. The patient should be referred to a genito-urinary medicine department so that the diagnosis can be confirmed. Sometimes the penis is so tender that it is impossible to take urethral swabs. In that case the patient's sexual partner should be examined and the diagnosis confirmed from her. If no infection is found, ice or 1% hydrocortisone cream applied twice a day can be helpful.

TREATMENT: PUBIC LICE

- Shaving the pubic hair is the simplest solution.
- 0.5% Malathion lotion (Derbac-M), 0.5% phenothrin lotion or 5% permethrin cream are applied to the pubic hair and washed off 12 hours later. Treatment is repeated after 7 days to kill any adult lice that have hatched since the first application. Alcoholic solutions are not suitable for applying to the pubic area.
- In individuals who are very hairy, pubic lice can also be found in the axillae, on the body hair and in the eyelashes. These areas should always be checked and, if involved, the whole body should be treated.
- Lice and nits on the eyelashes should be picked off with the fingers and petroleum jelly applied three or four times a day so that the lice cannot hold on!
- All sexual contacts must also be treated.

ANGIOKERATOMA OF FORDYCE

Numerous small, bright-red or purple non-itchy papules on the scrotum are quite common particularly in the elderly. They are usually asymptomatic, but occasionally they bleed. The diagnosis can be confirmed by skin biopsy. They are quite harmless.

FABRY'S DISEASE (ANGIOKERATOMA CORPORIS DIFFUSUM)

This is a very rare X-linked disorder in which tiny angiokeratomas occur on the skin in the area usually covered by the underpants. They occur just before puberty and are associated with excruciating pains in the limbs and with renal failure. If this diagnosis is suspected, a specialist opinion should be sought.

EPIDERMOID CYSTS AND IDIOPATHIC CALCINOSIS

Single or multiple white papules confined to the scrotal skin are most commonly due to epidermoid cysts. In women, similar cysts occur on the labia majora. Histologically they are identical to epidermoid cysts elsewhere, with a lining that looks like normal epidermis and the centre filled with keratin.

Sometimes lesions that look exactly the same as epidermoid cysts are found not to be cysts histologically but lumps of calcium lying in the dermis. There is no capsule around them and there is no indication of why they are there. They are not associated with hypercalcaemia or deposition of calcium elsewhere. If the diagnosis is thought of before excision, the calcification can be shown on X-ray. Both conditions are completely harmless.

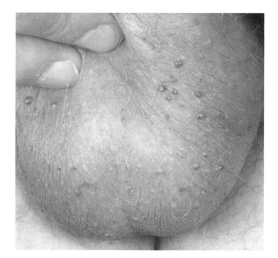

Fig. 11.21 Angiokeratoma of Fordyce on the scrotum

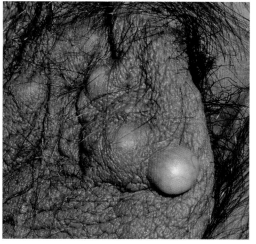

Fig. 11.22 Multiple epidermoid cysts on the scrotum

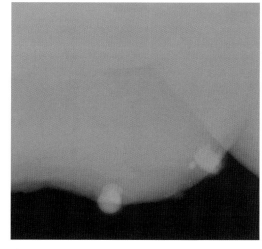

Fig. 11.23 X-ray showing idiopathic calcification of the scrotum

Vulva, perianal and perineal skin
Papules, plaques and nodules

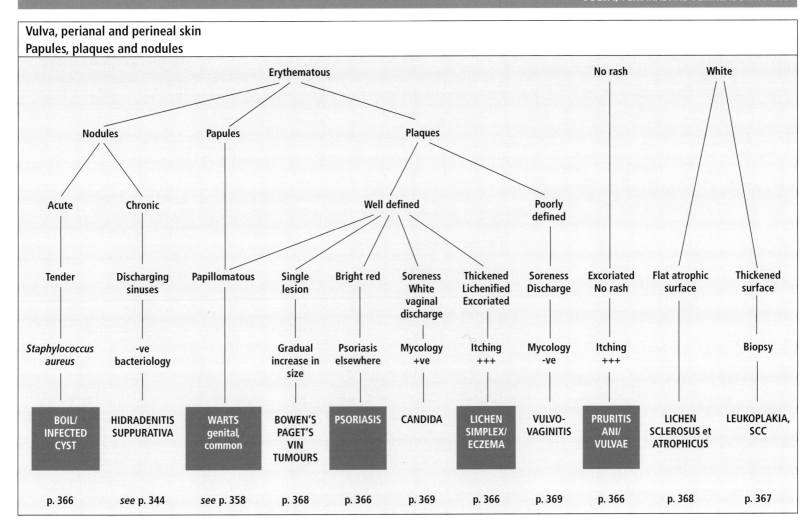

HIDRADENITIS SUPPURATIVA

This is an uncommon condition where painful papules, nodules, discharging sinuses and scars occur at sites where apocrine glands are present, i.e. in the axillae, pubic area, labia majora, scrotum, groins, perianal skin, buttocks or the areolae of the breasts. If such lesions are confined to the perianal skin, think of **Crohn's disease** and, much less commonly, **tuberculosis**. A biopsy will be needed to establish these diagnoses (*see* also p. 344).

BOILS AND INFECTED CYSTS

An acutely painful red nodule on the vulva, pubic area or scrotum may be an abscess of a hair follicle (boil) due to infection with *S. aureus* or in women a similar lesion can be an infection of a Bartholin gland due to gonorrhoea, *C. trachomatis* or *Gardnerella vaginalis*.

PRURITIS ANI OR VULVAE

When a patient complains of perianal, scrotal or vulval itching, you need to know whether there are any other symptoms such pain or vaginal discharge, whether a rash is present on the vulva or elsewhere, and whether anyone else in the family has the same or similar symptoms.

Rashes presenting with perianal, scrotal or vulval itch

Psoriasis

When psoriasis is itchy the diagnosis is often missed. If the plaque is bright red rather than pink or mauve, whether scaly or not, it is probably psoriasis. Look at the natal cleft, the rest of the skin, the scalp and the fingernails for other signs of psoriasis (*see* p. 225).

Lichen simplex

Lichen simplex is a single lichenified plaque with or without obvious excoriations caused by continual rubbing or scratching. The scrotum and vulva are common sites for this condition (*see* p. 219).

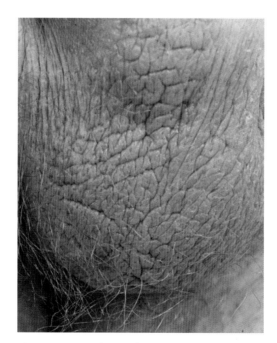

Fig. 11.24 Scrotal lichenifiction from persistent scratching

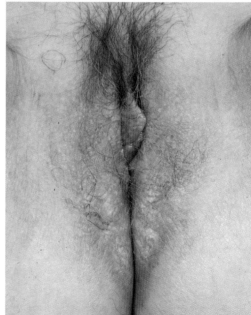

Fig. 11.25 Lichenification of vulva

Eczema

Atopic eczema or unclassifiable **endogenous eczema** may present with vulval itching. In the former, intolerable genital itching may be the final straw that makes it impossible for the patient to cope with her eczema. In the latter, sexual infidelity or anxiety about possible venereal disease may be the precipitating factor. Both conditions are clinically identical to eczema elsewhere, with poorly defined itchy pink papules and plaques with excoriations, scaling and no vesicles.

Contact irritant eczema occurs in babies (nappy/diaper rash, *see* p. 341); an identical rash can occur in the elderly if they are incontinent. Applied irritants can also cause an irritant eczema or an acute vulvitis.

Allergic contact dermatitis is often due to medicaments (containing lanolin, parabens, antibiotics or local anaesthetics bought over the counter or prescribed by a doctor), deodorants, contraceptives or other preparations. It usually presents acutely with vesicles, weeping and crusting, and it may be extremely sore rather than itchy. Patch testing once the acute reaction has settled down will sort out the cause.

Pubic lice

The diagnosis is confirmed by finding nits or adult lice on the pubic or labial hair (*see* p. 363).

Scabies

There should be an itchy rash all over the body except on the face, and the telltale burrows will be found between the fingers. Other members of the family or sexual contacts may also be itching (*see* p. 248).

Herpes simplex

This often causes pain as well as itching. Patients should be referred to the local department of genito-urinary medicine so that other sexually acquired diseases can be excluded (*see* p. 355).

Vaginal intra-epidermal neoplasia (VIN)

White plaques on the vulva that are thickened rather than atrophic may be due to VIN (leukoplakia). If in doubt, histology will distinguish between leukoplakia and lichen sclerosus et atrophicus.

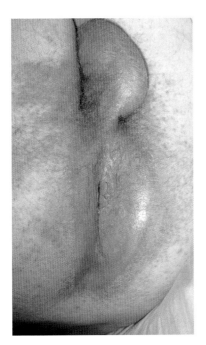

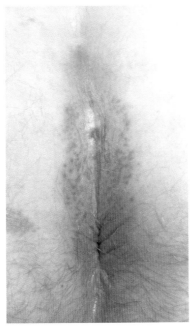

Fig. 11.26 Allergic contact dermatitis to a local anaesthetic cream

Fig. 11.27 Perianal eczema with erythema and excoriations

Lichen sclerosus et atrophicus

This is a very itchy condition that principally occurs on the vulva or perianal skin. It occurs in little girls or in middle-aged women. In children itching, soreness or blisters are the presenting symptoms; it gets better spontaneously at puberty. In older women, intolerable itching, soreness or dyspareunia are the reasons for seeking help. White atrophic papules and plaques with or without follicular plugging or haemorrhagic blisters are seen on the vulva and/or perianal skin. Occasionally lesions may occur elsewhere on the skin where they are very similar to lichen planus, with flat-topped, shiny, polygonal papules, but white in colour rather than mauve and with a wrinkled atrophic surface (*see* p. 285).

Tumours

A single red, scaly plaque unresponsive to treatment should be biopsied to exclude **Bowen's disease** (VIN), **extramammary Paget's disease** or a **squamous cell carcinoma**.

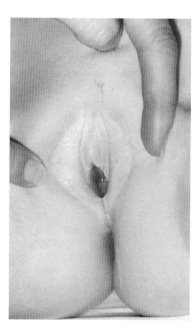

Fig. 11.28 Lichen sclerosus in a child

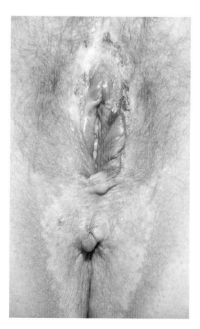

Fig. 11.29 Lichen sclerosus in an adult

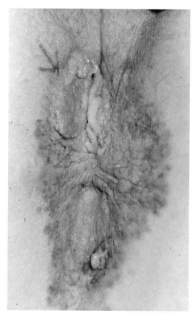

Fig. 11.30 Vulval intraepithelial neoplasia (biopsy sites marked)

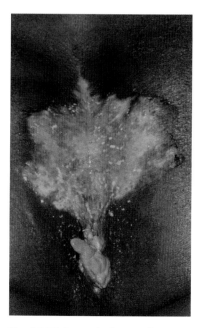

Fig. 11.31 Bowen's disease of perianal skin

Vulvo-vaginitis

This is inflammation of the vagina primarily with secondary involvement of the vulva. It can be caused by:

- *C. albicans*: soreness rather than itching is usually the presenting symptom on the vulva. An acute vulvitis with a red, glazed appearance is characteristic and there may be an associated thick, white vaginal discharge. The diagnosis can be confirmed by direct microscopy (*see* p. 343), or culture of the discharge. Remember to check for diabetes
- **bacterial vaginosis** due to *Gardnerella vaginalis* (a vaginal discharge with a fishy smell is usually the clue to the diagnosis); wet smears of the discharge show clue cells – multiple organisms stuck to the epithelial cells. Gram staining shows Gram-negative rods
- *Trichomonas vaginalis* infection (a frothy, greenish-white vaginal discharge); direct microscopy of the discharge will show the protozoae
- a **retained foreign body** in the vagina.

When no rash is present consider the following diagnoses

Threadworms

These usually cause pruritis ani in children, but in females they may wander forward to the vulva, causing itching there too. Scratching leads to the ova being transferred to the patient's fingers and fingernails and thence to the mouth (directly, or indirectly on food eaten with unwashed hands). Inside the patient's large bowel the ova mature and the cycle starts again. The diagnosis is made by seeing the worms wriggling out of the faeces (tell the patient or the mother to look), by seeing them on the perineum, or by the Sellotape test (apply some sticky transparent tape to the perianal skin, place on a glass slide and look for the eggs).

Anal discharge

A discharge or liquid faeces can cause itching due to the perianal area being continually wet. Mucous discharge, bleeding or diarrhoea can all cause problems and a rectal examination is essential to exclude haemorrhoids, a fistula-in-ano or carcinoma of the rectum. Patients with poor perianal hygiene, particularly if they have diarrhoea or soft stools, may itch because faeces are left on the skin after defecation. You can check for this by looking; if it is not obvious, try wiping the perianal skin with a gauze swab – any trace of brown or yellow indicates that the hygiene of the area is not ideal.

Idiopathic

Perianal and vulval itching is quite common and a specific cause may not be found.

VULVODYNIA AND SCROTODYNIA

Localised superficial dyspareunia and point tenderness within the vestibule at the 5 o'clock and 7 o'clock positions is termed **localised vulvodynia**, and occurs in young premenopausal women who experience discomfort on penetration. **Generalised vulvodynia** and **scrotodynia** presents as a burning pain. Symptoms can occur all the time, and may spread over all the genitalia and down the thighs; they are present without anything touching the area, and can worsen on sitting or climbing stairs. The appearance of the skin is normal. There may be associated depression, fibromyalgia or irritable bowel syndrome.

Patients should be referred to a dermatologist with a special interest in these conditions (*see* p. 370).

TREATMENT: PRURITIS ANI OR VULVAE

Any coexisting disease should be treated.

Psoriasis (*see* p. 340)
Eczema (*see* p. 339)
Lichen planus (*see* p. 198)
Scabies (*see* p. 248)
Pubic lice (*see* p. 363)
Genital warts (*see* p. 359)
Herpes simplex (*see* p. 355)

Lichen sclerosis et atrophicus. In little girls, 1% hydrocortisone cream or ointment applied twice a day is usually sufficient. In adult women, a very potent[UK]/group 1[USA] topical steroid cream will be required to dramatically improve the symptoms and make the patient believe that there is some hope for the future. It is applied twice a day to the affected area and produces a very rapid and dramatic improvement. Once the disease is under control, reduce the frequency of application to two to three times a week. Control of the disease is important to prevent the development of squamous cell carcinoma in the atrophic skin.

Candidiasis. An imidazole pessary placed high in the vagina at night: clotrimazole (500 mg) single dose or miconazole (1200 mg) single dose.

T. vaginalis infection. The patient should be given metronidazole 400 mg bid for 5–7 days, or 2 g as a single dose (alcohol must be avoided while taking metronidazole).

Bacterial vaginosis. Both the patient and her sexual partner should be given metronidazole 400 mg orally tid for 7 days (alcohol must be avoided while taking metronidazole).

Surgical problems. Haemorrhoids, fistula-in-ano or carcinoma of the rectum can all present with pruritis ani and will need dealing with surgically.

Threadworms. The whole family should be treated with mebendazole 100 mg orally as a single dose (except for pregnant women and children under the age of 2). If re-infection occurs, treatment can be repeated after 2–3 weeks. Children under the age of 2 are treated with piperazine 50 mg/kg body weight daily for 7 days. As well as the drug treatment, the patient should be told to wash the perianal skin first thing in the morning to remove any ova laid during the night, and to wash her hands and scrub under her fingernails with a nail brush after going to the toilet and before meals.

Idiopathic group. There remain a large number of patients for whom no physical cause can be found.

Pruritis ani. Whatever the original cause of the itching, scratching damages the skin and makes it itch more. Wearing loose-fitting cotton underpants to keep the area as cool as possible is often helpful, and it is important to pay particular attention to keeping the perianal skin clean and dry. He should wash his bottom with a mild soap and water after defecation. A bidet is very helpful in this respect and if the patient does not have one, he might find it helpful to buy a plastic one (from a boat shop or a surgical appliance department) that can be placed over the toilet. Meanwhile, the application of hydrocortisone (1%) or hydrocortisone-17-butyrate (Locoid) cream is likely to be helpful in stopping the itching. It is important to use this especially at night to break the itch scratch cycle, and to reassure the patient that 'something can be done'. Once the itching is controlled, the cream should only be used if required for intermittent itch. If these measures do not work he should be referred to a dermatologist so that any other diagnosis can be ruled out and patch testing carried out. Very often such patients become allergic to the numerous ointments and creams that they have used to treat the condition (especially local anaesthetics).

Pruritis vulvae. Like pruritis ani it may be due to some psychosexual problem. It is a mistake to think that it is just a question of finding the right cream or ointment to use. It is worth exploring with the patient whether there is some anxiety at the bottom of it (guilt about her own or her partner's adultery or impotence, a previous abortion or sexual abuse in childhood) and if possible sort this out.

Vulvodynia and **scrotodynia** are difficult to manage and are best referred to a specialist dermatology clinic. These patients require detailed counselling, and treatment with regular application of bland emollients. In localised vulvodynia, local anaesthetic applied before intercourse may be helpful. Antidepressants can sometimes be helpful.

Lower legs

12

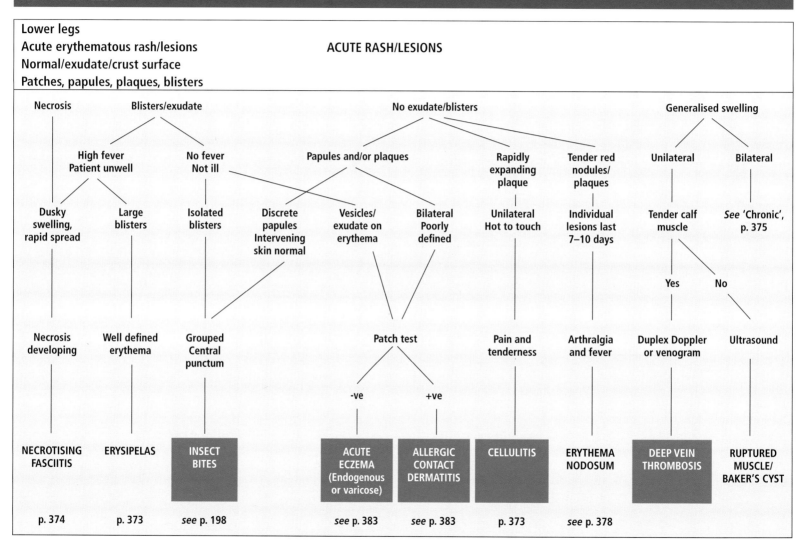

Lower legs
Acute erythematous rash/lesions
Normal/exudate/crust surface
Patches, papules, plaques, blisters

ACUTE RASH/LESIONS

Necrosis

Blisters/exudate

No exudate/blisters

Generalised swelling

High fever
Patient unwell

No fever
Not ill

Papules and/or plaques

Rapidly
expanding
plaque

Tender red
nodules/
plaques

Unilateral

Bilateral

Dusky
swelling,
rapid spread

Large
blisters

Isolated
blisters

Discrete
papules
Intervening
skin normal

Vesicles/
exudate on
erythema

Bilateral
Poorly
defined

Unilateral
Hot to touch

Individual
lesions last
7–10 days

Tender calf
muscle

See 'Chronic',
p. 375

Yes   No

Necrosis
developing

Well defined
erythema

Grouped
Central
punctum

Patch test

Pain and
tenderness

Arthralgia
and fever

Duplex Doppler
or venogram

Ultrasound

-ve   +ve

NECROTISING
FASCIITIS

ERYSIPELAS

INSECT
BITES

ACUTE
ECZEMA
(Endogenous
or varicose)

ALLERGIC
CONTACT
DERMATITIS

CELLULITIS

ERYTHEMA
NODOSUM

DEEP VEIN
THROMBOSIS

RUPTURED
MUSCLE/
BAKER'S CYST

p. 374   p. 373   *see* p. 198   *see* p. 383   *see* p. 383   p. 373   *see* p. 378

ERYSIPELAS

This is an infection of the upper half of the dermis with a group A β-haemolytic streptococcus (*Streptococcus pyogenes*). The patient becomes suddenly unwell with a high fever and rigors, associated with a well-defined red swollen area with central blistering. No obvious portal of entry for the bacteria is seen, which distinguishes it from cellulitis.

CELLULITIS

This is an infection of the lower half of the dermis by a group A, C or G β-haemolytic streptococcus. There is usually an obvious portal of entry for the organism such as a leg ulcer, tinea between the toes, or eczema on the feet or legs. It looks like erysipelas except the area of erythema is less well defined. There are *no blisters* and there is associated lymphangitis and lymphadenopathy. The patient is less unwell.

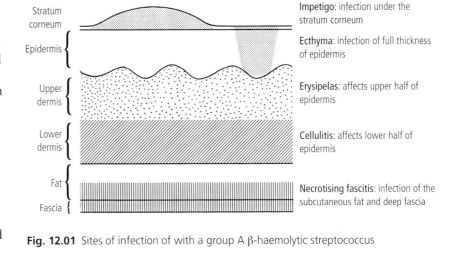

Fig. 12.01 Sites of infection of with a group A β-haemolytic streptococcus

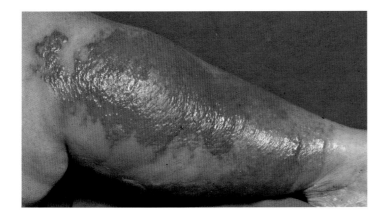

Fig. 12.02 Erysipelas: large bullae on well-demarcated erythema

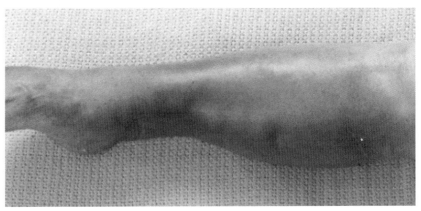

Fig. 12.03 Cellulitis: erythema with no blistering

TREATMENT: CELLULITIS AND ERYSIPELAS

β-haemolytic streptococci are always sensitive to penicillin, but as there may be associated infection with staphylococci, current practice is to give both intravenous benzyl penicillin, 600 mg and flucloxacillin 500 mg every 6 hours. As an outpatient, high-dose flucloxacillin (1 gm 6-hourly) may be used. Treat erysipelas for 7 days and cellulitis for at least 2 weeks, otherwise relapse is likely. For patients who are allergic to penicillin, oral erythromycin/clarithromycin 500 mg or clindamycin 300 mg 6-hourly can be used instead. Do not use ampicillin because it does not work. If the infection is slow to settle, check that the patient is not diabetic. Cellulitis is always slower to resolve than erysipelas, which usually responds within 24 hours.

As well as treating the cellulitis, you must also treat the co-existing eczema, tinea pedis or leg ulcer that has allowed entry of the streptococcus into the skin. Otherwise recurrent cellulitis will occur and this leads to chronic lymphoedema. If there have been more than two episodes of cellulitis within 6 months, long-term prophylactic penicillin is needed. You can use oral phenoxymethylpenicillin (penicillin V) 250 mg bid.

NECROTISING FASCIITIS

Necrotising fasciitis is an acute fulminant infection of the subcutaneous fat and deep fascia, usually by a group A β-haemolytic streptococcus. A toxin released from the organism causes thrombosis of the blood vessels in the skin and thence necrosis. Initially it looks like cellulitis or erysipelas but purple areas followed by frank necrosis occur within 2–3 days. The most important thing here is to think of the diagnosis in any patient who has what looks like erysipelas or cellulitis that does not begin to improve with penicillin or erythromycin after 24–48 hours, or who has dusky-purple areas appearing within the larger red, swollen area. Think of it in patients with co-morbidities such as immunosuppression, diabetes, alcohol excess, cancer or penetrating injury (e.g. road traffic accident) or orthopaedic surgery. High levels of anti-desoxyribonuclease B and anti-hyaluronidase in the patient's serum will confirm the diagnosis.

Measuring the antistreptolysin O titre is not helpful, as it is always normal.

It can be an acute fulminant illness, with the patient dying almost before you can think of the diagnosis, or it can be a much slower process, with the necrotic tissue gradually separating from the surrounding normal skin. In children and young adults, streptococci are the common pathogen, but in the elderly, especially after surgery, other organisms may be implicated such as staphylococci, *Escherichia coli* and clostridium.

TREATMENT: NECROTISING FASCIITIS

Patients should be admitted urgently to hospital so that wide surgical debridement of the affected skin can be carried out. Antibiotics alone are not sufficient treatment. This is because the streptococci produce a toxin, which causes the blood vessels in the affected area to thrombose. This not only causes the necrosis of the skin, which is the hallmark of the disease, but also prevents the antibiotics from getting to where they are needed. Without surgery some patients with necrotising fasciitis will die and others will spend many months in hospital.

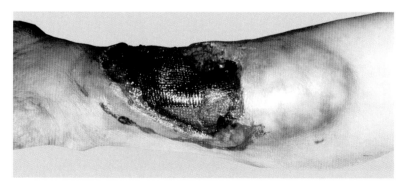

Fig. 12.04 Necrotising fasciitis

Lower legs
Chronic erythematous rash/lesions
Normal surface
Patches, papules, pustules, plaques, nodules and swelling

CHRONIC RASH/LESIONS

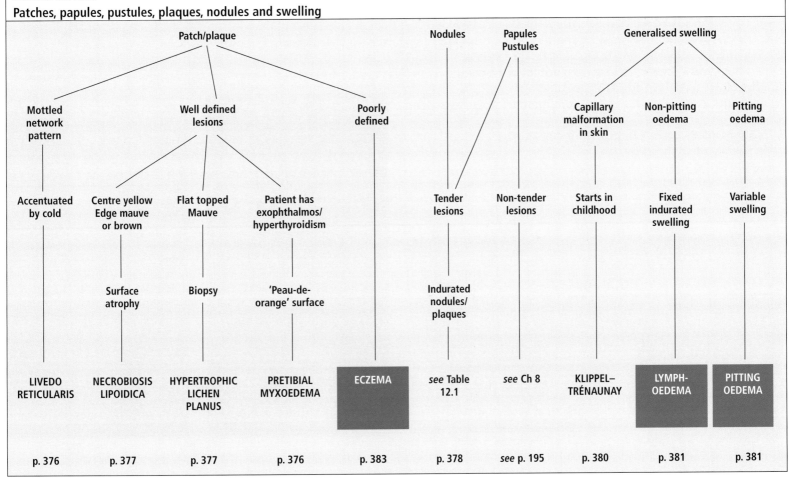

LIVEDO RETICULARIS

Livedo reticularis is a mottled reticular discolouration of the skin, usually on the legs, but can be seen on arms and trunk. It is due to stagnation of blood in capillaries of the skin at the margins of supply between adjacent arterioles. Any reduction in the blood flow of skin arterioles may cause this pattern. The causes are:

1. congenital – cutis marmorata telangiectasia congenita
2. physiological – seen in children and adults in the cold
3. idiopathic – occurs in adults, cause unknown
4. vasculitic – polyarteritis nodosa, autoimmune connective tissue diseases
5. intravascular – cryoglobulins, thrombocytopenia, hypercoagulability states.

Patients should be referred to a specialist to rule out vasculitic and intravascular causes.

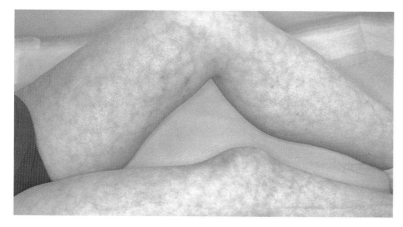

Fig. 12.05 Livedo reticularis

PRETIBIAL MYXOEDEMA

Pink, skin-coloured or yellow, waxy plaques or nodules are seen on the anterior shins of around 10% of patients with hyperthyroidism. It is associated with diffuse thyroid enlargement, exophthalmos, and thyroid acropachy. The surface of the skin has a 'peau d'orange' effect.

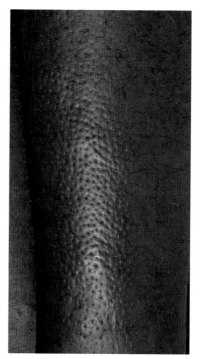

Fig. 12.06 Pretibial myxoedema in black skin

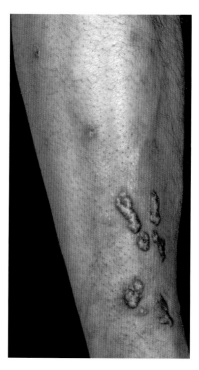

Fig. 12.07 Hypertropic lichen planus in Asian skin

TREATMENT: PRETIBIAL MYXOEDEMA

Treat the skin with a very potent[UK]/group 1–2[USA] topical steroid under occlusion. The thyroid disease will need to be treated with antithyroid drugs or thyroidectomy.

HYPERTROPHIC LICHEN PLANUS

Multiple itchy, thickened, pink-purple, violaceous or hyperpigmented plaques on the lower legs may be due to lichen planus (*see* Fig. 12.07). The surface may be slightly scaly or warty. The presence of typical lichen planus elsewhere will suggest the diagnosis, but an isolated plaque needs to be distinguished from lichen simplex by skin biopsy.

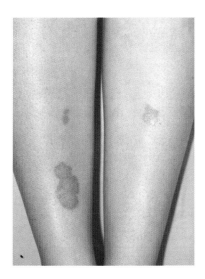
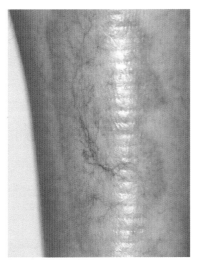

Fig. 2.08 Necrobiosis lipoidica

Fig. 2.09 Necrobiosis lipoidica (close up)

TREATMENT: HYPERTROPHIC LICHEN PLANUS

Hypertrophic lichen planus on the legs may last for years rather than months and is often extremely itchy. A very potent[UK]/group 1[USA] topical steroid cream or ointment, such as 0.05% clobetasol propionate (Dermovate[UK]/Temovate[USA]), will frequently be effective when less potent topical steroids have not helped. Occasionally steroids will have to be injected intralesionally in order to be effective (triamcinolone 10 mg/mL).

NECROBIOSIS LIPOIDICA

Well-defined round or oval plaques on the front of the shins are characteristic of necrobiosis lipoidica. The plaques have a raised mauve or brown edge, while the centre is yellow in colour with obvious telangiectasia. Seventy per cent of patients with this condition are diabetic but there seems to be no relationship between the appearance or spread of the skin disease and control of the diabetes. The affected areas of skin are atrophic and occasionally may ulcerate after trauma (usually obvious trauma such as being kicked or knocked with a supermarket trolley).

TREATMENT: NECROBIOSIS LIPOIDICA

Always check for underlying diabetes mellitus. Treatment is aimed at stopping the plaques from enlarging. If the disease is active (raised mauve border), treat with a potent[UK]/group 2–3[USA] topical steroid cream twice a day until the edge has flattened off. The patient should be warned that the treatment will not get rid of the marks altogether. If the edge is not raised, and the area of skin merely discoloured, treatment with topical steroids will not help.

It can be very difficult to get ulceration to heal. The legs should be carefully protected from further trauma, and a non-stick hydrocolloid or foam dressing applied (*see* Table 2.05, p. 43, and Table 2.08, p. 46). The dressings can be changed twice a week until the ulcer(s) heal.

(cont.)

Systemic steroids such as prednisolone 30 mg/day for a few weeks may induce healing but may upset diabetic control. Alternatively, a skin graft may be required but with a poor cosmetic result. If an area of necrobiosis lipoidica has been ulcerated in the past, the patient should take every care to protect the legs from further injury in the future. This may involve wearing shin pads under the trousers and avoiding trauma.

TENDER RED NODULES (PLAQUES) ON LEGS

One or several tender red nodules or indurated plaques on the lower legs are distinguished by a careful history, examination and a biopsy. A referral to a specialist is usually necessary except for erythema nodosum.

Table 12.1 Causes of **tender** nodules and plaques on the lower legs

Erythema nodosum	Tender red nodules on front of shins Individual lesions only last 7–14 days Associated fever and arthralgia, mainly young women
Panniculitis	Single or multiple red nodules, mainly on lower legs but can be any area of subcutaneous fat Lesions last weeks or months Heal with scarring
Nodular vasculitis	Impossible to distinguish from panniculitis except on biopsy of an early lesion Mainly lower legs, lesions last weeks or months
Polyarteritis nodosa	Benign cutaneous form associated with livedo reticularis and/or ulceration on lower legs Generalised form: patient unwell with involvement of lungs and kidneys; high erythrocyte sedimentation rate
Superficial thrombophlebitis	Red papules over superficial veins No deep involvement

ERYTHEMA NODOSUM

Tender red nodules (plaques) appear on the front of the shins mainly in young women. Individual lesions are 1–10 cm in diameter and initially bright red in colour but fading through the colour changes of a bruise over 7–10 days. Lesions come in crops for 3–6 weeks. There may be associated general malaise, fever and arthropathy.

Common causes of erythema nodosum:
- drugs, e.g. sulphonamides and the oral contraceptive pill
- pregnancy
- streptococcal sore throat
- sarcoidosis
- ulcerative colitis
- Crohn's disease
- tuberculosis
- numerous other viral, bacterial and fungal infections.

TREATMENT: ERYTHEMA NODOSUM

First, treat the underlying cause. Non-steroidal anti-inflammatory drugs (NSAIDs) such as indomethacin 50 mg qid are the most useful treatment. Give regular oral analgesics for the pain (paracetamol, co-codamol) if required. Tell the patient to rest with the feet up as much as possible, and to wear elastic support stockings when walking around.

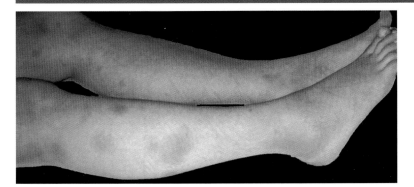

Fig. 12.10 Erythema nodosum: multiple tender nodules and plaques on the lower legs

NODULAR VASCULITIS/PANNICULITIS

One or several red nodules/indurated plaques on the lower legs that persist for weeks or months are due to a nodular vasculitis (inflammation around the blood vessels in the deep dermis or subcutaneous fat) or a panniculitis (inflammation in the subcutaneous fat itself). These can be distinguished by a deep biopsy of an early lesion.

Panniculitis can be caused by:
- cold, especially in the newborn
- trauma to heavy breasts and buttocks
- release of enzymes by pancreatic disease (e.g. pancreatitis or carcinoma of pancreas)
- discoid lupus erythematosus (**lupus profundus**)
- artefact from self-injection of oily liquids (look for the needle mark in the centre!).

In nodular vasculitis, look for a focus of infection such as tuberculosis.

TREATMENT: NODULAR VASCULITIS/PANNICULITIS

Look for the cause and treat that. Where none is found, treatment is symptomatic with analgesics or NSAIDs and compression stockings. Systemic steroids may be needed, starting with prednisolone 30 mg daily and gradually reducing as soon as the disease comes under control to a maintenance dose of 7.5–10 mg daily. Ciclosporin, azathioprine or cyclophosphamide can be tried as steroid-sparing agents. It is often a case of trial and error to find something that will work for a particular individual.

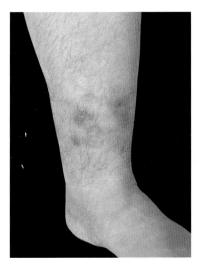

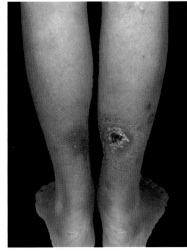

Fig. 12.11 Nodular vasculitis in a patient with tuberculosis

Fig. 12.12 Panniculitis

KLIPPEL–TRÉNAUNAY SYNDROME

Limb enlargement is associated with congenital vascular abnormalities such as a capillary malformation (port wine stain), deeper cavernous vessels, arteriovenous fistulae or venous-lymphatic malformations. The limb enlargement is due to increased blood flow resulting in soft tissue and sometimes bone overgrowth. Typically, a port wine stain is obvious at birth or in early childhood. The limb hypertrophy occurs gradually later on.

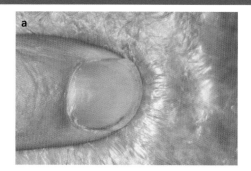
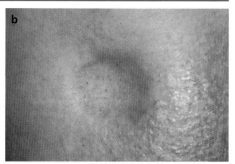

Fig. 12.13 Pitting oedema: (a) firm pressure; (b) slow filling of indentation

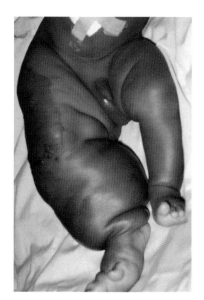

Fig. 12.14 Klippel–Trénaunay syndrome

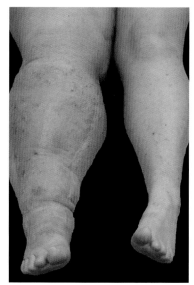

Fig. 12.15 Congenital lymphoedema in the right leg

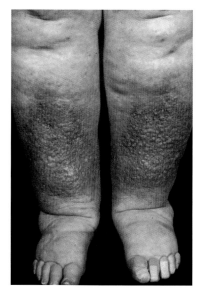

Fig. 12.16 Lymphoedema with secondary polypoid hyperplasia and pigmentation

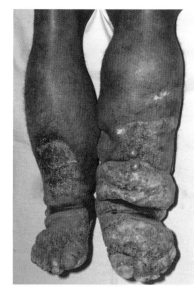

Fig. 12.17 Chronic lymphoedema due to filariasis

PITTING OEDEMA

Oedema is due to accumulation of fluid in the dermis and is demonstrated clinically by firm pressure producing a depression in the surface that only slowly fills in again (*see* Fig. 12.13). Pitting oedema is seen in the most dependent areas – ankles in someone who is ambulant, and over the sacrum in someone who is bedridden. It will resolve with diuretics or if the affected area is elevated.

Unilateral oedema can be due to:
- a deep vein thrombosis
- chronic venous disease (*see* p. 387)
- severe skin disease (e.g. eczema, psoriasis, cellulitis, erysipelas).

Bilateral oedema can be due to:
- cardiac failure
- hypoproteinaemia
- obesity
- nephrotic syndrome
- early lymphoedema
- immobility
- drugs causing salt and water retention (e.g. hormones, antihypertensives, calcium-channel blockers, monoamine oxidase inhibitors, systemic steroids)
- venous outflow obstruction in pregnancy and abdominal masses.

TREATMENT: LYMPHOEDEMA

Because the lymphatics are permanently absent or damaged, the condition is incurable. Simple hygiene measures such as washing with soap and water and moisturising the skin can prevent recurrent bacterial infections. Deep breathing for 10 minutes before getting out of bed in the morning helps to empty the lymphatics in the chest and abdomen. Massaging the limb regularly and applying a compression bandage is helpful (*see* p. 389). It is important to keep the limb moving and when seated to elevate the limb. Complications should be prevented by the use of prophylatic penicillin V (250 mg bid) and antifungals applied every night between the toes. Hyperkeratosis can be treated with 5% salicylic acid ointment and excessive papillomatosis can be removed by curettage (*see* p. 391).

LYMPHOEDEMA

Damage to lymphatics results in retention of protein-rich interstitial fluid in the affected limb, leading to swelling (*see* Fig. 12.15) and fibrosis, so that the oedema becomes non-pitting and non-dependent (i.e. will not improve with diuretics or on elevation of the limb). The skin becomes thickened (you will not be able to pinch a fold of skin over the base of the second toe) with accentuated skin creases. Hyperkeratosis and papillomatosis occur after a few years (*see* Fig. 12.32). Secondary complications of lymphoedema include discomfort and 'heaviness' in the limb, reduced mobility, leakage of fluid from breaks in the skin, secondary streptococcal infection (cellulitis) and tinea pedis between the toes.

Causes of primary lymphoedema:
- absence or hypoplastic lymphatics.

The age the lymphoedema becomes apparent is determined by other factors such as infection and venous insufficiency.

Causes of secondary lymphoedema:
- Infection: recurrent streptococcal infections
- Filariasis: *Wuchereria bancrofti* microfiliariae are transmitted by mosquito bites; they mature into adult worms, which obstruct the lymphatics – think of it in patients from the tropics (*see* Fig. 12.17)
- Inflammation: chronic eczema or psoriasis
- Neoplasia: cancer infiltrating lymph nodes
- Trauma:
  — surgical removal of lymph nodes
  — radiotherapy to lymph nodes
  — artefactual – restrictive band applied to leg.

Lower legs
Chronic erythematous rash/lesions
Scale, crust or exudate on surface
Large patches and plaques (>2 cm diameter)
(For lesions <2 cm size *see* Chapter 8, pp. 202 and 245)

SCALE, CRUST, EXUDATE

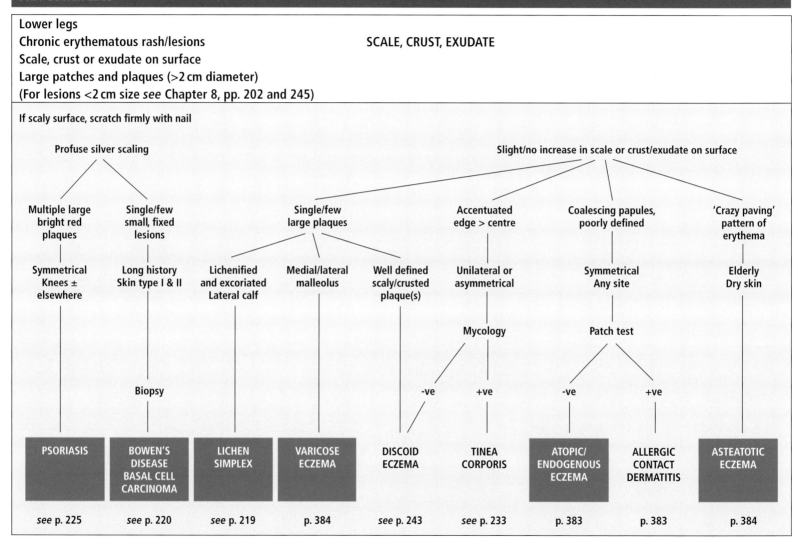

If scaly surface, scratch firmly with nail

Profuse silver scaling

Slight/no increase in scale or crust/exudate on surface

Multiple large bright red plaques

Single/few small, fixed lesions

Single/few large plaques

Accentuated edge > centre

Coalescing papules, poorly defined

'Crazy paving' pattern of erythema

Symmetrical Knees ± elsewhere

Long history Skin type I & II

Lichenified and excoriated Lateral calf

Medial/lateral malleolus

Well defined scaly/crusted plaque(s)

Unilateral or asymmetrical

Symmetrical Any site

Elderly Dry skin

Mycology

Patch test

Biopsy

-ve   +ve

-ve   +ve

PSORIASIS	BOWEN'S DISEASE BASAL CELL CARCINOMA	LICHEN SIMPLEX	VARICOSE ECZEMA	DISCOID ECZEMA	TINEA CORPORIS	ATOPIC/ ENDOGENOUS ECZEMA	ALLERGIC CONTACT DERMATITIS	ASTEATOTIC ECZEMA
see p. 225	*see* p. 220	*see* p. 219	p. 384	*see* p. 243	*see* p. 233	p. 383	p. 383	p. 384

ECZEMA ON THE LOWER LEGS

Poorly defined, red scaly papules or plaques on the lower legs are likely to be due to eczema. It is possible to classify the eczema by the distribution and appearance.

- Acute weeping eczema suggests an allergic contact dermatitis.
- Varicose eczema occurs around the malleoli in patients with other evidence of venous disease.
- Asteototic eczema is seen in elderly patients where the skin has been allowed to dry out (*see* p. 384).
- Atopic eczema elsewhere (previous or present flexural eczema in the antecubital or popliteal fossae or on the front of wrists).
- Symmetrical eczema that does not fit any of the above is an unclassifiable endogenous eczema.

Well-defined plaques may be due to:

- varicose eczema around medial or lateral malleoli
- discoid eczema – either the wet type, if surface exudate and crust present, or the dry type, if scaly (*see* p. 243)
- lichen simplex if situated on the lateral calf or ankle and associated with itching and excessive scratching (*see* p. 219).

These will need to be distinguished from psoriasis (scratching the surface leads to profuse silver scaling).

ALLERGIC CONTACT DERMATITIS

Allergic contact dermatitis on the lower legs is usually due to medicaments applied in the treatment of venous eczema or ulcers. The common sensitisers are various antibiotics (neomycin, soframycin, fucidin), lanolin in various ointments, parabens and MCI (methylchloroisothiazolinone) in creams and paste bandages, and occasionally the rubber in elastic support bandages.

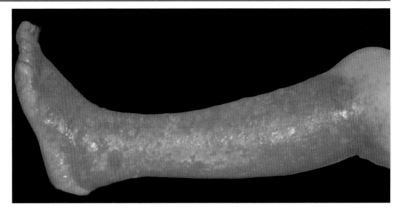

Fig. 12.18 Acute allergic contact dermatitis from bandages: erosions and exudate but no ulceration

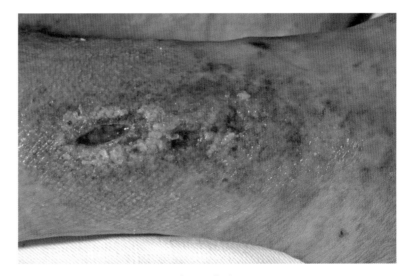

Fig. 12.19 Varicose eczema around a small ulcer

TREATMENT: ACUTE ALLERGIC CONTACT DERMATITIS

Dry up the exudate with potassium permanganate^UK or aluminium acetate^USA soaks (*see* p. 30). Treat the eczema with a potent^UK/group 2–3^USA topical steroid ointment twice a day (not a cream, as the preservative in a cream can itself be the causative allergen). Once the rash is better, identify the allergen by patch testing so that it can be avoided in the future.

ASTEATOTIC ECZEMA (ECZEMA CRAQUELÉ)

Asteatotic eczema is due to drying out of the skin especially in the elderly. It occurs in winter or when patients are hospitalised and made to bathe more frequently than they are used to. The skin is dry or scaly with irregular erythematous fissures like 'crazy paving'. The associated itching usually brings it to the attention of the doctor.

TREATMENT: ASTEATOTIC ECZEMA

The patient should either bathe less often or use one of the dispersible bath oils in the bath water each day and a greasy (water-in-oil) emollient (*see* p. 26) can then be applied to the dry scaly skin twice a day. Occasionally a weak^UK/group 7^USA topical steroid such as 1% hydrocortisone ointment may be needed.

VARICOSE/STASIS ECZEMA

Eczema may occur in patients with venous hypertension (*see* p. 387). It is distinguished from other types of eczema by being confined to the lower legs in a patient with other signs of venous disease. Acute-on-chronic varicose eczema should suggest a superadded allergic contact dermatitis rather than cellulitis, which is unilateral and feels hot.

Fig. 12.20 Asteatotic eczema

TREATMENT: VARICOSE ECZEMA

More important than what is put onto the eczema itself is treatment of the underlying problem (chronic venous stasis due to incompetent valves in the deep veins of the calf) with proper elastic support. It is probably best to use bandages (*see* p. 389) until the eczema is better and then change to elastic stockings, because the treatment for the eczema may otherwise ruin the stockings.

For the eczema itself, a moderately potent^UK/group 4–5^USA topical steroid ointment can be applied twice a day. The patient may prefer a cream to an ointment, particularly since that will make less of a mess of his or her bandages. This should be resisted though, because many patients are allergic to parabens (from the use of creams or paste bandages). All patients with varicose eczema should be patch tested to make sure that you do not make things worse by applying ointments, dressings and bandages that they are allergic to.

Lower legs, feet (any site)

Ulcerated surface

1. Acute – rapid onset

2. Chronic: surrounding skin affected

ULCERS: ACUTE, & CHRONIC (surrounding skin abnormal)

Rapid (acute) onset
Dusky discolouration of skin
→ large necrotic ulcer

Chronic (>2 weeks) slow onset — *Surrounding skin normal*, see *next page*

Surrounding skin *abnormal*

Unwell Toxic	Patient feels well	Child, malnourished	Associated purpuric papules/ vesicles	Surrounding erythema, scaling, pigmentation		Yellow plaque telangiectasia	Skin atrophic telangiectasia
Lower legs, hands, face	Any site ? Associated systemic disease	Legs and feet Tropical climate	Legs and feet BIOPSY	Around ankles Large, shallow painless (usually)	Afro-Caribbean +ve sickle cell	Front of shin BIOPSY	Previous therapy
NECROTISING FASCIITIS	PYODERMA GANGRENOSUM	TROPICAL ULCER	VASCULITIS/ POLYARTERITIS NODOSUM	VENOUS/STASIS ULCER	SICKLE CELL ULCER	NECROBIOSIS LIPOIDICA	STEROIDS or RADIOTHERAPY
see p. 374	p. 396	p. 397	p. 401	p. 387	p. 397	*see* p. 377	p. 396

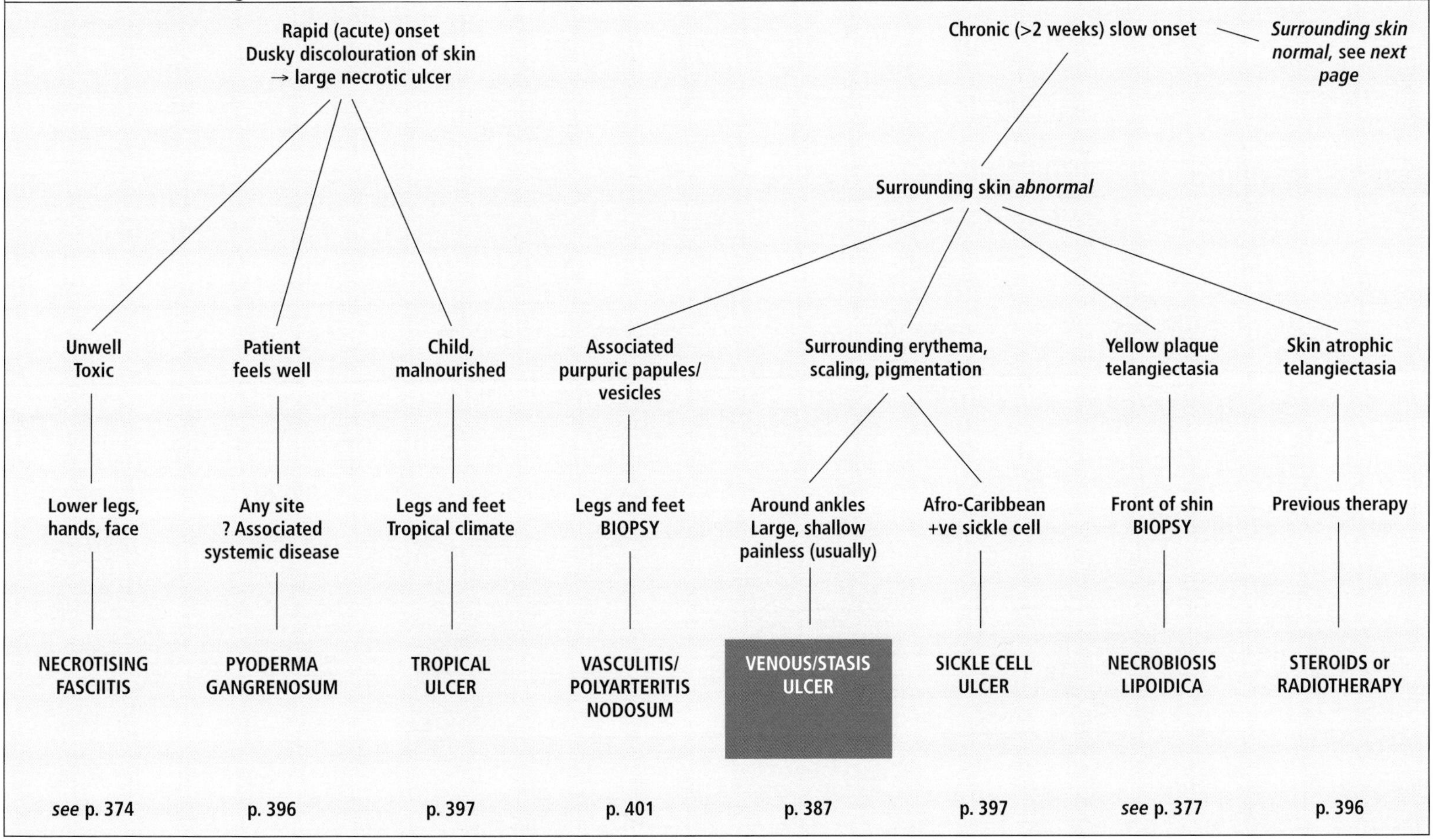

Lower legs, feet (any site)
Ulcerated surface
Surrounding skin normal

CHRONIC ULCERS – surrounding skin normal

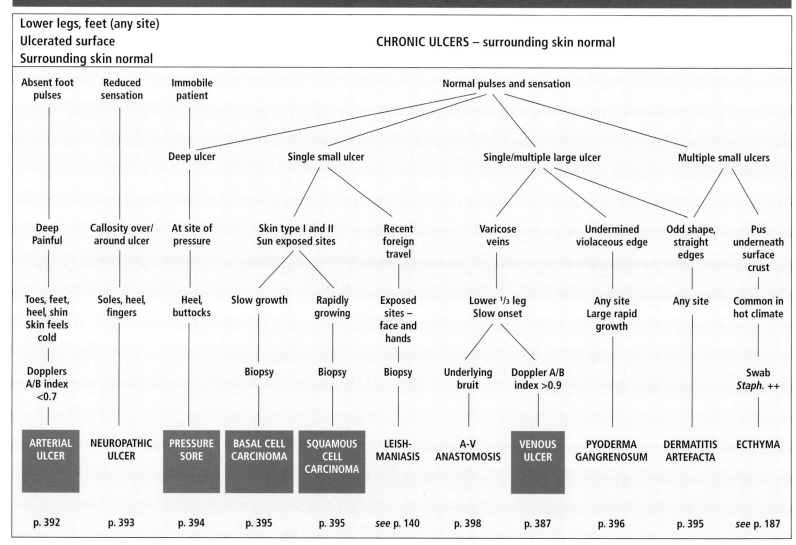

Absent foot pulses	**Reduced sensation**	**Immobile patient**				**Normal pulses and sensation**				
		Deep ulcer	**Single small ulcer**			**Single/multiple large ulcer**		**Multiple small ulcers**		
Deep Painful	Callosity over/ around ulcer	At site of pressure	Skin type I and II Sun exposed sites		Recent foreign travel	Varicose veins	Undermined violaceous edge	Odd shape, straight edges	Pus underneath surface crust	
Toes, feet, heel, shin Skin feels cold	Soles, heel, fingers	Heel, buttocks	Slow growth	Rapidly growing	Exposed sites – face and hands	Lower ⅓ leg Slow onset	Any site Large rapid growth	Any site	Common in hot climate	
Dopplers A/B index <0.7			Biopsy	Biopsy	Biopsy	Underlying bruit / Doppler A/B index >0.9			Swab *Staph.* ++	
ARTERIAL ULCER	**NEUROPATHIC ULCER**	**PRESSURE SORE**	**BASAL CELL CARCINOMA**	**SQUAMOUS CELL CARCINOMA**	**LEISH-MANIASIS**	**A-V ANASTOMOSIS** / **VENOUS ULCER**	**PYODERMA GANGRENOSUM**	**DERMATITIS ARTEFACTA**	**ECTHYMA**	
p. 392	p. 393	p. 394	p. 395	p. 395	*see* p. 140	p. 398 / p. 387	p. 396	p. 395	*see* p. 187	

VENOUS ULCERS

The cause of venous ulceration is loss of the valves in the deep or perforating veins. The venous blood returns from the lower legs back to the heart by the calf muscle pump. Compression of the calf muscles (by walking or running) squeezes blood up the legs. Blood is drawn from the superficial veins and pushed upwards by valves, which prevent back flow. Loss or incompetence of these valves results in enormous pressure (venous hypertension) in the superficial veins that is transmitted back to the capillaries, resulting in venous disease and ulceration.

Venous ulcers occur on the lower third of the leg, over either the medial or the lateral malleolus. They are large, superficial and painless; if painful, then there may be an element of arterial insufficiency. There will be other evidence of venous disease such as oedema, varicose veins (see Fig. 12.22), venous flare (see Fig. 12.26), pigmentation (orange brown due to haemosiderin or dark brown due to melanin, see Figs 12.27 and 12.28), eczema (see Fig. 12.19), atrophie blanche (white scars with telangiectasia on the surface, see Fig. 12.25) and fibrosis around the ankle (lipodermatosclerosis, see Fig. 12.23), which results in narrowing around the ankle with lack of skin mobility (the opposite to oedema).

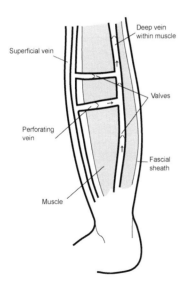

Fig. 12.21 Anatomy of veins in lower leg showing deep, superficial and perforating veins with one-way valves

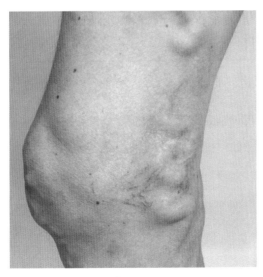

Fig. 12.22 Varicose veins

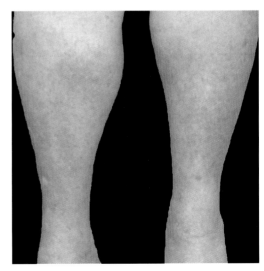

Fig. 12.23 Lipodermatosclerosis (inverted champagne bottle shape)

Complications of venous ulceration are relatively rare and include cellulitis, haemorrhage, soft tissue calcification (*see* p. 391) and malignant change (*see* p. 395). Infection of the ulcer itself is of little consequence and mixed organisms are often present. Taking swabs for bacteriology should be discouraged, as this tempts the physician to treat with potentially sensitising topical antibiotics. Cellulitis should be treated promptly, but this diagnosis is made on clinical grounds (*see* p. 373). Venous ulcers may be complicated by arterial insufficiency; pain and poor healing with compression bandages suggest this.

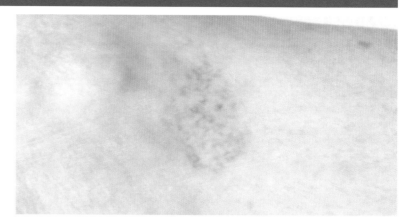

Fig. 12.25 Atrophie blanche around the ankle

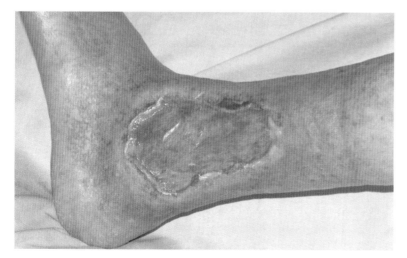

Fig. 12.24 Venous leg ulcer: large, superficial and painless, situated on the lower third of the lower leg – note both post-inflammatory hyperpigmentation and haemosiderin pigmentation around the ulcer

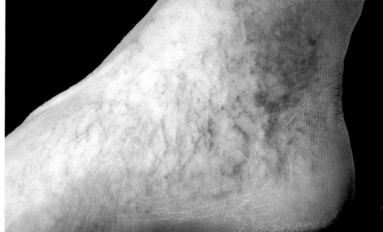

Fig. 12.26 Venous flare: tiny dilated veins visible on the surface

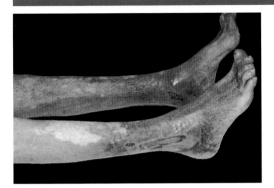

Fig. 12.27 Post-inflammatory hyperpigmentation secondary to venous disease and varicose eczema

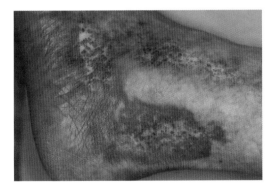

Fig. 12.28 Haemosiderin pigmentation on lower leg, secondary to venous stasis with areas of atrophie blanche

TREATMENT: VENOUS LEG ULCERS

1. Clean and debride the ulcer (*see* Table 2.05, p. 43)
2. Apply an emollient to the skin around the ulcer (*see* Table 2.01a, p. 26)
3. Apply a dressing to absorb any exudate (*see* Table 2.07, p. 45) and protect the ulcer during healing (*see* Table 2.08, p. 46)
4. Assess arterial blood flow to leg (feel pulses and do Dopplers, p. 393)
5. Compression bandaging or stockings – *see* next box
6. Treat any associated complications and consider skin grafting
7. Elevate the leg when at rest; the ankle should be at the level of the pelvis

Compression bandaging

The only effective way of treating venous hypertension is by external compression of the leg by bandaging or support stockings. This compresses the superficial veins so that blood must flow in the deep veins (*see* Fig. 12.21).

Two-layer bandaging (*see* Fig. 12.29) has replaced four-layer bandaging because the dressings are less expensive and patients can wear normal footwear, improving compliance. A tubular stockinette is applied over the skin and any ulcer dressings and the two layers are as follows.
1. Orthopaedic wool: it is applied as a spiral with 50% overlap. This is absorbent and pads out any bony protuberances.
2. Compression bandage: **short-stretch** bandages, where the bandage is pulled to full stretch (e.g. Actico, Comprilan), are preferred – this is easier for patients to apply themselves but should be used only in mobile patients; **long-stretch** bandages, where the bandage is pulled to 50% stretch (e.g. Tensopress, Setopress, Surepress), can be used on mobile or non-mobile patients.

Four-layer bandaging (*see* Fig. 12.30) is best used in immobile patients, as it provides constant pressure to the leg. It needs to be applied by a nurse with the appropriate training. It will remain in place and be effective for a full week.

The four layers come as a pack (Ultra Four, Profore) and consist of the following:
1. orthopaedic wool (Ultra Soft, Profore#1) as a spiral with 50% overlap
2. crepe bandage (UltraLite, Profore#2) as spiral at mid-stretch
3. high-compression long-stretch bandage (Ultraplus, Profore#3)
4. cohesive lightweight elastic bandage (UltraFast, Profore#4).

Profore is the only system available for calf size of 25–30 cm and above.

(cont.)

Once the ulcer has healed, bandaging should be continued for at least 4 weeks to allow the healed skin to stabilise. Dopplers should be repeated every 6 months if compression is continued.

Elastic support in the form of **compression stockings** is necessary for the rest of the patient's life, since the missing leg valves cannot be replaced. Support is achieved by wearing a below-knee elastic stocking. Decide on the compression level required (*see* Table 12.02). For treatment of venous disease, UK class 2 (EU/US class 1) is usual. Table 12.03 gives an indication of the size the patient requires. Styles of stocking vary. Pulling on stockings can be helped by using a glide sheet, which is put on the leg first, over which the stocking then easily slides, and is then removed; alternatively, a metal stocking donner aid can be used.

Table 12.02 Compression levels for stockings

Indication	Prolonged sitting, pregnancy	Varicose veins, healed leg ulcers	Moderate lymphoedema, severe varicose veins	Severe lymphoedema
Compression UK Class EU/US class	Light Class 1	Moderate Class 2 Class 1	Firm Class 3 Class 2	Extra-firm Class 3
UK range (mmHg)	14–17	18–24	25–35	
US range (mmHg)		15–20	20–30	30–40
EU range (mmHg)		18–21	23–32	34–46

Table 12.03 Measuring for compression stockings

Measure circumference at calf and ankle					
Stocking size	Small	Medium	Large	X-Large	XX-Large
Calf circumference (cm)	30–37	33–40	35–43	37–46	40–49
Ankle circumference (cm)	19–23	22–25	24–28	28–30	30–34
Measure height below kneecap to floor					
Floor to below-knee height (cm)	<42 = Regular			>42 = Long	

Note: sizes are approximate, as individual brands vary.

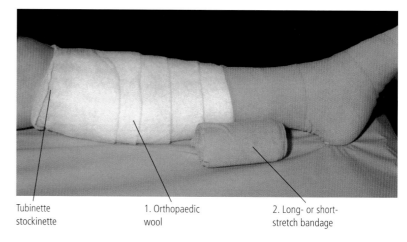

Tubinette stockinette — 1. Orthopaedic wool — 2. Long- or short-stretch bandage

Fig. 12.29 Two-layer bandaging

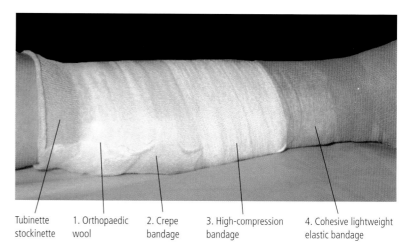

Tubinette stockinette — 1. Orthopaedic wool — 2. Crepe bandage — 3. High-compression bandage — 4. Cohesive lightweight elastic bandage

Fig. 12.30 Four-layer bandaging

Skin grafting

Pinch grafts or partial thickness skin grafts can be used to hasten the healing process. Small islands of skin are placed on the clean ulcer bed and the area covered with a non-adherent dressing. The patient will need to remain on bed rest for 2 weeks with leg elevation to allow the graft to take.

TREATMENT: COMPLICATIONS

- Associated **arterial disease** (*see* pp. 393–4).
- **Overgranulation** of the ulcer: too much granulation tissue will delay healing. This can be removed by applying a silver nitrate stick to the area before applying compression. Some patients find this extremely painful, and if this is the case apply a gauze swab soaked in 0.25% silver nitrate solution instead. Alternatively, granulation tissue can be curetted off.
- **Secondary infection** of the ulcer. Only two infections in leg ulcers matter:
  —Pseudomonas infection causes an unpleasant smell. This can be eradicated with 5% acetic acid (use ordinary household vinegar diluted 50% in water). Cut a piece of gauze to the size of the ulcer and soak it in the vinegar. Apply the gauze daily to the ulcer until the smell goes. Alternatively, a 0.25% solution of silver nitrate can be used (*see* Table 2.06, p. 44). These are much more effective than intravenous piperacillin or ticarcillin and clavularic acid.
  —Group A β-haemolytic streptococci in an ulcer causes cellulitis. This is diagnosed clinically. Taking swabs from leg ulcers is to be discouraged. Treat with intravenous benzyl penicillin (*see* p. 374).
- **Eczema** around the ulcer (*see* p. 384).
- **Nodular polypoid hyperplasia**: the excess tissue can be scraped off using a curette (*see* Fig. 12.32). No anaesthetic is needed. It will not reoccur if the patient wears compression bandages.
- **Subcutaneous calcification**: some venous ulcers will not heal because of calcium deposition in the subcutaneous fat, which can be confirmed by X-ray (*see* Fig. 12.50). Because it is difficult to treat, refer to a dermatologist.

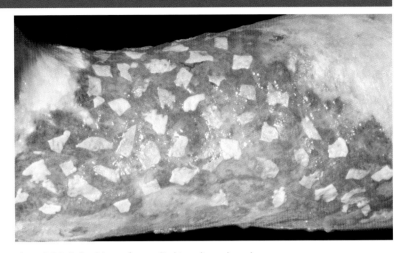

Fig. 12.31 Split skin grafts applied to a large leg ulcer

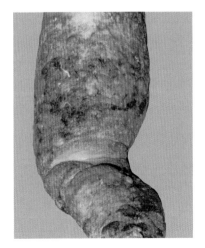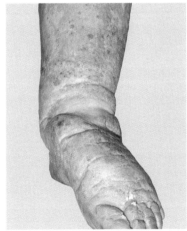

Fig. 12.32 (a) Nodular polypoid hyperplasia associated with lymphoedema; (b) after excess tissue removed by curettage

ARTERIAL ULCERS

These are due to a reduction in arterial blood supply to the lower limb usually due to atherosclerosis. They are typically painful, punched out and relatively deep (sometimes revealing the underlying tendons). They occur where the arterial supply is poorest – on the tips of toes, the dorsum of the foot, the heel and the front of the shin. The absence of peripheral pulses and a history of intermittent claudication will confirm the diagnosis. Other signs to look for are cold feet, blotchy erythema of the feet, loss of hair and thickened toenails. Untreated, gangrene will eventually follow. The patient may have evidence of more widespread arterial disease, e.g. a past history of coronary thrombosis or stroke.

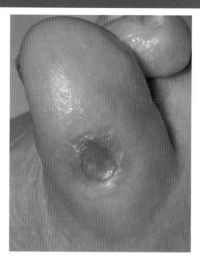

Fig. 12.34 Arterial ulcer on side of toe

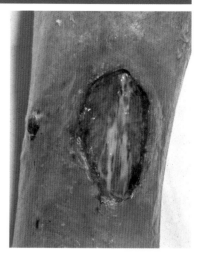

Fig. 12.35 Arterial ulcer on front of shin with tendon visible

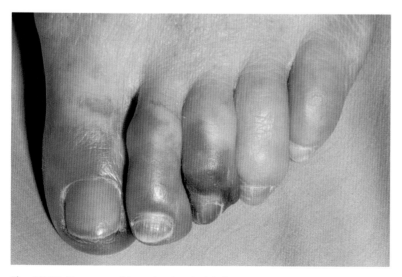

Fig. 12.33 Gangrene of toes due to arterial disease

TREATMENT: ARTERIAL LEG ULCERS

A patient with an arterial ulcer should be referred to a vascular surgeon. If it is not possible to improve the arterial blood supply, it is very unlikely that the ulcer will heal, and gangrene will eventually occur. Early rather than late amputation is advised before the pain becomes intolerable.

Treatment of the ulcer itself. If there is any slough present, it should be removed either with a pair of sharp scissors or a scalpel or with a desloughing agent (*see* p. 43). Once the ulcer is clean it should be covered with a non-adhesive dressing (*see* p. 46). This can be left in place for a week at a time so that any new epithelial cells will not be removed as soon as they have formed. The dressing is covered with a light bandage simply to keep it in place. Do not apply tight bandages or any kind of elastic support, because they can impede the arterial supply further. Adequate analgesics must also be given during the healing process since these ulcers are always painful.

NEUROPATHIC ULCERS

These ulcers result from trauma to anaesthetic feet, so occur over bony prominences, particularly the first metatarsophalangeal joint, the metatarsal heads or the heel, or at any other site of injury. Classically they are deep, painless, and often covered with thick callous. The diagnosis is confirmed by finding sensory loss and some associated disorder that has caused it, e.g. diabetes, leprosy, paraplegia, peripheral nerve injury, polyneuropathy, syringomyelia.

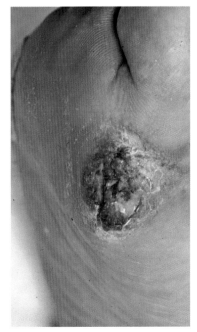

Fig. 12.37 Neuropathic ulcer over first metatarsal head

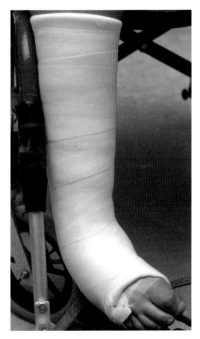

Fig. 12.38 Treatment of a neuropathic ulcer by protecting it in a plaster cast

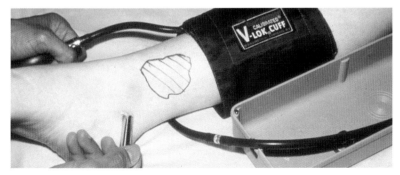

Fig. 12.36 Measurement of the systolic blood pressure at the ankle using a Doppler probe: shaded area usual site for venous ulcers – place cuff above this on calf

TREATMENT: NEUROPATHIC ULCERS

Loss of sensation means that patients may not notice an injury to their anaesthetic feet or legs. Rubbing from shoes, treading on a nail, being bumped into by a supermarket trolley, having the toes accidentally trodden on, or burning by hot water are some of the common sources of injury. If the patient does not notice what has happened and does not protect the area from further damage, an ulcer can form. On the sole of the foot, callous often builds up around the injury, making an ulcer seem smaller than it really is or sometimes completely covering it. It is essential to remove the callous with a scalpel to see how big the ulcer is. If nothing is done at this stage, repeated trauma will cause the ulcer to enlarge, and secondary infection is likely to occur (sometimes leading to osteomyelitis). The foot should be X-rayed and bacteriology swabs taken. If osteomyelitis is present the patient should be admitted to hospital so that high doses of intravenous antibiotics can be given.

To get the ulcers healed, further injury/friction must be avoided. The simplest way of achieving this is by the patient resting in bed but this is not usually practical. An alternative is to apply a below-knee walking plaster for 2 months at a time (*see* Fig. 12. 38). This removes any friction and allows the ulcer to heal. After 2 months when the plaster is removed the ulcer is usually healed; if it is not, it is put back on for a further 2 months. If the ulcer is very dirty and there is a lot of exudate, the plaster can have a window cut in it to allow the ulcer to be cleaned regularly and to minimise the unpleasant smell for the patient.

Removing the slough (*see* p. 43) and applying non-adherent dressings (*see* p. 46) is the same as for venous ulcers. There is no need for elastic support. The idea is simply to keep the ulcer clean and free of friction while it heals.

The same principles apply to the treatment of pressure sores. Pressure on bony areas should be minimised by frequent changes of position and the use of a wool fleece or ripple bed.

ULCERS IN A DIABETIC PATIENT

Patients with diabetes mellitus can have both arterial and neuropathic ulcers. It is important to sort out which of the two is the main culprit and treat accordingly. The arterial disease can be due to atherosclerosis of the major limb vessels or small vessel disease (in which case the treatment options may be limited). Either type of ulcer (or both) can be complicated by bacterial infection. It is important to deal with this promptly with systemic antibiotics. Necrobiosis lipoidica (*see* p. 377) can also ulcerate.

PRESSURE SORES

Sustained pressure over pressure points in immobile patients leads to localised ischaemia and eventual ulceration.

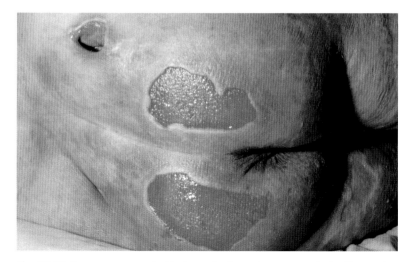

Fig. 12.39 Pressure sores on buttocks: note deep ulcer over posterior iliac crest

SKIN NEOPLASM

Basal cell carcinomas (*see* p. 330) are a common cause of leg ulcers in the elderly with fair skin. They are usually small, slow growing and can be anywhere on the lower legs (*see* Fig. 12.41). A squamous cell carcinoma (*see* p. 332) can arise in sun-damaged skin but also in a chronic venous ulcer or burn scar. Occasionally a tumour around the ankles can be misdiagnosed as a venous ulcer and can be treated for a long time by compression bandaging. Any chronic non-healing ulcer, especially one with a proliferative base (*see* Fig. 12.40) should be biopsied to exclude a skin tumour. Any red or pigmented lesion that ulcerates should be urgently biopsied to exclude a malignant melanoma.

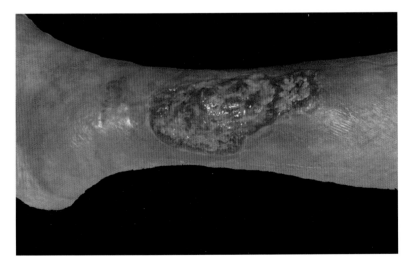

Fig. 12.40 A large squamous cell carcinoma that had been treated as a venous ulcer for over a year: note the proliferation of tissue in the centre (compare with Fig. 12.24)

DERMATITIS ARTEFACTA

Any ulcer with straight edges (linear, square or triangular), or at an unusual site is likely to be artefactual unless proven otherwise (*see* p. 260). Treatment depends on preventing the patient damaging the site, e.g. by covering it with a bandage or plaster cast.

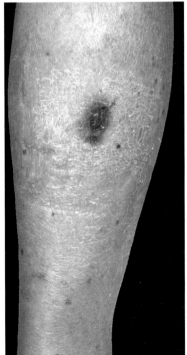

Fig. 12.41 Basal cell carcinoma on the shin: biopsy confirms diagnosis

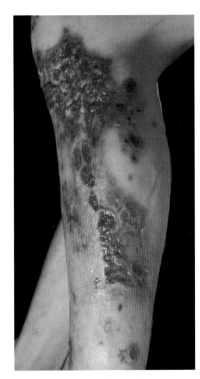

Fig. 12.42 Dermatitis artefacta: bizarre straight edges

PYODERMA GANGRENOSUM

A rapidly growing ulcer with a violaceous overhanging edge and a yellow, honeycomb-like base should make you think of pyoderma gangrenosum. It is associated with ulcerative colitis, Crohn's disease, rheumatoid arthritis and multiple myeloma. In patients with ulcerative colitis, the activity of the pyoderma gangrenosum reflects the activity of the bowel problem, but with the other diseases the two conditions seem to behave independently of each other.

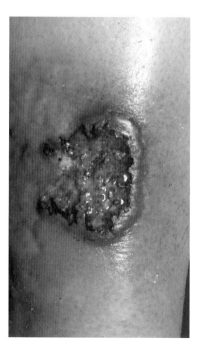

Fig. 12.43 Pyoderma gangrenosum with violaceous overhanging edge

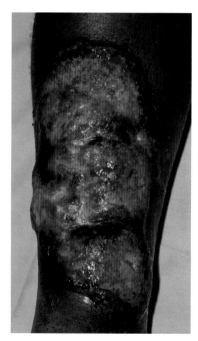

Fig. 12.44 Pyoderma gangrenosum in black skin

TREATMENT: PYODERMA GANGRENOSUM

Patients with pyoderma gangrenosum should be referred urgently to a dermatologist or gastroenterologist for investigation of the underlying cause. The ulcer is treated with large doses of systemic steroids, beginning with prednisolone 60 mg daily. Once the ulcer is healed the dose can gradually be reduced, and eventually the patient will be able to come off the steroids. Other immunosuppressive agents such as ciclosporin 3–5 mg/kg/day or azathiaprine 3 mg/kg/day can also be tried in addition to or instead of oral steroids.

Other possible treatments are a very potent[UK]/group 1[USA] topical steroid such as 0.05% clobetasol propionate applied twice a day to the ulcer, oral clofazamine, dapsone or minocycline. Biologics such as the anti-TNF therapies (see p. 56) can be trialled in severe recalcitrant cases.

STEROIDS OR RADIOTHERAPY

Topical or systemic steroids used over a long period, or previous radiotherapy, may result in thinning of dermal collagen and ulceration after minor trauma.

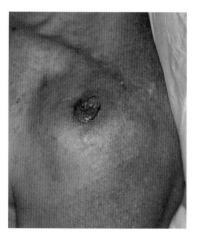

Fig. 12.45 (right) Ulcer on shoulder at site of previous radiotherapy

TROPICAL AND BURULI ULCERS

The most likely cause of ulcers developing in a tropical climate is **ecthyma**, a staphylococcal infection of the epidermis and dermis from an insect bite or scratch (*see* p. 187).

A **tropical phagedenic ulcer** is a fast-growing, painful ulcer on the lower legs and feet in malnourished children from Africa, India, South East Asia, Central and South America or the Caribbean. It can grow 5 cm or larger in 2–3 weeks and usually has a rolled edge. It is due to fusiform bacilli and treponemes.

A **Buruli ulcer** begins as a firm, painless, subcutaneous nodule that either heals spontaneously or ulcerates. Ulcers can remain small and heal without treatment, or spread rapidly undermining the skin over large areas, even an entire limb. It is due to *Mycobacterium ulcerans*, which is found in water bugs in swamps. The organism enters the skin through a cut or abrasion, usually in children who play in and around swamps in tropical Africa or Mexico. The diagnosis can be confirmed by taking a smear from the necrotic base of the ulcer and finding acid-fast bacilli on Ziehl–Neelsen stain.

TREATMENT: TOPICAL ULCERS

- Ecthyma: *see* p. 188.
- Phagedenic ulcer: clean the ulcer and give antibiotics orally for 1–2 weeks (phenoxymethylpenicillin, erythromycin or metronidazole).
- Buruli ulcer: rifampicin at 10 mg/kg body weight by mouth daily for 8 weeks and streptomycin at 15 mg/kg body weight by intramuscular injection daily for 8 weeks (contraindicated in pregnancy) remains the World Health Organization's recommended standard antibiotic treatment.

SICKLE CELL ULCERS

Patients with sickle cell anaemia who are homozygous for the sickle cell gene develop ischaemic ulcers on the legs and feet in childhood and early adult life. They look like venous ulcers but are due to blockage of small arterioles in the legs and feet by the sickled red blood cells. Confirm the diagnosis by haemoglobin electrophoresis. Keep the ulcer clean until it heals.

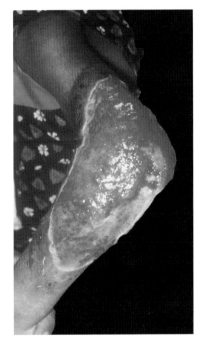

Fig. 12.46 Buruli ulcer

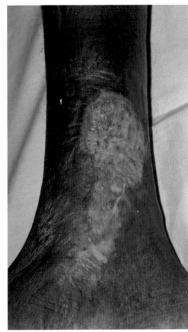

Fig. 12.47 Sickle cell ulcer: looks like an ordinary venous leg ulcer but the patient is Afro-Caribbean and has no evidence of venous disease

ATYPICAL ULCERS

Leg ulcers are most commonly due to venous disease, arterial insufficiency or sensory loss. If an ulcer on the leg (or elsewhere) is not healing with recognised treatments or does not fit any of the common patterns or appearances, it should be biopsied to exclude a skin tumour or one of the rare causes illustrated on this page.

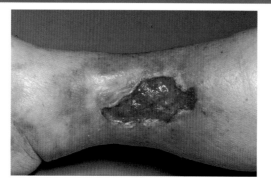

Fig. 12.48 Leg ulcer over an arteriovenous anastomosis: warm leg with an obvious bruit – can be congenital or follow a fracture

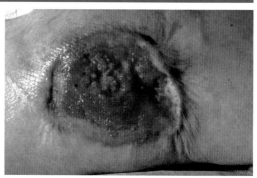

Fig. 12.49 Very rapidly growing ulcer due to tertiary syphilis

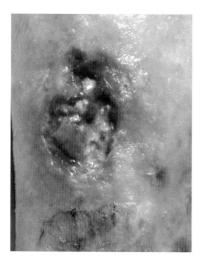
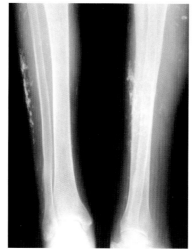

Fig. 12.50 (a) Non-healing ulcer on calf found to be full of calcium; (b) X-ray to demonstrate subcutaneous calcification beneath ulcer

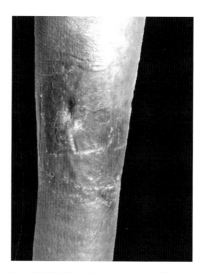
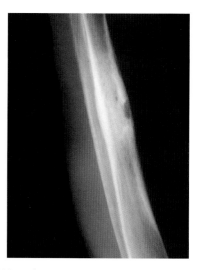

Fig. 12.51 This ulcer looked as if it should have been a venous ulcer but it is situated on the front of the shin: biopsy revealed tuberculosis with involvement of the tibia on X-ray (right)

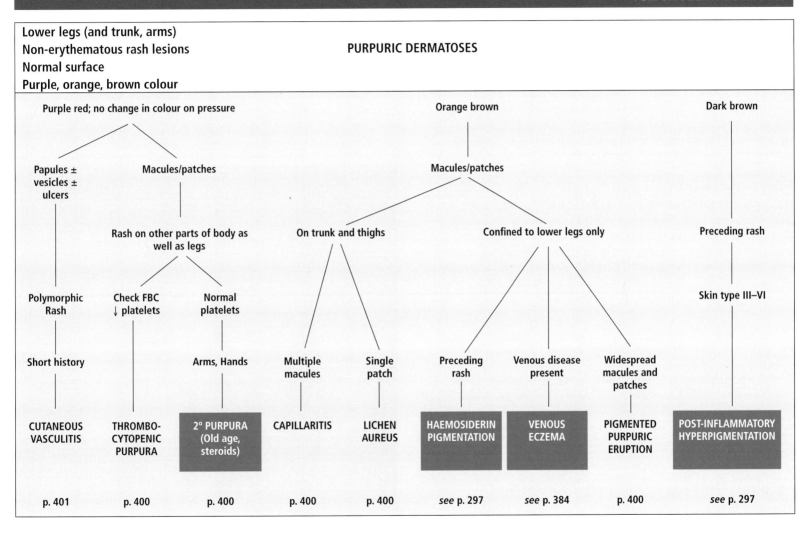

PURPURA

Purpura is due to leakage of red blood cells from blood vessels into the skin. When compressed with the finger, the red colour does not disappear as it would if the blood were still inside the blood vessels (as in erythema, *see* Figs. 1.60 and 1.61, p. 14). The extravasated blood is broken down to haemosiderin, causing the colour to change from purple to orange brown. Purpura may be due to a platelet disorder (thrombocytopenic) or a vascular disorder (non-thrombocytopenic).

Thrombocytopenic purpura

If the platelet count falls below 50000/mm³ bleeding may occur. In the skin this is seen as tiny purpuric macules and papules (petechiae) and larger patches (ecchymoses). There may be bleeding elsewhere too. Thrombocytopenia may be due to bone marrow disease (pancytopenia, leukaemia, drug-induced marrow failure), systemic infections, splenomegaly or idiopathic thrombocytopenic purpura.

Non-thrombocytopenic purpura

Non-thrombocytopenic purpura can be due to the following:
- leaky blood vessels (**capillaritis**) – uniformly small, orange-brown macules occur anywhere on the skin; the cause is unknown and no treatment is available; when this is localised to a single area it is known as **lichen aureus**
- lack of connective tissue support for blood vessels, occurring in old age (**senile purpura**) or after topical or systemic corticosteroid therapy; bruising occurs after minor trauma; large purpuric patches are seen, especially on the forearms and dorsum of the hands (*see* Figs. 12.54 and 2.05, p. 33)
- **pigmented purpuric eruption**
- **cutaneous vasculitis** (*see* p. 401).

PIGMENTED PURPURIC ERUPTION

This presents as rusty-brown pigmentation, starting on the feet and gradually working its way up the lower leg over a period of months to years. If you look carefully you will see tiny purpuric macules within the pigmented areas, which are the result of deposition of haemosiderin following the purpura. There is no obvious cause for the condition and no effective treatment.

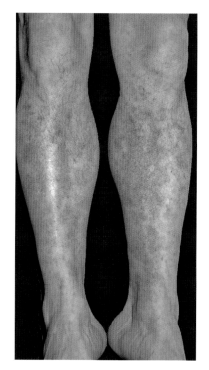 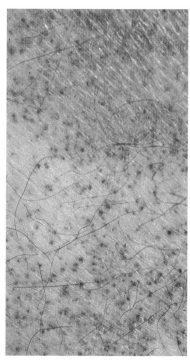

Fig. 12.52 Pigmented purpuric eruption

Fig. 12.53 Close-up of pigmented purpuric eruption

PURPURIC DRUG RASH

Some drugs cause **thrombocytopenia** with purpura and larger ecchymoses. All such patients should be referred urgently to hospital for investigation. Drugs that can cause a fall in platelet count include:

- all cytotoxic drugs
- co-trimoxazole
- gold
- rifampicin.
- chlorpromazine
- furosemide
- indomethacin

Other drugs can cause a **non-thrombocytopenic** purpura due to an underlying vasculitis. This is likely to be mainly on the lower legs. Drugs that do this include:

- allopurinol
- thiazide diuretics
- barbiturates
- carbimazole.

VASCULITIS

Vasculitis is an inflammation of the blood vessels in the skin, usually due to deposition of immune complexes in their walls. There are several different patterns dependent on the size and site of the vessels involved:

- capillaries in the superficial and mid dermis (**leucocytoclastic vasculitis; Henoch–Schönlein purpura**, *see* p. 402); there will be a polymorphic rash with palpable purpura as well as macules, papules, vesicles and pustules (*see* Fig. 12.56)
- arteries at the junction of the dermis and subcutaneous fat (**cutaneous polyarteritis nodosa**); there will be livedo reticularis, nodules and/or ulceration on the lower legs (*see* p. 378)
- arteries and veins in the subcutaneous fat (**nodular vasculitis; erythema nodosum**); there will be tender red nodules or plaques deep in the subcutaneous fat (*see* p. 378).

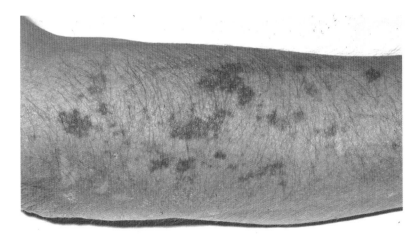

Fig. 12.54 Steroid purpura on forearm

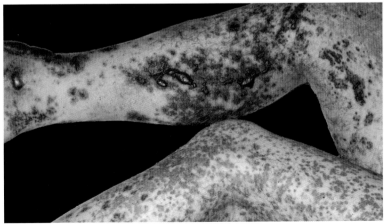

Fig. 12.55 Severe vasculitis: rash with blisters and early skin necrosis

Causes of cutaneous vasculitis:
- distant focus of infection, e.g. streptococcal infection
- collagen vascular disease (systemic lupus erythematosus, rheumatoid, systemic sclerosis)
- plasma protein abnormality, e.g. cryoglobulinaemia
- drugs (*see* p. 401)
- idiopathic (no cause found).

TREATMENT: CUTANEOUS VASCULITIS

Look for an underlying cause and treat this if possible. It is worth checking the urine for protein, blood and casts, and the blood urea and creatinine to make sure that the kidneys are not involved. If there is renal damage, specialist help should be sought, because treatment with systemic steroids or cyclophosphamide may be needed. If no cause can be found the patient can be reassured that it is a self-limiting condition that will get better after 3–6 weeks. Bed rest will stop new lesions from developing on the skin. Treatment is symptomatic, with analgesics for pain.

HENOCH–SCHÖNLEIN PURPURA

This form of leucocytoclastic vasculitis occurs mainly in young children and is associated with arthralgia and abdominal pain. Leucocytoclastic is a histological term describing dead white blood cells seen around blood vessels. The rash consists of erythematous and purpuric macules and papules together with vesicles and pustules. It should be thought of in any child with purpura and a normal platelet count. It may follow a streptococcal sore throat.

TREATMENT: HENOCH–SCHÖNLEIN PURPURA

If it follows a streptococcal throat infection, treat with phenoxymethyl penicillin. Otherwise, bed rest will stop new lesions from occurring, and most cases will get better spontaneously after 3–6 weeks. Use analgesics (paracetamol syrup) for the joint and abdominal pain. Renal involvement may be more serious. Proteinuria or microscopic haematuria without impairment of renal function will normally get better spontaneously in less than 4 weeks. If acute nephritis or progressive renal failure occur, the patient should be referred urgently to a renal physician.

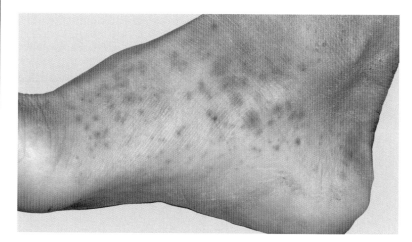

Fig. 12.56 Henoch–Schönlein purpura: note polymorphic nature of lesions, macules, papules, vesicles and crusts

Hands and feet

13

HANDS

Hands

Dorsum and palm

HANDS – ACUTE

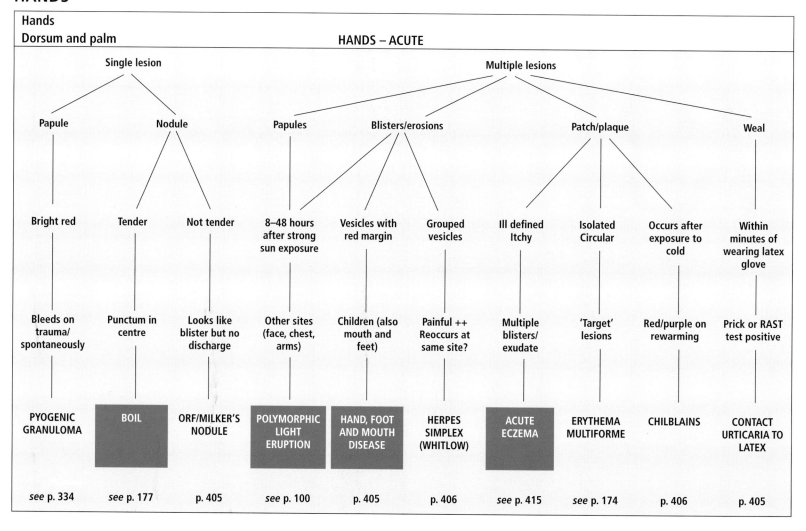

Single lesion

Papule — Bright red — Bleeds on trauma/ spontaneously — **PYOGENIC GRANULOMA** — *see* p. 334

Nodule — Tender — Punctum in centre — **BOIL** — *see* p. 177

Nodule — Not tender — Looks like blister but no discharge — **ORF/MILKER'S NODULE** — p. 405

Multiple lesions

Papules — 8–48 hours after strong sun exposure — Other sites (face, chest, arms) — **POLYMORPHIC LIGHT ERUPTION** — *see* p. 100

Blisters/erosions — Vesicles with red margin — Children (also mouth and feet) — **HAND, FOOT AND MOUTH DISEASE** — p. 405

Blisters/erosions — Grouped vesicles — Painful ++ Reoccurs at same site? — **HERPES SIMPLEX (WHITLOW)** — p. 406

Patch/plaque — Ill defined Itchy — Multiple blisters/ exudate — **ACUTE ECZEMA** — *see* p. 415

Patch/plaque — Isolated Circular — 'Target' lesions — **ERYTHEMA MULTIFORME** — *see* p. 174

Patch/plaque — Occurs after exposure to cold — Red/purple on rewarming — **CHILBLAINS** — p. 406

Weal — Within minutes of wearing latex glove — Prick or RAST test positive — **CONTACT URTICARIA TO LATEX** — p. 405

ORF AND MILKER'S NODULE

Orf is a pox virus infection of lambs. It causes sores around the mouth so that they have difficulty in suckling. It can be transmitted to those bottle-feeding affected lambs, especially if they have a cut on the finger. A red, purple, or white round nodule develops on the finger and looks like a blister, but when pricked with a needle no fluid comes out. It gets better spontaneously after 3–4 weeks and the patient is then immune for the rest of his or her life.

Milker's nodules are another pox infection, acquired from the teats of cows or the mouths of calves. It is seen as small papules or vesicles on the fingers of those involved in milking cows or feeding calves. Like orf, it gets better spontaneously and confers immunity for the future.

HAND, FOOT AND MOUTH DISEASE

This is a mild infection due to Coxsackie A16 virus that occurs in children, where small grey vesicles with a red halo occur on the fingers and toes together with small erosions in the mouth (*see* Fig. 6.02, p. 143). It gets better spontaneously after a few days so no treatment is necessary.

CONTACT URTICARIA TO LATEX

Natural latex is the sap from the rubber tree (*Hevea brasiliensis*). Latex gloves or condoms are made from water-based natural rubber latex (NRL) emulsions, and these can cause type I hypersensitivity (contact urticaria, angio-oedema, asthma or anaphylaxis). Powdered NRL gloves cause more problems than the non-powdered ones. Contact urticaria presents with weals within a few minutes at the site of contact with the rubber.

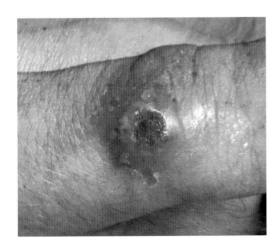

Fig. 13.01 Orf on side of finger

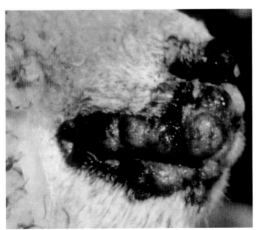

Fig. 13.02 Orf on a lamb's mouth (courtesy of Coopers Animal Health)

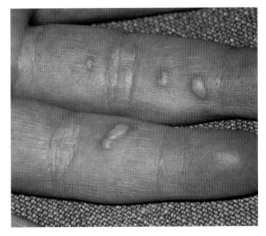

Fig. 13.03 Hand, foot and mouth disease

Patients who react in this way may also get problems with eating bananas, avocado pears, kiwifruit and/or chestnuts. NLR used to be responsible for intra-operative anaphylactic reactions, but widespread use of non-latex gloves has made this less likely. The diagnosis can be confirmed by a positive prick test, or if this is negative and the history is suggestive, by a 'use test' – wearing a finger from a NLR glove on wet skin for 15 minutes. Dry rubber latex (in household rubber gloves, elasticated bandages, balloons, shoes, car tyres, and so forth) cause a type IV hypersensitivity reaction, i.e. allergic contact dermatitis, from chemicals used to cure the latex. This must not be confused with true latex allergy, which is an *immediate* hypersensitivity reaction.

TREATMENT: CONTACT URTICARIA TO LATEX

Avoid direct contact with NRL gloves and condoms. Use non-latex gloves instead of latex gloves and use condoms made of polyurethane. It is essential to warn surgeons of the possibility of latex sensitivity before surgery is undertaken.

HERPETIC WHITLOW

Pain, swelling and vesicles on the fingers are usually due to a herpes simplex infection, which may be the result of inoculation of virus in medical or dental personnel (type 1) or from genital contact (type 2). It may be confused with a fixed drug reaction if recurrent (*see* p. 181).

CHILBLAINS

Tender mauve papules or nodules occurring on the hands or feet from the cold, which become painful on rewarming (*see* p. 161).

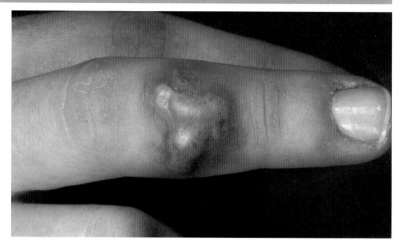

Fig. 13.04 Herpetic whitlow on finger

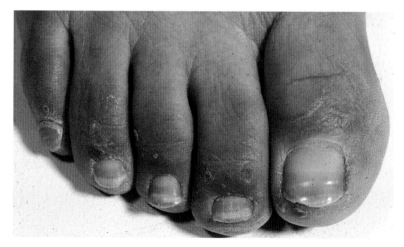

Fig. 13.05 Chilblains on the toes

Dorsum hands and wrist
Chronic erythematous rash/lesions
Papules, plaques, erosions and blisters

DORSUM HANDS – CHRONIC RASH/LESIONS

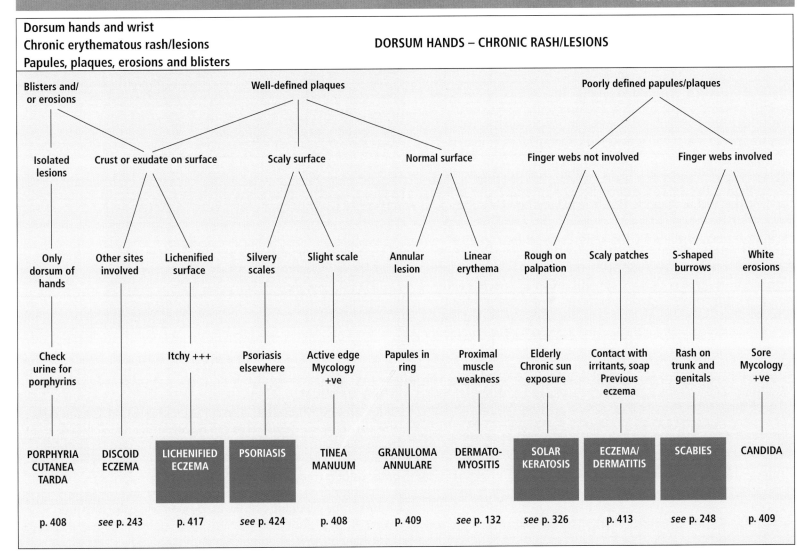

Blisters and/or erosions	Well-defined plaques				Poorly defined papules/plaques			
Isolated lesions	Crust or exudate on surface	Scaly surface	Normal surface		Finger webs not involved		Finger webs involved	
Only dorsum of hands	Other sites involved / Lichenified surface	Silvery scales / Slight scale	Annular lesion	Linear erythema	Rough on palpation	Scaly patches	S-shaped burrows	White erosions
Check urine for porphyrins	Itchy +++	Psoriasis elsewhere / Active edge Mycology +ve	Papules in ring	Proximal muscle weakness	Elderly Chronic sun exposure	Contact with irritants, soap Previous eczema	Rash on trunk and genitals	Sore Mycology +ve
PORPHYRIA CUTANEA TARDA	**DISCOID ECZEMA** / **LICHENIFIED ECZEMA**	**PSORIASIS** / **TINEA MANUUM**	**GRANULOMA ANNULARE**	**DERMATO-MYOSITIS**	**SOLAR KERATOSIS**	**ECZEMA/DERMATITIS**	**SCABIES**	**CANDIDA**
p. 408	*see* p. 243 / p. 417	*see* p. 424 / p. 408	p. 409	*see* p. 132	*see* p. 326	p. 413	*see* p. 248	p. 409

PORPHYRIA CUTANEA TARDA

This is an acquired porphyria and the one most likely to be seen in clinical practice. It is due to reduced levels of uroporphyrinogen decarboxylase in the liver resulting in increased levels of uroporphyrins in the urine and plasma. It is caused by excessive alcohol intake (2% of alcoholics develop porphyria cutanea tarda), hepatitis C, subclinical haemochromatosis or the use of oestrogens or hormone replacement therapy. The patient is usually a middle-aged or elderly male (less common in females), who presents with blisters, scars and milia on sun-exposed skin – dorsum of hands and forearms, face and bald scalp. There may also be hypertrichosis on the face. The patient rarely associates the development of skin lesions with sunlight. The diagnosis is made by finding increased porphyrins in the urine. The urine can be screened using a Wood's (ultraviolet) lamp when a coral-pink fluorescence is seen. Acidifying the urine or adding talc to it makes the fluorescence more obvious. Detailed analysis of the various porphyins by a specialist laboratory will confirm the type of porphyria. Check also the liver enzymes, hepatitis C antibodies, serum ferritin and look for the haemochromatosis gene mutation.

TREATMENT: PORPHYRIA CUTANEA TARDA

Stop alcohol or the contraceptive pill (the most likely causes). If symptoms do not improve, remove 500 mL blood fortnightly until the serum ferritin is back to normal or symptoms abate, usually after 2–3 months. The patient should avoid sun exposure (even through window glass – porphyrins absorb long-wave ultraviolet [UVA] radiation), wear a long-sleeved shirt, hat and opaque sunscreen. Oral chloroquine 200 mg bid improves the skin fragility within 6 months by complexing the porphyrins and promoting excretion.

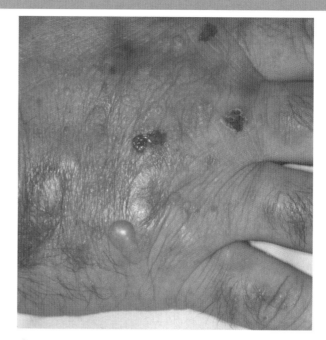

Fig. 13.06 Porphyria cutanea tarda: blisters and erosions on dorsum of hand

TINEA MANUUM

Ringworm infection should be considered in any red, scaly rash affecting only one hand. This can be confirmed or excluded by mycology (*see* p. 20). The source of the infection is often the patient's own toe webs or nails, so look at the feet as well. Three patterns of infection can occur:

1. an annular plaque on the dorsum of the hand (*see* Fig. 13.07)
2. fine scaling picking out the creases on one palm only (*see* Fig. 13.49)
3. scaling or vesicles on one hand only.

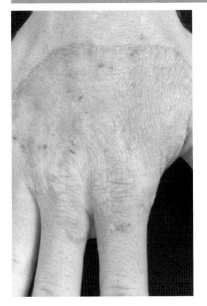

Fig. 13.07 Tinea manuum

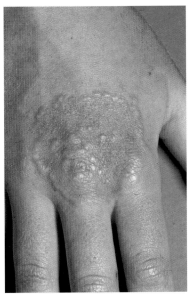

Fig. 13.08 Granuloma annulare

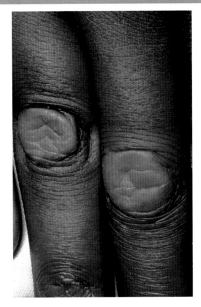

Fig. 13.09 Knuckle pads

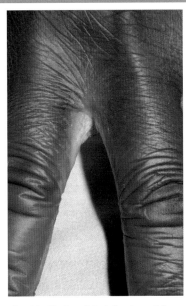

Fig. 13.10 Candida infection of finger webs

CANDIDA INFECTION OF FINGER WEB

Infection with *Candida albicans* occurs in the finger webs as well as the toe webs, especially if the hands are always in water. The finger webs become macerated and are usually white in colour.

TREATMENT: CANDIDA

> Dry the hands thoroughly after washing, especially in the finger webs. Apply a topical antifungal such as nystatin ointment or an imidazole cream or 0.5% gentian violet paint twice daily until it is better.

GRANULOMA ANNULARE

Small, skin-coloured or mauvish-pink papules form rings on the dorsum of the fingers, hand or foot. It is usually asymptomatic, although it can be tender if knocked. It is distinguished from ringworm by not being scaly (*see* also p. 210).

KNUCKLE PADS

These are thickened plaques that occur over the interphalangeal joints in young adults for no apparent reason. There is no treatment.

Dorsum of wrist, hand, fingers
1. Chronic erythematous
2. Non-erythematous
(Acute erythematous, *see* p. 404)

DORSUM HAND – NODULES

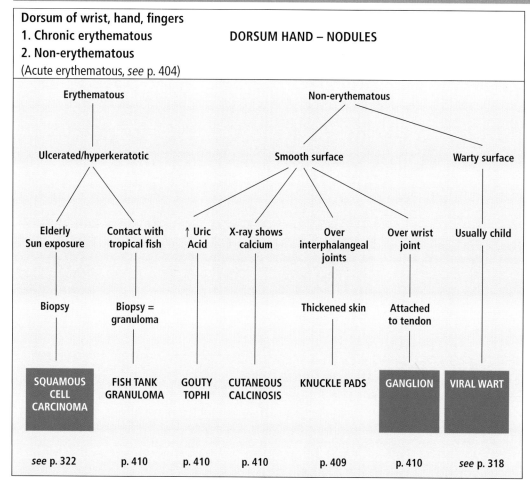

see p. 322   p. 410   p. 410   p. 410   p. 409   p. 410   *see* p. 318

NODULES ON DORSUM OF HAND

White, hard papules or nodules containing calcium (**cutaneous calcinosis**, p. 276 and Fig. 13.13) can occur on the fingers or dorsum of the hand in patients with scleroderma

or dermatomyositis. The diagnosis can be confirmed by X-ray. Gout results in **tophi** (deposits of uric acid crystals, associated with joint deformity. A **ganglion** is a synovial cyst associated with the wrist joint (*see* Fig. 13.14).

Myxoid cysts (*see* p. 448) are seen on the dorsum of the fingers, as soft cystic papules due to herniation of the interphalangeal joint capsule.

FISH TANK GRANULOMA

Tropical fish infected with *Mycobacterium marinum* die. In removing the dead fish the owner can scrape the back of his or her hand on the gravel at the bottom of the tank and so implant the atypical mycobacterium into the skin. Pink/purple nodules occur at the site of implantation. Occasionally the lesions may ulcerate. Similar lesions can occur proximally up the arm due to spread along the lymphatics (*see* Fig. 13.11b).

TREATMENT: FISH TANK GRANULOMA

Treatment is with co-trimoxazole 960 mg bid, or minocycline 100 mg bid until the skin heals (usually 6–12 weeks). Advise the patient to wear rubber gloves when removing dead fish in the future.

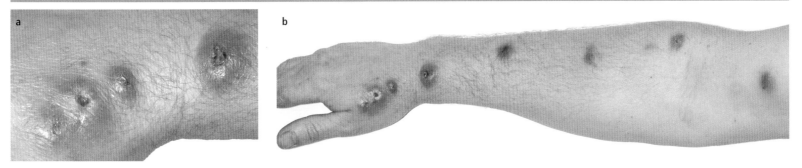

Fig. 13.11 Fish tank granuloma: (a) on dorsum of hand and wrist; (b) lesions spreading up arm proximally (sporotrichoid spread)

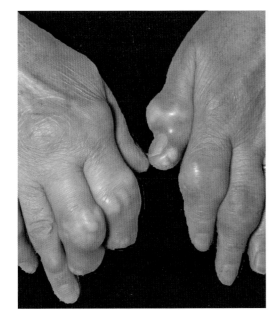

Fig. 13.12 Gouty tophi over interphalangeal joints

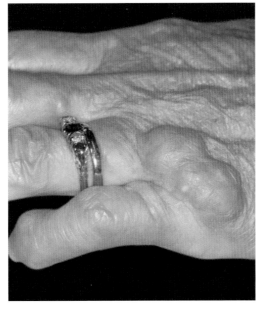

Fig. 13.13 Cutaneous calcinosis

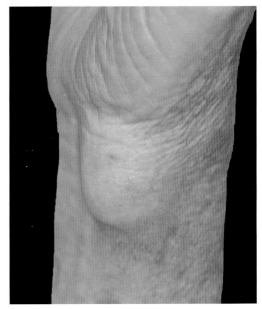

Fig. 13.14 Ganglion

Palms

1. Chronic erythematous rash/multiple lesions (for single/few lesions, *see* Chapter 8, p. 195)   PALMS
2. Non-erythematous rash with scaling, peeling or increased skin markings
3. Sweating, *see* p. 59

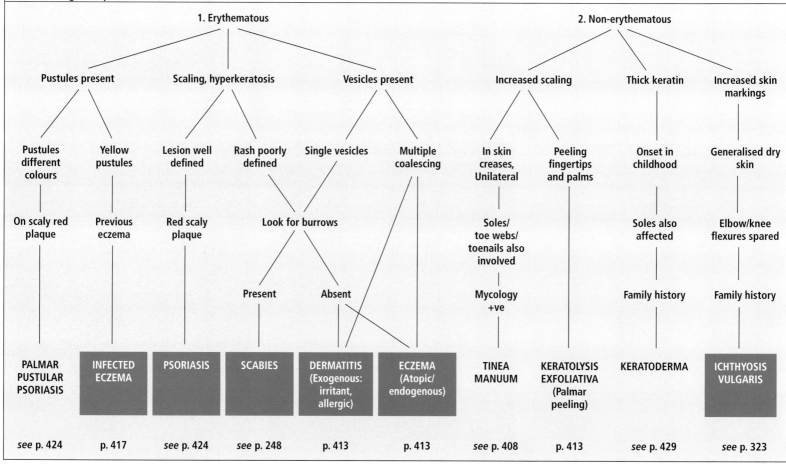

1. Erythematous				2. Non-erythematous		

Pustules present — Scaling, hyperkeratosis — Vesicles present — Increased scaling — Thick keratin — Increased skin markings

Pustules different colours | Yellow pustules | Lesion well defined | Rash poorly defined | Single vesicles | Multiple coalescing | In skin creases, Unilateral | Peeling fingertips and palms | Onset in childhood | Generalised dry skin

On scaly red plaque | Previous eczema | Red scaly plaque | Look for burrows | | | Soles/toe webs/toenails also involved | | Soles also affected | Elbow/knee flexures spared

Present — Absent

Mycology +ve

Family history | Family history

PALMAR PUSTULAR PSORIASIS	INFECTED ECZEMA	PSORIASIS	SCABIES	DERMATITIS (Exogenous: irritant, allergic)	ECZEMA (Atopic/endogenous)	TINEA MANUUM	KERATOLYSIS EXFOLIATIVA (Palmar peeling)	KERATODERMA	ICHTHYOSIS VULGARIS
see p. 424	p. 417	*see* p. 424	*see* p. 248	p. 413	p. 413	*see* p. 408	p. 413	*see* p. 429	*see* p. 323

KERATOLYSIS EXFOLIATIVA (PALMAR PEELING)

Peeling of the palms and fingers is common, often occurring about once a month. It is usually asymptomatic but there may be increased sensitivity to touch. The cause is not known and there is no specific treatment.

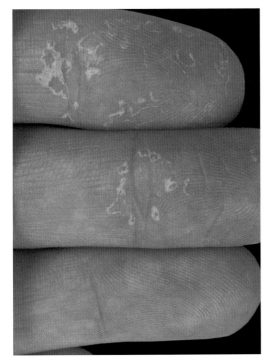

Fig. 13.15 Keratolysis exfoliativa

HAND ECZEMA/DERMATITIS

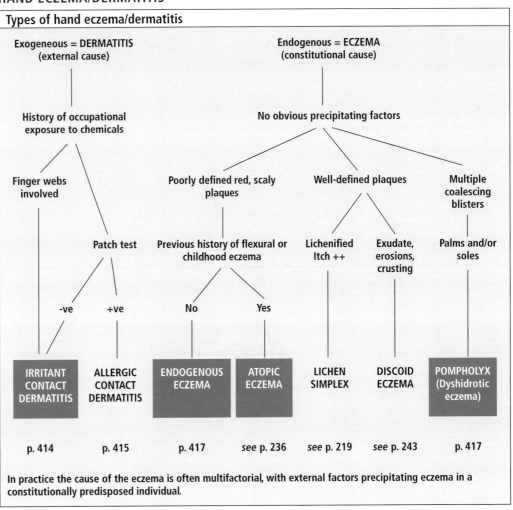

Types of hand eczema/dermatitis

In practice the cause of the eczema is often multifactorial, with external factors precipitating eczema in a constitutionally predisposed individual.

DERMATITIS = EXOGENEOUS ECZEMA

1. Irritant contact dermatitis

Irritant contact dermatitis is due to weak acids or alkalis (e.g. in detergents, shampoos, cleaning materials, cutting oils, cement dust) coming into contact with the skin. It occurs in everyone who has enough contact with these. It is the commonest type of hand eczema. Poorly defined pink scaly patches or plaques with a dry, chapped surface occur at the site of contact with the irritant. Usually there are no vesicles or crusts.

In women, detergents are the main culprit. The rash begins under a ring or in the finger webs, where the alkaline detergent particles get trapped. A lot of young mothers will get eczema on their hands when their children are small. Hairdressers commonly develop this kind of eczema when they first begin work because of the frequent shampooing. Cooks and nurses are also at risk because of repeated hand washing.

In men this kind of eczema is mainly on the dorsum of the hands from contact with cement dust or soluble oils used for cooling the moving parts of machinery in the engineering industries.

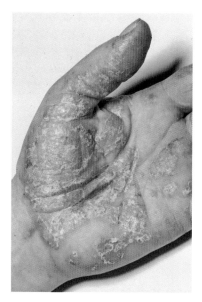

Fig. 13.16 Irritant contact dermatitis from paint stripper

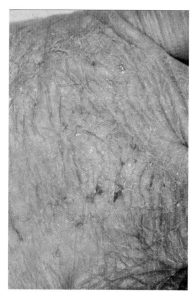

Fig. 13.17 Irritant dermatitis on dorsum of hand: dry, chapped surface

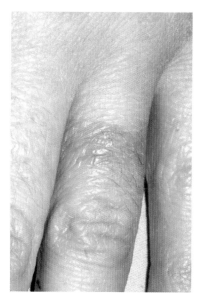

Fig. 13.18 Irritant contact dermatitis under a ring

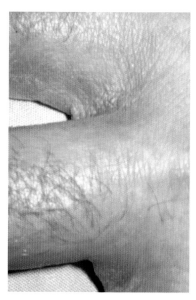

Fig. 13.19 Irritant contact dermatitis in finger webs

2. Allergic contact dermatitis

Allergic contact dermatitis is a type IV allergic reaction and affects only a very small proportion of the population. The rash occurs at the site of contact with the allergen, but on the hands it is difficult to predict the cause from the site involved because the hands come into contact with so many things during the day.

Nevertheless there are several well-recognised patterns:
- **fingertips** – from formalin in laboratory workers and secretaries (from formaldehyde resins in cardboard folders), local anaesthetics in dentists, garlic and onion in cooks, tulip bulbs and less commonly Balsam of Peru in orange peel
- **centre of palm** and flexor aspects of **fingers** – from rubber, nickel or plastic handle grips
- **whole hand** (palm, dorsum and wrist) – from rubber gloves
- **in lines** on flexor aspect of wrist or dorsum of hand and forearm – from the leaves of the plants (*see* p. 182)
- **flexor aspect of the wrist** from nickel in watch buckle or PTBP formaldehyde resin in the watch strap.

It is probably wise to patch test (*see* p. 21) anyone with hand eczema who does not get better quickly with topical steroids.

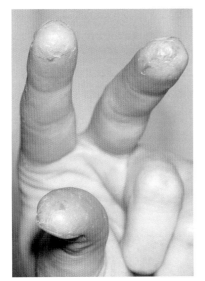
Fig. 13.20 Allergic contact dermatitis on fingertips from garlic (usually on the non-dominant hand)

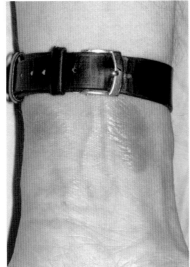
Fig. 13.21 Allergic contact dermatitis from PTBP formaldehyde resin in the watch strap

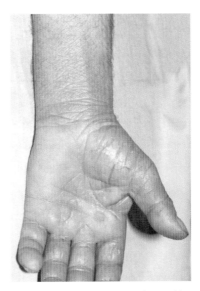
Fig. 13.22 Allergic contact dermatitis from rubber gloves, extending onto the wrist

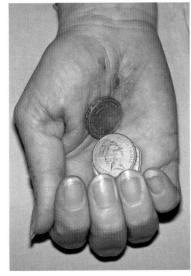
Fig. 13.23 Allergic contact dermatitis on palm from the nickel in coins

Allergic contact eczema may develop explosively with vesicles, exudate and crusting. If it develops more slowly, then the rash is a poorly defined red, scaly rash just like eczema elsewhere.

Occupational dermatitis has medico-legal implications. The assessment of each patient depends on whether the patient could have reasonably expected to have developed eczema if he or she had not been engaged in that particular job or occupation.

Patients with atopic eczema in childhood should be discouraged from going into hairdressing or jobs that involve contact with cutting oils or cleansing agents.

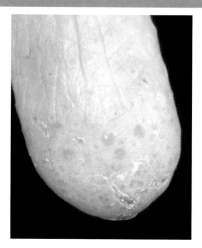

Fig. 13.25 Pompholyx on fingertip

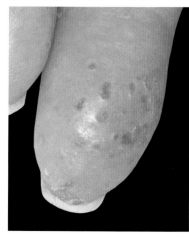

Fig. 13.26 Pompholyx: tiny erosions on fingertips where the vesicles have broken

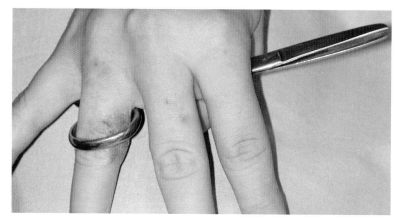

Fig. 13.24 Allergic contact dermatitis from nickel in scissors in a hairdresser

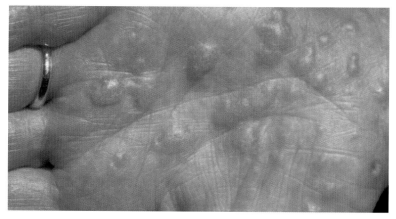

Fig. 13.27 Pompholyx: intact vesicles under the thick stratum corneum of the palm

POMPHOLYX ECZEMA

Acute eczema resulting in blistering on the palms and soles is termed **pompholyx** (or **dyshidrotic eczema**[USA]). Because of the thickened stratum corneum, the epidermal blisters persist and appear as tiny grey-white 'grains' within the skin. Eventually they burst and erosions occur. Sometimes pompholyx can occur as an isolated episode that then resolves spontaneously.

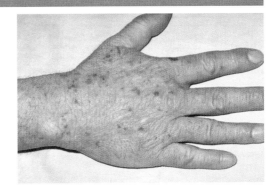

Fig. 13.29 Endogenous eczema on dorsum of hand: note lichenification and excoriations

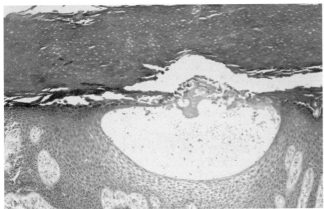

Fig. 13.28 Histology of pompholyx: epidermal blister underneath the thick stratum corneum

ENDOGENOUS ECZEMA

Endogenous eczema can occur on both the palm and dorsum of the hand. You should think of this diagnosis if the patient has symmetrical eczema, particularly if there is a past history of atopic eczema in childhood. The eczema is itchy and continual scratching and rubbing will lead to lichenification. If it becomes secondarily infected with bacteria (*Staphylococcus aureus*), pustules may occur. On the palms this differs from pustular psoriasis because all the pustules are the same colour (yellow). Some hand eczema becomes hyperkeratotic, resulting in fissures over the finger joints, along the skin creases and over fingertips. These are painful and can be very disabling.

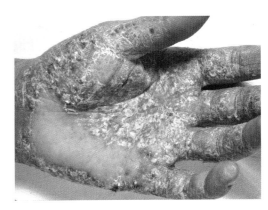

Fig. 13.30 Infected eczema on palm

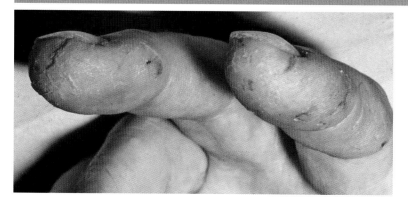

Fig. 13.31 Fissures on fingers that can be treated with Haelan tape

TREATMENT: HAND AND FOOT ECZEMA

With eczema on the hands it is always worth doing patch tests, because the hands touch a lot of things during the course of a day. If the cause can be found and contact with it stopped, the eczema may be cured. Otherwise, the patient will be condemned to using ointments or creams indefinitely.

- **Acute weeping eczema.** Initially rest will be required to get the eczema better. For the hands stop washing up, cleaning, shampooing, and so forth. Resting the feet in practice means bed rest. Dry up the exudate by soaking the hands/feet for 10 minutes twice a day in an astringent such as 1:10 000 potassium permanganate solution[UK] or aluminium acetate (Burow's solution[USA]), see p. 30. After drying the skin apply a moderate[UK]/group 4–5[USA] topical steroid ointment that does not contain lanolin. Always use an ointment rather than a cream until the cause of the eczema is sorted out. Once the eczema is better, try to find the cause by patch testing (see p. 21).
- **Pompholyx eczema.** A potent[UK]/group 2–3[USA] topical steroid ointment will be needed to penetrate the thick stratum corneum, which should be applied twice a day. When the vesicles break, potassium permanganate soaks may be needed to dry any exudate.

- **Chronic eczema.** The patient will require a potent[UK]/group 2–3[USA] topical steroid ointment or cream applied once or twice a day. It will often be a question of trial and error to find the one that will suit this particular patient best. If the skin is very dry or there are a lot of fissures, start with an ointment. If it is not too scaly the patient may prefer to use a cream. If the eczema is on the hands, prevent further damage by wearing cotton gloves for doing housework and rubber gloves or cotton-lined PVC gloves for all wet work. Manual labourers also will need to protect their hands from irritants as much as possible by wearing surgical latex gloves, which should be provided at work. Often wearing gloves is not practicable, and it may be necessary to have time off work if the eczema will not settle down. In many cases, once the dermatitis is established, it will not resolve without a change in occupation (e.g. trainee hairdressers, machine workers, chefs and nurses may have to change jobs). If the eczema is on the feet, white cotton socks and leather shoes are likely to be more comfortable than man-made fibres, unless of course the eczema is an allergic contact eczema due to chromate in leather.
- **Hyperkeratotic eczema.** Both the eczema and the hyperkeratosis need treating. The thickened keratin will prevent applied topical steroids getting through the skin, and any fissures will be painful when the hyperkeratosis cracks. The hyperkeratosis can be reduced by 2-5% salicylic acid ointment, either applied alone or mixed with a topical steroid, e.g. Diprosalic ointment. If the salicylic acid is used alone, it can be applied either in the morning or at night, and a topical steroid ointment used alone the other time. One of the potent[UK]/group 2–3[USA] steroid ointments will be required. Haelan tape may also be useful for hyperkeratotic or fissured eczema on the fingers and feet. Patients like it because it is not messy. A strip of tape is applied to the area and left on for 12 hours at a time. This usually results in the cracks healing. Applying superglue (bought from a hardware store) to the cracks is another good way of healing the fissures and reducing pain. Once the fissure has healed, the superglue will fall out.

FAILURE OF TOPICAL TREATMENT

Severe disabling hand or foot eczema may require treatment with systemic immunosuppressive agents such as azathioprine (see p. 54) or ciclosporin (see p. 53). Alitretinoin 30 mg daily (see p. 50) given for a 2-month trial may be useful in hyperkeratotic eczema.

FEET

Dorsum of the foot
Erythematous rash/lesions

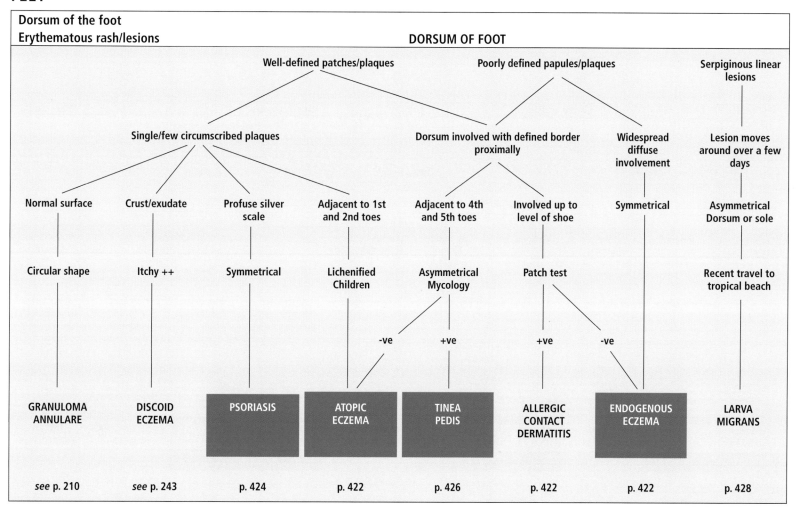

DORSUM OF FOOT

Well-defined patches/plaques

Poorly defined papules/plaques

Serpiginous linear lesions

Single/few circumscribed plaques

Dorsum involved with defined border proximally

Widespread diffuse involvement

Lesion moves around over a few days

Normal surface

Crust/exudate

Profuse silver scale

Adjacent to 1st and 2nd toes

Adjacent to 4th and 5th toes

Involved up to level of shoe

Symmetrical

Asymmetrical Dorsum or sole

Circular shape

Itchy ++

Symmetrical

Lichenified Children

Asymmetrical Mycology

Patch test

Recent travel to tropical beach

-ve   +ve

+ve   -ve

GRANULOMA ANNULARE

DISCOID ECZEMA

PSORIASIS

ATOPIC ECZEMA

TINEA PEDIS

ALLERGIC CONTACT DERMATITIS

ENDOGENOUS ECZEMA

LARVA MIGRANS

see p. 210   see p. 243   p. 424   p. 422   p. 426   p. 422   p. 422   p. 428

Soles: instep and weight-bearing area
Scaling, hyperkeratosis, maceration
SOLES: SCALING, MACERATION

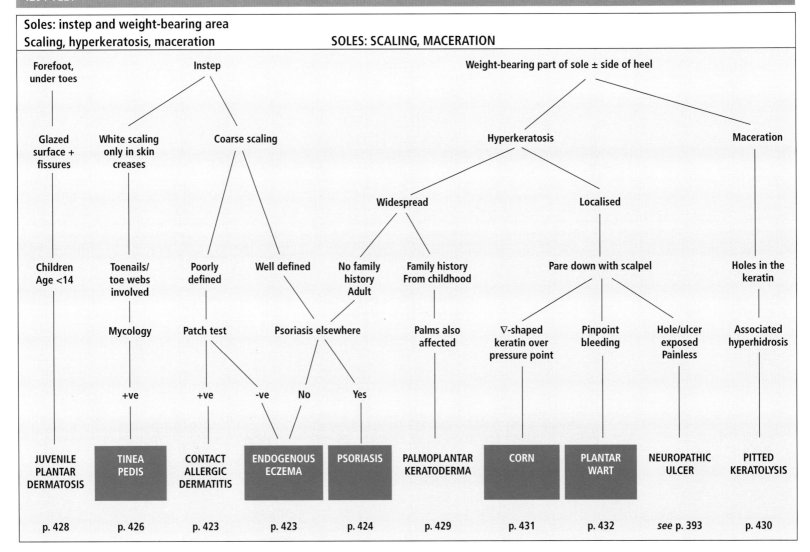

Forefoot, under toes	Instep		Weight-bearing part of sole ± side of heel	

Forefoot, under toes → Glazed surface + fissures → Children Age <14 → **JUVENILE PLANTAR DERMATOSIS** — p. 428

Instep:
- White scaling only in skin creases → Toenails/toe webs involved → Mycology → +ve → **TINEA PEDIS** — p. 426
- Coarse scaling:
  - Poorly defined → Patch test → +ve → **CONTACT ALLERGIC DERMATITIS** — p. 423
  - Well defined → Psoriasis elsewhere → -ve → **ENDOGENOUS ECZEMA** — p. 423
    - No → **ENDOGENOUS ECZEMA** — p. 423
    - Yes → **PSORIASIS** — p. 424

Weight-bearing part of sole ± side of heel:
- Hyperkeratosis:
  - Widespread:
    - No family history / Adult → Psoriasis elsewhere → **PSORIASIS** — p. 424
    - Family history / From childhood → Palms also affected → **PALMOPLANTAR KERATODERMA** — p. 429
  - Localised → Pare down with scalpel:
    - ∇-shaped keratin over pressure point → **CORN** — p. 431
    - Pinpoint bleeding → **PLANTAR WART** — p. 432
    - Hole/ulcer exposed Painless → **NEUROPATHIC ULCER** — *see p. 393*
- Maceration → Holes in the keratin → Associated hyperhidrosis → **PITTED KERATOLYSIS** — p. 430

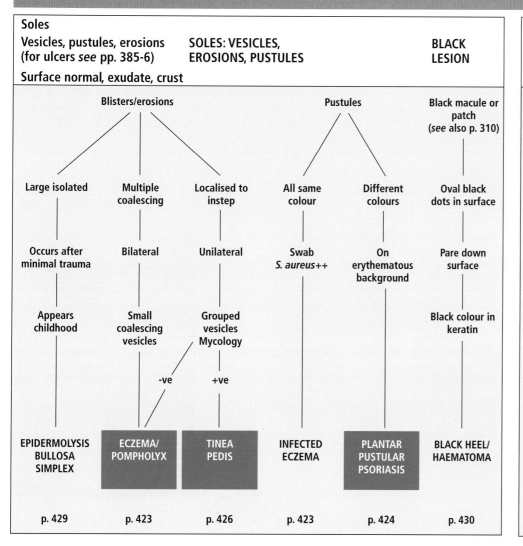

Soles

Vesicles, pustules, erosions
(for ulcers *see* pp. 385-6)

Surface normal, exudate, crust

SOLES: VESICLES,
EROSIONS, PUSTULES

BLACK
LESION

Blisters/erosions

- Large isolated
  - Occurs after minimal trauma
    - Appears childhood
      - **EPIDERMOLYSIS BULLOSA SIMPLEX**
      - p. 429

- Multiple coalescing
  - Bilateral
    - Small coalescing vesicles
      - -ve
        - **ECZEMA/ POMPHOLYX**
        - p. 423

- Localised to instep
  - Unilateral
    - Grouped vesicles Mycology
      - +ve
        - **TINEA PEDIS**
        - p. 426

Pustules

- All same colour
  - Swab *S. aureus*++
    - **INFECTED ECZEMA**
    - p. 423

- Different colours
  - On erythematous background
    - **PLANTAR PUSTULAR PSORIASIS**
    - p. 424

Black macule or patch
(*see* also p. 310)

- Oval black dots in surface
  - Pare down surface
    - Black colour in keratin
      - **BLACK HEEL/ HAEMATOMA**
      - p. 430

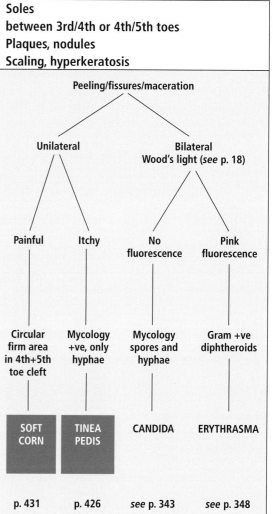

Soles

between 3rd/4th or 4th/5th toes
Plaques, nodules
Scaling, hyperkeratosis

Peeling/fissures/maceration

- Unilateral
  - Painful
    - Circular firm area in 4th+5th toe cleft
      - **SOFT CORN**
      - p. 431
  - Itchy
    - Mycology +ve, only hyphae
      - **TINEA PEDIS**
      - p. 426

- Bilateral
  Wood's light (*see* p. 18)
  - No fluorescence
    - Mycology spores and hyphae
      - **CANDIDA**
      - *see* p. 343
  - Pink fluorescence
    - Gram +ve diphtheroids
      - **ERYTHRASMA**
      - *see* p. 348

ECZEMA ON THE FOOT

A symmetrical, red scaly rash on the foot in which vesicles have been present at some stage is likely to be eczema (for treatment, *see* p. 418).

Dorsum of the foot

Eczema here can be due to the following.

- **Atopic eczema**: eczema affecting the dorsum of the big toe in a child aged 7–10 years is one of the patterns of atopic eczema. Note tinea pedis affects the fourth and fifth toes, not the big toe.

- **Allergic contact dermatitis**: a rash up to the level of the shoe and sparing the toe webs is usually due to an allergic contact dermatitis to chrome in the leather of the shoe uppers, or azo dyes in nylon socks/stockings. A rash at the site of contact with flip-flops is due to mercaptobenzothiazole, a rubber additive.
- **Endogenous eczema**: symmetrical eczema on the dorsum of the foot can be due to endogenous eczema. Patch testing is negative.
- **Discoid eczema** presents as a well-defined, round or oval, red scaly plaque with obvious vesiculation and crusting (*see* p. 243).

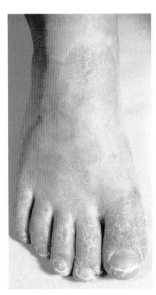

Fig. 13.32 Atopic eczema on the dorsum of the foot in a child

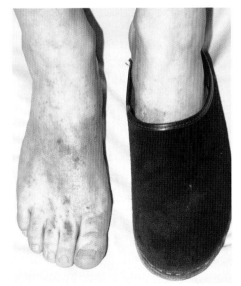

Fig. 13.33 Allergic contact dermatitis from shoe uppers, note the cut-off at the level of the shoe

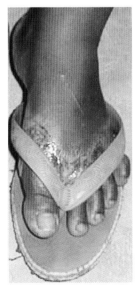

Fig. 13.34 Allergic contact dermatitis to the rubber in flip-flops

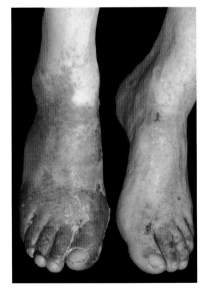

Fig. 13.35 Endogenous foot eczema; symmetrical distribution

Sole of the foot

Hyperkeratosis occurs when eczema affects the weight-bearing areas of the soles. Painful fissures occur if the thickened keratin splits. The causes of eczema on the soles are as follows.

- **Allergic contact dermatitis**: symmetrical eczema on the weight-bearing area of the soles is due to an allergic contact dermatitis until proven otherwise. It is usually due to rubber in the soles of shoes, PTBP formaldehyde resin (the glue used to stick layers of leather together) or the azo dyes in nylon socks/stockings. The diagnosis can be confirmed by patch testing.
- **Endogenous eczema**: an identical rash can occur in endogenous eczema or psoriasis. Because of the thick layer of keratin on the soles, rashes are much more difficult to distinguish from one another at this site. Eczema tends to have a less well-defined border. There may be evidence of eczema or psoriasis elsewhere. Often both hands and feet are involved, which suggests an endogenous cause.
- **Pompholyx (dyshidrotic eczema)**: vesicles often remain intact for days or weeks on the soles and look like tapioca. When they are present alone with no redness or scaling it is called pompholyx (*see* hands, p. 417). This is usually due to endogenous or atopic eczema but can occur as a reaction to tinea between the toes ('id' reaction). Unilateral vesicles on one instep are usually due to tinea (*see* p. 426).

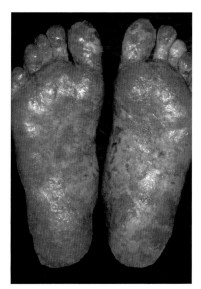

Fig. 13.36 Allergic contact dermatitis due to PTBP resin

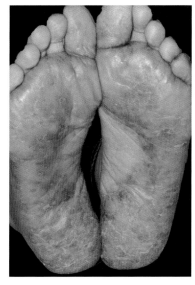

Fig. 13.37 Allergic contact dermatitis to shoe rubber sparing the insteps

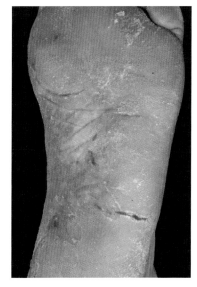

Fig. 13.38 Hyperkeratotic foot eczema with deep fissures

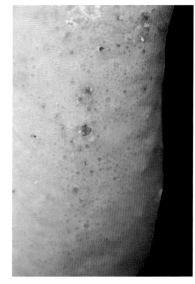

Fig. 13.39 Pompholyx; vesicles on the sole

PSORIASIS OF HANDS AND FEET

Psoriasis of the hands and feet can be of four different patterns.

1. **Plaque psoriasis**: there are well-defined, bright-red scaly plaques with silver scaling just like psoriasis elsewhere (*see* p. 225).
2. **Hyperkeratosis** of the central palm or weight-bearing area of the sole (*see* Fig. 13.45). There is no redness to give you a clue to the diagnosis, although the plaques are often well defined. Usually there is more typical psoriasis elsewhere.
3. **Pustular psoriasis**, where there are pustules of different colours. Individual pustules dry out as they pass through the keratin layer, changing in colour from white to yellow to orange brown to dark brown before peeling off in the scale. There may or may not be a background erythema and scaling. It differs from eczema or tinea that has become secondarily infected, because in these conditions the pustules will all be the same colour (yellow).
4. **Rupioid psoriasis** affects the ends of the fingers and toes. There are bright-red, thickened scaly plaques with involvement of the nails as well.

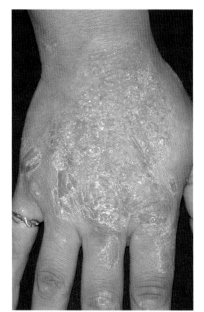

Fig. 13.40 Psoriasis on dorsum of hand

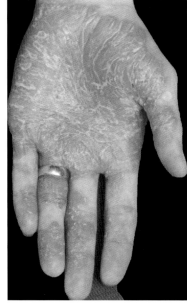

Fig. 13.41 Psoriasis affecting the central palm: note well-defined border

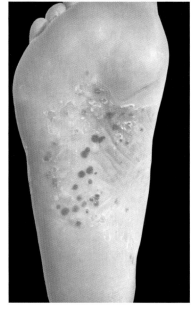

Fig. 13.42 Pustular psoriasis on the instep: pustules of different colours

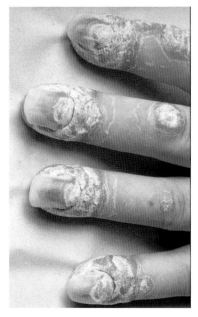

Fig. 13.43 Rupioid psoriasis affecting ends of fingers and nails

TREATMENT: PSORIASIS OF HANDS AND FEET

- Ordinary plaque psoriasis on the palms and soles: the treatment of this is the same as treatment of plaque psoriasis anywhere else (*see* p. 226).
- Thick hyperkeratotic psoriasis: treatment is the same as for hyperkeratotic eczema (*see* p. 418). Use the keratolytic agent (*see* p. 36) at night, if necessary under occlusion, and white soft paraffin/petrolatum in the daytime. Once the thick keratin has been removed, use a specific psoriatic agent during the day. You can try coal tar and salicylic acid ointment but the tar will make a mess so may not be tolerated. Alternatively, try a vitamin D_3 analogue ointment, a potent[UK]/group 2–3[USA] topical steroid ointment or a combination of both (Dovobet).
- Pustular psoriasis of the palms and soles is a very difficult condition to help. A potent[UK]/group 2–3[USA] topical steroid ointment or cream applied twice a day may provide relief. If it does not, then referral to a dermatologist may help.

FAILURE OF TOPICAL TREATMENT FOR HAND AND FOOT PSORIASIS
Sometimes no topical agents will help patients with hand or foot psoriasis, in which case either patients have to learn to live with it or you will need to refer to a dermatologist for a systemic treatment.

- Acitretin (*see* p. 49).
- PUVA. There are special hand and foot machines for PUVA, with small banks of light tubes (emitting UVA) about the size of an X-ray viewing box. The patient takes the 8-methoxypsoralen as he or she would for ordinary PUVA treatment and 2 hours later puts the hands or feet on the box emitting the UVA. He will still need to protect both his eyes and his skin in the same way as if he had been irradiated all over, because of the circulating psoralens. For details about the precautions to be taken with PUVA and the side effects *see* pp. 61–3.
- Topical PUVA is an alternative: the hands and/or feet are soaked in a 1% solution of 5-methoxypsoralen for 15 minutes, patted dry and then irradiated with UVA using a hand and foot machine.
- One of the cytotoxic drugs: methotrexate, ciclosporin, azathioprine or hydroxycarbamide. Obviously the disease will need to be seriously interfering with the patient's life to consider using drugs like these. For how to use them, *see* pp. 52–5.

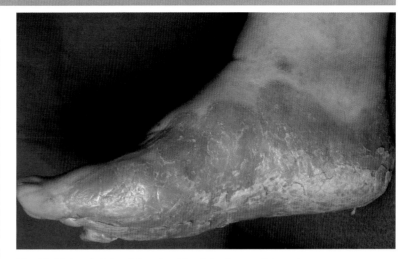

Fig. 13.44 Psoriasis involving the side of the foot and the sole

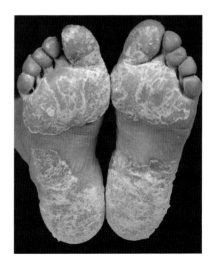

Fig. 13.45 Hyperkeratotic psoriasis on soles: note sparing of insteps

TINEA PEDIS

There are five different patterns of tinea on the feet.

1. **Scaling or maceration between the toes**, usually between the fourth and fifth toes. Here the web spaces are narrow and the humidity high. It begins on one foot only and results in itching. With time it may spread medially but never as far as the space between the first and second toes. Later it may spread to the other foot and/or the toenails.
2. **Typical plaques** of tinea on the dorsum of one foot with a raised scaly edge (*see*, for example, Fig. 13.07, on the hand). It usually starts laterally near to the fourth and fifth toe cleft.
3. **Scaling on the sides** of the foot in the shape of a 'moccasin' shoe.

4. **White scaling on the soles**: this may be unilateral or bilateral, and is often associated with discolouration and thickening of the toenails; it is due to one particular fungus, *Trichophyton rubrum*. It may be found by chance when examining a patient's feet, or the patient may complain of burning or itching of the soles. Rarely a similar pattern can be found on the palm, in which case it is usually on one side only.
5. **Vesicles on the instep**: unilateral vesicles are due to tinea until proven otherwise. Sometimes they may be present on both feet, but usually there will be more on one foot than the other. The fungus is in the roof of the blisters. To confirm the diagnosis, cut off the roof of the blister with a pair of fine scissors and examine under the microscope for fungal hyphae (*see* p. 337) or send the blister roof for mycology culture (*see* p. 20).

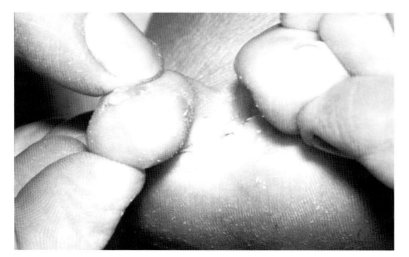

Fig. 13.46 Tinea pedis: maceration of cleft between fourth and fifth toes – the same pattern may also be due to candida or erythrasma

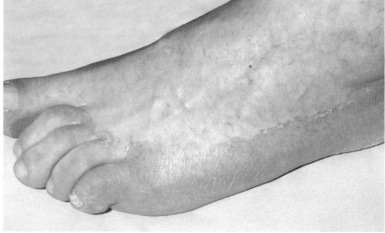

Fig. 13.47 Tinea pedis: 'moccasin' pattern on side of foot

TREATMENT: TINEA PEDIS

For tinea **between the toes** or for **blisters on the instep**, use an imidazole cream twice a day for 2 weeks, or 1% terbinafine cream daily for 7–10 days.
For the **white scaling** on the soles due to *T. rubrum*, terbinafine 250 mg orally once a day for 2 weeks should clear it up. Often the nails will be involved and these should be treated by continuing with terbinafine for a further 3 months (*see* p. 443).

CANDIDA AND ERYTHRASMA

Symmetrical maceration or scaling between the lateral toe webs may be due to candida or erythrasma and not a dermatophyte fungus. Erythrasma will fluoresce bright pink under a Wood's (ultraviolet) light (*see* p. 348). If there is no fluorescence, then take scrapings to examine under the microscope (*see* Fig. 10.15, p. 342) and for culture, which will distinguish tinea from candida. (For treatment of candida, *see* p. 343; for treatment of erythrasma, *see* p. 348.)

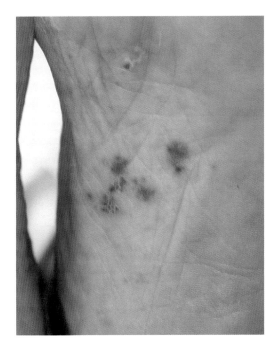

Fig. 13.48 Tinea pedis: unilateral vesicles on the instep

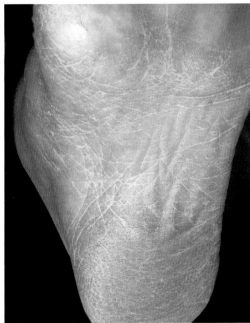

Fig. 13.49 Tinea pedis: white scaling of the skin creases due to *Trichophyton rubrum*

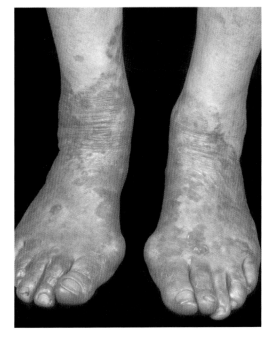

Fig. 13.50 Tinea incognito: tinea treated with topical steroids causing a symmetrical red rash

LARVA MIGRANS

The larva of the dog hookworm (*Ancylostoma braziliense*) burrows into the skin and migrates under the skin producing a serpiginous track. Sometimes blistering can occur within the track. The patient notices itching and can see the track extend over a period of a few days. It is acquired by walking or sitting on a tropical beach where dogs have been defecating (Africa or West Indies, usually). The tracks can be found on the feet, buttocks, back of legs or back.

TREATMENT: LARVA MIGRANS

Oral albendazole 400 mg daily for 4 days or a single dose of ivermectin 200 µg/kg body weight will cure it.

JUVENILE PLANTAR DERMATOSIS

This condition occurs only in children, usually between the ages of 7 and 14. The plantar surface of the forefoot is bright red and shiny, and children complain of itching or painful fissures. It is thought to be due to modern footwear – nylon socks and synthetic soles, which do not allow sweat to escape through the shoe. It gets better spontaneously after puberty.

TREATMENT: JUVENILE PLANTAR DERMATOSIS

Nylon socks and trainers should be discouraged, and cotton socks and leather shoes worn if possible. Charcoal or cork insoles inside the shoes will also help the sweat to evaporate. Medical treatment on the whole is unsatisfactory. Topical steroids are not usually of any help. Try one of the following:
- white soft paraffin applied two or three times a day; alternatively, use one of the less greasy moisturisers (*see* p. 26)
- a mild keratolytic agent, e.g. 10% urea cream (Calmurid) or 2% salicylic acid ointment applied twice a day.

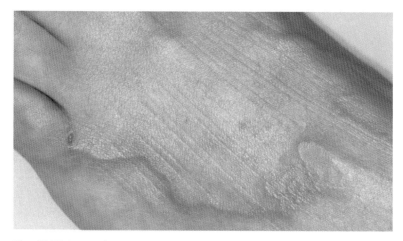

Fig. 13.51 Larva migrans

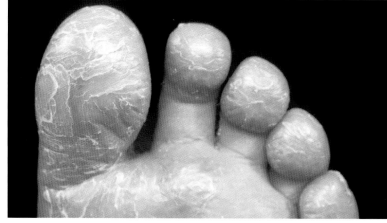

Fig. 13.52 Juvenile plantar dermatosis

EPIDERMOLYSIS BULLOSA SIMPLEX

Epidermolysis bullosa (EB) is a group of inherited conditions where blisters occur in response to trauma. There are three main types, depending on where the site of the split is in the skin. EB simplex is the mildest form, and blisters appear on the feet spontaneously or after minimal trauma, e.g. on wearing a new pair of shoes or joining the Army and having to march. Junctional EB is usually lethal in the first 2 years of life. Dystrophic EB (*see* p. 259) results in recurrent blisters and erosions throughout life.

TREATMENT: EPIDERMOLYSIS BULLOSA SIMPLEX

Apply a moisturiser such as aqueous cream to the feet twice a day to keep the skin soft. Gradually wear in new shoes and avoid excessive walking. Cotton socks are more comfortable than nylon ones. Most patients can lead a normal life.

PALMOPLANTAR KERATODERMA

This is a genetically determined condition inherited as an autosomal dominant trait. Thickening of the keratin on the palms and soles is present from birth or early infancy. There are many variants of this condition, some with striate or punctate patterns.

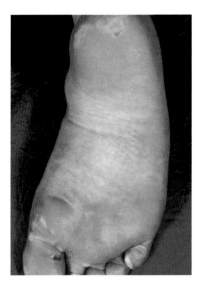

Fig. 13.53 Epidermolysis bullosa simplex: blisters on the soles

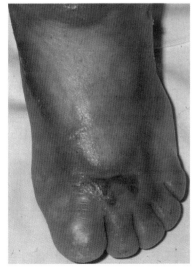

Fig. 13.54 Dystrophic epidermolysis bullosa with loss of toenails and webbing of toes

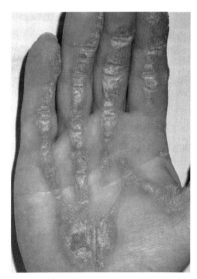

Fig. 13.55 Striate keratoderma

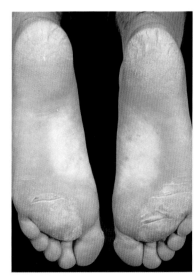

Fig. 13.56 Plantar keratoderma

TREATMENT: PALMOPLANTAR KERATODERMA

Salicylic acid ointment (5%–20%) applied at night may keep the hyperkeratosis down. Regular chiropody will almost certainly be needed. If it is very severe it may be necessary to use acitretin by mouth. This is only available in hospitals. The dosage is the same as in psoriasis (*see* p. 49).

PITTED KERATOLYSIS

Pitted keratolysis is a condition that only occurs in patients with sweaty feet. A corynebacterium eats into the keratin on the sole, which becomes covered with shallow pits.

TREATMENT: PITTED KERATOLYSIS

Treating the sweaty feet works better than specifically removing the causative organism (*see* p. 59). Alternatively, apply 3% fusidic acid cream or clindamycin lotion (Dalacin T) twice a day.

BLACK HEEL/HAEMATOMA

It is quite common for bleeding to occur into the skin on the back of the heel or the sole in teenagers and young adults engaged in sporting activities. It is due to rubbing from shoes or direct trauma. A painless dark-red or black patch is seen over the heel. The sudden appearance may alarm the patient and make the patient think that he or she has a malignant melanoma. When pared down, dried blood is seen within the keratin layer. Reassurance is all that is needed.

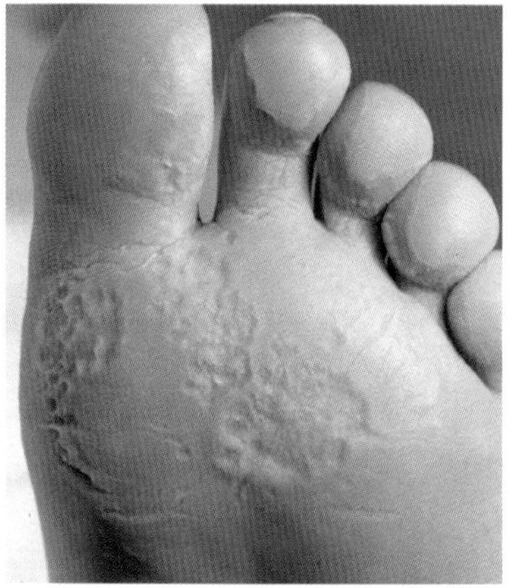

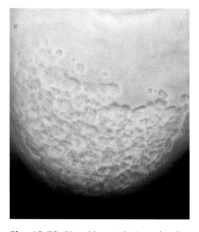

Fig. 13.57 Pitted keratolysis on forefoot

Fig. 13.58 Pitted keratolysis on heel

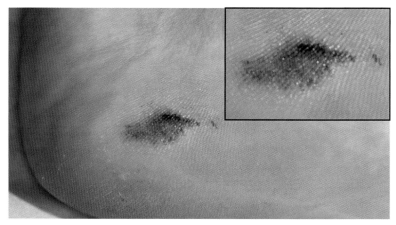

Fig. 13.59 Black heel due to bleeding into the keratin layer (inset shows close-up) (compare with Fig. 13.60)

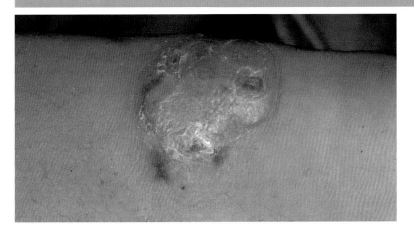

Fig. 13.60 Acral lentiginous melanoma on sole of foot: note pigment at edge and ulceration

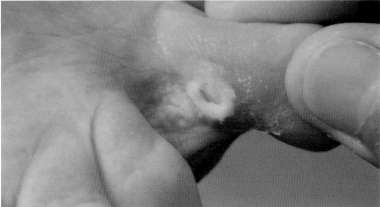

Fig. 13.61 Soft corn: maceration on medial aspect of fifth toe

CORN

A corn is a localised ∇-shaped area of hyperkeratosis over a pressure point on the foot. When pared down with a scalpel, no bleeding points are seen (*see* Fig. 13.66b and c, p. 433).

SOFT CORN

Scaling between the fourth and fifth toes on one foot may be due to a soft corn (*see* Fig. 13.61). If you remove the surface keratin with a scalpel you will quickly come to firmer keratin underneath, just like a corn elsewhere. Soft corns are due to wearing shoes that are too tight around the toes. The problem can be explained very simply to the patient by making him or her stand on a piece of paper on the floor in bare feet. Draw around the affected foot with a pencil and then put the patient's shoe on the drawing. It will be immediately obvious that the shoe is too tight for the foot (*see* Fig. 13.62).

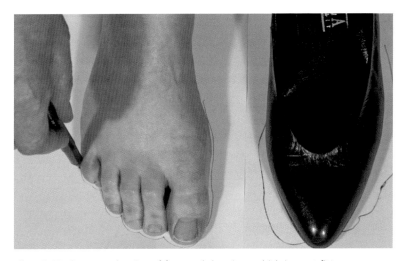

Fig. 13.62 Compare the size of foot and shoe into which it must fit!

TREATMENT: CORN

If a bony exostosis is present or there is an obvious anatomical abnormality of the foot, the help of an orthopaedic surgeon may be needed.

The patient should wear shoes that fit properly.

The area of hyperkeratosis can be pared down regularly with a scalpel by the patient or a podiatrist and the central core of keratin removed. Alternatively, 5%–10% salicylic acid ointment can be applied every night to soften the keratin and make it easier to remove. Salicylic acid plasters left on for a week at a time will do the same thing. Wearing a corn pad or circle of orthopaedic felt around the corn will take the pressure off it and make walking more comfortable. Alternatively, a proper orthotic appliance can be made to fit into the shoe.

For **soft corns**, keep the affected toes apart with a piece of foam or a silicone wedge to reduce the sideways pressure. It is most important that the patient wears shoes that are not too small around the toes.

PLANTAR WART (VERRUCA)

Verruca is the proper name for a wart. In common usage, warts on the hands are called warts and those on the feet verrucae. On the feet individual lesions are discrete, round papules with a rough surface surrounded by a collar of hyperkeratosis. They may be very numerous and join together to form mosaic warts (*see* Fig. 13.67). If the diagnosis is in doubt, pare down the surface with a scalpel and very soon tiny bleeding points will be seen (*see* Fig. 13.66a).

Two problems arise from warts on the feet.
1. They hurt. This is not due to the wart growing into the foot when it is situated on weight-bearing areas, but to the hyperkeratosis that occurs around the wart. This grows outward and causes pain just as a stone in the shoe does. Less commonly, very severe pain occurs if the blood vessels in the wart thrombose – this causes the wart to go black and within a few days drop off.
2. Children with verrucae are not allowed to swim. This may be overcome by wearing a sock on the affected foot to prevent spread of virus from one person to another.

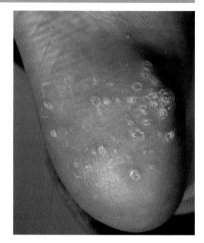

Fig. 13.63 Multiple plantar warts

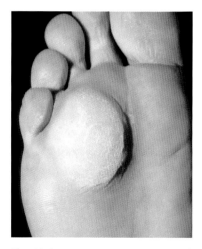

Fig. 13.64 Large corn over metatarsal heads

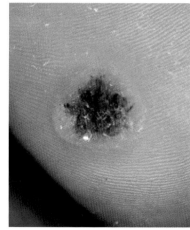

Fig. 13.65 Thrombosed wart causing pain

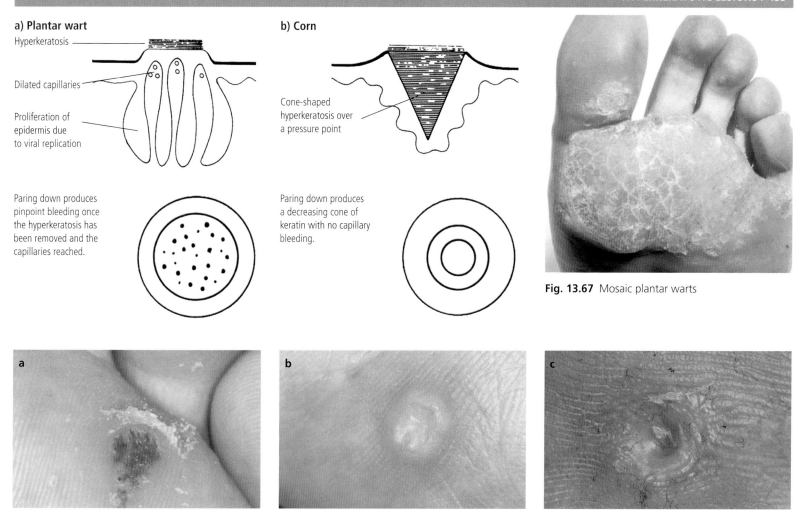

a) Plantar wart

Hyperkeratosis

Dilated capillaries

Proliferation of epidermis due to viral replication

Paring down produces pinpoint bleeding once the hyperkeratosis has been removed and the capillaries reached.

b) Corn

Cone-shaped hyperkeratosis over a pressure point

Paring down produces a decreasing cone of keratin with no capillary bleeding.

Fig. 13.67 Mosaic plantar warts

Fig. 13.66 Differentiation between plantar wart and corn by paring down the surface keratin: (a) plantar wart showing bleeding points; (b) corn before paring; (c) corn showing cone of solid keratin in centre

TREATMENT: PLANTAR WARTS

SINGLE/FEW PLANTAR WARTS
Keratolytic agents
These work by reducing pain from the hyperkeratosis that forms around a verruca. **They do not on their own get rid of the wart**, so the patient needs to be aware of this. The verruca will only go if the body's immunity gets rid of it.

The most important thing is for the patient to pare down the hard skin every night with a scalpel or to rub it flat with a pumice stone so that it does not hurt. A wart paint or gel is then applied carefully just to the warts, left to dry and then covered with a plaster overnight. In the morning the plaster is removed to allow the wart to harden up again before the wart is pared down the next night.

Wart paints (suitable for use on the feet) are:
- salicylic acid 50% in paraffin (Verrugon)
- salicylic acid/lactic acid mixtures in collodion (Cuplex, Duofilm, Salactol, Salatac); 26% salicylic acid only (Occlusal)
- podophyllotoxin preparations (Warticon cream)
- 10% glutaraldehyde solution (Glutarol).

Whichever paint (or gel) is chosen, it should be used each night before the patient goes to bed. A fair trial of a treatment is to use it for 12 weeks before giving up and changing to something else. If the plaster is left on for too long the wart becomes soggy and painful. If this occurs, treatment will have to be left off for a few days. One of the reasons why the treatment does not work is that the patient stops using it if the foot becomes sore.

Freezing with liquid nitrogen
This is not a good treatment for plantar warts, because you need to freeze for quite a long time to produce a blister (because of the thick layer of keratin on the sole of the foot) and this will be too painful for the patient.

Surgery
Any kind of surgery *is contraindicated* on the feet. The most likely outcome is recurrence of the wart, and there is always the risk that scarring will lead to the formation of permanent callosities, especially over pressure points.

MOSAIC WARTS
These do not respond as well to treatment as single warts. You can try the following options.
- One of the salicylic and lactic acid paints applied every night.
- Formalin or glutaraldehyde soaks. Get the patient to soak the affected part of the foot in a 5% solution of formaldehyde BP or Glutarol once a day. First apply a thickish layer of white soft paraffin (Vaseline) around the warts, so that the formalin does not make the normal skin sore. Then pour the formalin into a saucer or shallow bowl and soak the warts in it for 10 minutes each day. The next day, rub down any hard skin with a pumice stone or foot scraper before repeating the treatment.
- Apply 40% salicylic acid plasters cut to the same size as the warts. These are stuck onto the warts shiny side down, taped securely in place with Hypafix (or something similar), and left for a week at a time. When they are removed the soggy keratin is removed with a sharp scalpel blade before putting on a new plaster. This can be done once a week by the nurse or podiatrist until no wart is left.

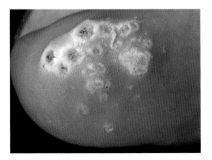

Fig. 13.68 Verruca treated with a keratolytic agent

Nails

14

ANATOMY OF THE NAIL

Nails are keratin produced by a modified epidermis called the nail matrix. From this grows the nail plate, which lies on the nail bed. Nails protect the end of the digits and on the fingers they are useful for picking up small objects and for scratching. Abnormalities can arise from any part of the nail apparatus.

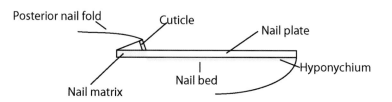

Fig. 14.01 Anatomy of the nail

EXAMINATION OF THE NAIL

When looking at nails, examine the following in turn.

1. The nail from above

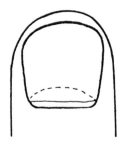

SURFACE OF THE NAIL
- Pitting, p. 437
- Transverse ridging, p. 437
- Longitudinal ridging, p. 438
- Shiny, *see* p. 236

COLOUR OF THE NAIL
- Discolouration of the nail bed, p. 439
- Discolouration of the nail plate, p. 440

NAIL FOLD AND CUTICLE
- Loss of cuticle – paronychia, p. 445
- Nail fold telangiectasia, *see* p. 132

2. The nail from end on

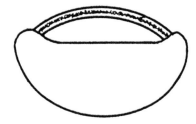

THICKNESS OF THE NAIL
- Thickening of nail plate, p. 442
- Splitting of nail plate, p. 443
- Subungual hyperkeratosis, p. 445

DETACHMENT OF THE NAIL from nail bed
- Onycholysis, p. 444

3. The nail from the side

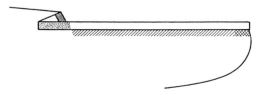

SHAPE OF THE NAILS
- Overcurvature, p. 446
- Spoon-shaped nails, p. 446
- Wedge-shaped nails, p. 446
- Ingrowing toenails, p. 447

LOSS OF NAILS
- Without scarring, p. 447
- With scarring (permanent), p. 447

LUMPS AND BUMPS AROUND THE NAILS, p. 448

ABNORMALITIES OF THE NAIL MATRIX

PITTING

Inflammatory conditions affecting the matrix cause abnormal keratin to be formed, which becomes detached from the nail plate leaving pits or ridges. Pits are more easily seen in the fingernails than in toenails.

Causes of pitting:
1. Psoriasis – small regular pits
2. Eczema – larger and more irregular pits, associated with eczema on the skin around the nail
3. Alopecia areata – small, regular pits may be a poor prognostic sign for regrowth of the hair
4. Twenty-nail dystrophy – all finger- and toenails have parallel pitting, which may merge to form ridges; cause unknown
5. Normal finding – isolated pits may be found in normal nails.

TRANSVERSE RIDGING

Causes of transverse ridging:
1. Eczema – some pits are so broad as to form transverse ridges
2. Chronic paronychia due to pressure on the nail matrix (*see* Fig. 14.05 and Fig. 14.32).
3. Beau's lines – a single line at the same place in all the nails is due to cessation of growth of the nail matrix at the time of a severe illness; when this is over, the matrix will begin to function normally again and the nail will grow out with a line in it; fingernails grow at a rate of approximately 1 mm/week (toenails at about a third of that speed), so you can tell how long ago the illness was (*see* Fig. 14.08).

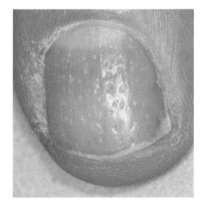

Fig. 14.02 Nail pitting in psoriasis

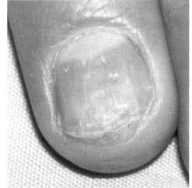

Fig. 14.03 Larger and more irregular pits and ridging in eczema

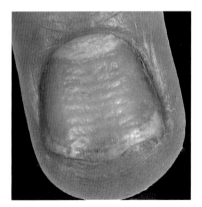

Fig. 14.04 Twenty-nail dystrophy

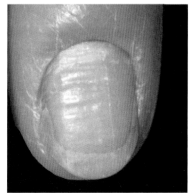

Fig. 14.05 Transverse ridging secondary to paronychia

LONGITUDINAL RIDGING

Causes when all nails are affected:
1. A few ridges are seen in normal nails
2. **Lichen planus** – fine regular lines (*see* also p. 447, pterygium)
3. **Darier's disease** – regular fine lines with V-shaped notching at the end of the nails (*see* also p. 247).

Causes when a single nail is affected:
1. **Median nail dystrophy** looks like an upside-down Christmas tree; it is a temporary abnormality and gets better spontaneously after a few months; the cause is unknown
2. **Habit-tic deformity** – here there is a broader groove made up of numerous concave transverse ridges; it is due to picking or biting the cuticle, which damages the nail plate as it grows out
3. A single wide groove may be due to **myxoid cyst** or **fibroma** over the posterior nail fold that presses on the underlying matrix (*see* p. 448).

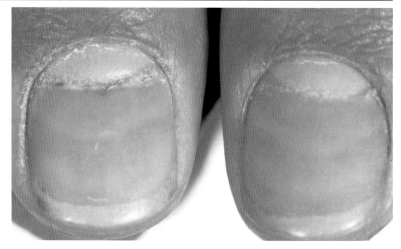

Fig. 14.08 Beau's lines: a transverse ridge in all nails due to interruption of nail growth secondary to a systemic illness

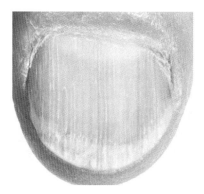

Fig. 14.06 Longitudinal ridging seen in lichen planus

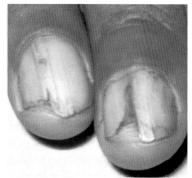

Fig. 14.07 Darier's disease: longitudinal ridging with V-shaped notches

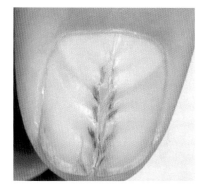

Fig. 14.09 Medial nail dystrophy

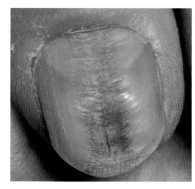

Fig. 14.10 Habit-tic deformity on a thumbnail

ABNORMALITIES OF THE NAIL BED
DISCOLOURATION UNDER THE NAIL

The nail bed is the epidermis underneath the nail. In normal circumstances it does not produce keratin. Problems in the nail bed cause areas of discolouration under the nail.

White

Pallor of the nail bed occurs in hypoalbuminaemia or chronic renal failure.

Orange-brown

This is due to psoriasis in the nail bed (salmon patches).

Brown

A round or oval area is a junctional naevus of the nail bed. If it is growing or made up of different colours, consider a malignant melanoma (*see* Figs 14. 17 and 14.18, p. 440).

Red, purple, black

1. **Splinter haemorrhages** are small, red, longitudinal streaks classically seen in subacute bacterial endocarditis. In fact, they are very common so are an unreliable clinical sign.

2. **Subungual haematoma** results from bleeding under the nail following trauma. It can occur on finger- or toenails. Initially, the area is exquisitely painful and dark-red or purple in colour. With time, if the blood is not released immediately by puncturing the nail, the area is discoloured black or brown. It can be distinguished from a subungual malignant melanoma by making a small horizontal nick on the nail plate at the distal end of the discolouration and watching for a week. A subungual haematoma will grow out at the same rate as the nail so the nick will still be at the distal end of the discolouration; a melanoma does not grow at such a regular rate.

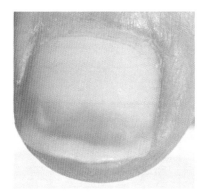

Fig. 14.11 White nail bed due to hypoalbuminaemia

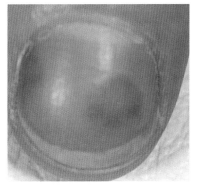

Fig. 14.12 Salmon patch due to psoriasis

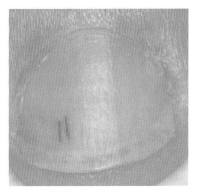

Fig. 14.13 Splinter haemorrhages

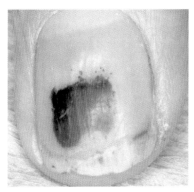

Fig. 14.14 Subungual haematoma

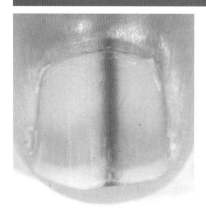

Fig. 14.15 Thin brown line due to a junctional naevus in the nail matrix

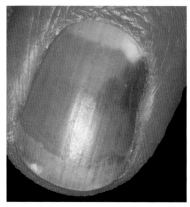

Fig. 14.16 Subungual pigmentation resulting from a low-grade haematoma under the nail due to minor trauma

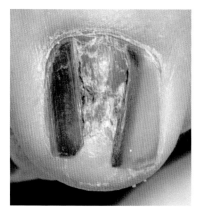

Fig. 14.17 Malignant melanoma arising in nail bed with destruction of the nail plate

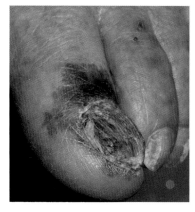

Fig. 14.18 Malignant melanoma in nail bed and involving the nail fold

3. **Malignant melanoma** arising in the nail bed or nail fold is very uncommon. There will be secondary signs, such as destruction of the nail plate (*see* Fig. 14.17) or spread of pigment into the adjoining nail fold (*see* Fig. 14.18).

Pink, mauve

A **glomus tumour** is a rare benign tumour that presents as a mauve area under the nail that is tender, particularly on pressure or in the cold.

ABNORMALITIES OF THE NAIL PLATE
DISCOLOURATION OF THE NAIL PLATE

The following are causes of discolouration of the nail plate.

1. **External staining**, especially from nicotine and medicaments (e.g. $KMnO_4$ [*see* Fig. 2.02 p. 30] and dithranol). It occurs less commonly from hair dyes or nail varnish.

2. **Drugs**: all the nails will be equally affected, e.g.
● chloroquine, azidothymidine (AZT) and gold stains nails blue-grey
● penicillamine stains nails yellow.

3. **Brown lines** in a nail: a thin line down the entire length of the nail is due to a **junctional naevus** of the nail matrix. A broad line under the nail plate that is expanding in width or extending up through the nail should make you think of a **malignant melanoma**. Light-brown pigmentation, especially at the edge of the nail plate, is likely to be due to a low-grade **haematoma** from minor trauma or pressure from footwear (*see* Fig. 14.16).

4. **White nails**:
- small white streaks due to **minor trauma** occur in most people at some time
- in **familial leuconychia** the whole of the nail is white; this is inherited as an autosomal dominant trait
- white discolouration that affects nails irregularly is often due to **tinea** infection (*see* p. 442).

5. **Green** discolouration occurs with pseudomonas infection.

6. **Blue** discolouration occurs in patients with HIV/AIDS infection and this may be a useful indicator of the disease. Similar discolouration can be due to AZT.

7. **Yellow nails**:
- **yellow nail syndrome** – all the nails are yellow or green in colour and are excessively curved in both longitudinal and transverse directions; the rate of growth is slowed almost to a standstill and sometimes onycholysis can also occur; it is thought to be due to a congenital abnormality of the lymphatics, although the nail changes do not occur until adult life and often not until middle or old age; there may be other abnormalities of the lymphatics, such as lymphoedema of the legs or bilateral pleural effusions
- localised yellow or brown discolouration can be due to **tinea**.

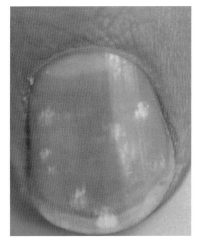

Fig. 14.19 White streaks in nail plate due to minor trauma

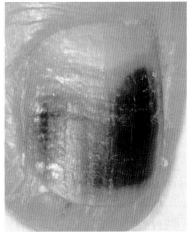

Fig. 14.20 Green discolouration due to pseudomonas infection

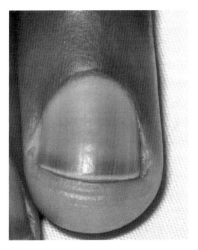

Fig. 14.21 Blue discolouration due to HIV infection

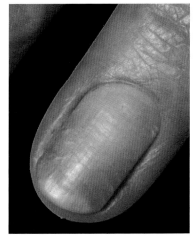

Fig. 14.22 Yellow nail syndrome

THICKENING OF THE NAIL PLATE

1. **Tinea unguium** – dermatophyte fungi live on keratin so multiply within the nail plate, causing it to become thickened and discoloured white or yellow. They can only become established in nails that are growing slowly, so they affect toenails much more readily than fingernails. Once established, the rate of growth slows down even more, so that cutting the affected nails becomes an infrequent necessity. It can be difficult on the feet to distinguish clinically between thickening of the nails due to tinea and onycholysis and subungual hyperkeratosis due to psoriasis. First look at the fingernails: the changes of psoriasis will be more obvious there with associated pits, salmon patches and onycholysis. If the fingernails are not involved, tinea is more likely. On the toes, tinea does not affect all the nails and usually affects one foot before the other. You can also look between the toes or on the instep for other evidence of tinea of the feet (*see* p. 426). Nail clippings for direct microscopy (*see* Fig. 10.03, p. 337) or fungal culture will confirm the diagnosis.
2. **Chronic trauma** to toenails (in patients who play football, tennis, etc.) can produce thickened nails.
3. In **old age** the nails become thickened, curved and difficult to cut.
4. Wedge-shaped nails occur in **pachyonychia congenita** (*see* p. 446).
5. **Chronic malalignment** of big toenails. A congenital disorder where the big toenails become thickened, ridged and over-curved, growing at an angle laterally. This condition is probably quite common and leads to ingrowing toenails.

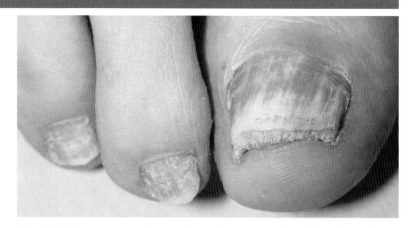

Fig. 14.23 Tinea unguium showing thickening and discolouration of nail plate

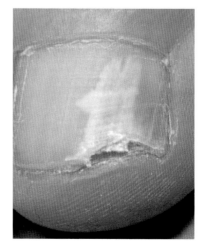

Fig. 14.24 Tinea unguium with yellow discolouration and patchy involvement

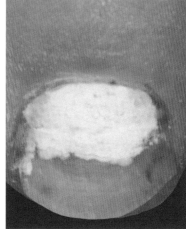

Fig. 14.25 White nail due to tinea unguium

TREATMENT: TINEA UNGUIUM

Many patients have tinea of their toenails without being aware of it. Treatment is only needed if the patient is complaining of the problem or if he or she is getting recurrent tinea infections elsewhere (feet, groin, body). Cure rates from treatment may be as low as 30%.

Topical treatment with 5% amorolfine (Loceryl) nail lacquer applied once or twice a week after nail filing is suitable if there are only two or three nails involved, with no more than 50% of the distal nail plate affected and lack of matrix involvement. Other indications for topical treatment are children, if systemic therapy is contraindicated and for prophylaxis. Amorolfine also works for toenail infections with the saprophytic moulds, *Hendersonula toruloidea* and *Scopulariopsis brevicaulis*.

Systemic treatment is recommended when:
- more than 50% of the plate is involved
- there is involvement of the matrix
- multiple nails are involved.

Terbinafine 250 mg is given once daily by mouth for 6 weeks for fingernails and 3–4 months for toenails. Liver function tests should be checked at baseline and every 4–6 weeks. An alternative is itraconazole 200 mg orally/day. This can be given continuously (as for terbinafine) or 400 mg/day pulsed (1 week on and 3 weeks off). It is contraindicated in heart failure and liver disease. Liver function tests should be monitored if given continuously (but not for pulsed treatment). Terbinafine gives a better cure rate (55% at 72 weeks).

The efficacy of oral therapy can be improved by combination with amorolfine topically. Failure of oral treatment necessitates the removal of the affected toenail(s) plus oral terbinafine 250 mg daily for 3–6 months.

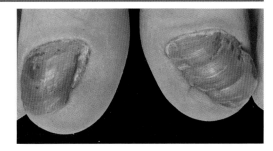

Fig. 14.26 Chronic malalignment of the big toenails

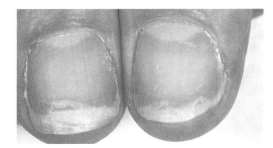

Fig. 14.27 Lamellar splitting at the distal end of the nail plate

SPLITTING OF THE ENDS OF THE NAILS

1. **Lamellar splitting** occurs when the distal portion of the nail plate splits into horizontal layers. It is mainly seen in women who have their hands wet for long periods of time. Water and detergents damage the keratin. It is treated by keeping the hands out of water or by wearing rubber gloves.
2. **Longitudinal splitting** may occur along a longitudinal ridge, especially in Darier's disease (*see* Fig. 14.07).

ABNORMALITIES OF THE HYPONYCHIUM

ONYCHOLYSIS

Onycholysis is separation of the nail plate from the nail bed. It is due to an abnormality of the hyponychium where the nail plate is less firmly stuck down onto the nail bed. It can be due to:

1. **Trauma** – on the hands the commonest cause is over-manicuring; the hyponychium is damaged by cleaning underneath the nails with a nail file; on the feet it usually follows a subungual haematoma
2. **Psoriasis** – onycholysis is more obvious on fingernails than toenails; once the nail has lifted off, subungual hyperkeratosis occurs and it may be difficult to distinguish from thickening of the nail plate due to tinea (compare Fig. 14.29 with Fig. 14.23)
3. **Poor peripheral circulation**
4. **Thyrotoxicosis**
5. **Allergic contact dermatitis** to substances that penetrate through the nail plate (e.g. methacrylate used as a glue for sticking on artificial nails)
6. **Doxycycline** taken orally can cause a photo-onycholysis in the summer; the patient experiences severe pain in all fingernails, and then the nails lift off; this is becoming more common since doxycycline is being used for malaria prophylaxis; it can occur simultaneously in the toenails if the patient is wearing open-toed sandals.

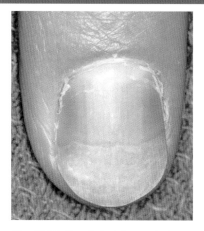

Fig. 14.28 Onycholysis in psoriasis

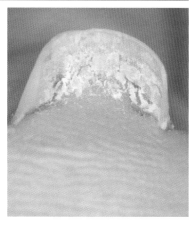

Fig. 14.29 Subungual hyperkeratosis: note the nail plate is of normal thickness

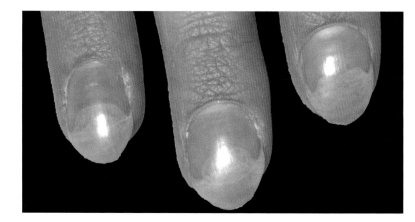

Fig. 14.30 Photo-onycholysis due to doxycycline: all fingernails involved equally

SUBUNGUAL HYPERKERATOSIS

This is a build-up of keratin under the end of the nail. It needs to be distinguished from nail thickening. The cause is usually **psoriasis**.

TREATMENT: PSORIASIS OF THE NAILS

There is no topical treatment that will help psoriatic nail changes (pitting, salmon patches, onycholysis or subungual hyperkeratosis). Coloured nail varnish will hide onycholysis in a woman, and keeping the nails cut short will stop onycholysis getting worse. Fortunately, patients do not often ask for treatment for their nails. If the skin psoriasis is bad enough to be treated with a systemic agent (*see* pp. 227 and 230), the nails will also improve.

ABNORMALITIES OF THE CUTICLE

PARONYCHIA

The cuticle is an area of keratin joining the posterior nail fold to the nail plate, preventing bacteria and yeasts from getting into the soft tissues around the nail. If the cuticle is lost (usually due to chronic trauma to hands that are continually wet, or to eczema), infection can occur under the posterior or lateral nail folds to cause paronychia. There are two types.

Acute paronychia: this is due to infection with *Staphylococcus aureus* (less commonly *Streptococcus pyogenes*). There is exquisite pain, a bright-red swelling and pus formation. Rarely herpes simplex may be the cause, but grouped vesicles over the distal phalanx will be seen.

Chronic paronychia: *Candida albicans* produces a more chronic infection with less swelling, a duller red colour and no pus. The nail plate may show transverse or longitudinal ridges from chronic pressure on the matrix (*see* Fig. 14.32).

TREATMENT: PARONYCHIA

Acute: flucloxacillin or erythromycin, 250 mg qid for 7 days. If there is obvious pus present, it should be lanced to let it out.

Chronic: the real cause is the loss of the cuticle. The paronychia will only get better permanently if a new cuticle can be induced to grow. The patient must keep the hands dry by wearing rubber or cotton-lined rubber or PVC gloves for all wet work until a new cuticle has grown (3–4 months). A protective film of Vaseline can be applied around the nail several times a day to keep water out.

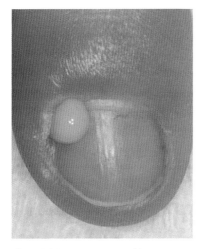

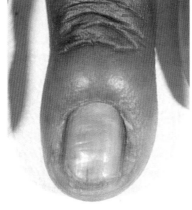

Fig. 14.31 Acute paronychia

Fig. 14.32 Chronic paronychia with associated nail dystrophy

ABNORMALLY SHAPED NAILS

OVERCURVATURE

This can be due to:

1. **Clubbing** – this is an apparent overcurvature of the nail due to loss of the angle between the posterior nail fold and the nail plate; if there is any doubt, put the distal phalanges of the two thumbs together and there should be a diamond-shaped gap between them – this disappears if the nails are clubbed; clubbing is due to chronic chest disease, carcinoma of the bronchus or congenital heart disease
2. Resorption of the distal phalanx in **hyperparathyroidism** – the nail curves over the end of the finger
3. **Yellow nail syndrome**, *see* p. 441
4. **Malalignment** of big toenails, *see* p. 442.

SPOON-SHAPED NAILS (KOILONYCHIA)

Spoon-shaped nails are most often seen in association with iron deficiency anaemia (although most patients with iron deficiency do not have this change). It may be a normal finding in young children.

WEDGE-SHAPED NAILS

Pachyonychia congenita is a rare genetic abnormality present from birth. The nail grows both vertically and horizontally, causing a thick, wedge-shaped nail that is unsightly on the fingers and causes pain from pressure of shoes on the toes.

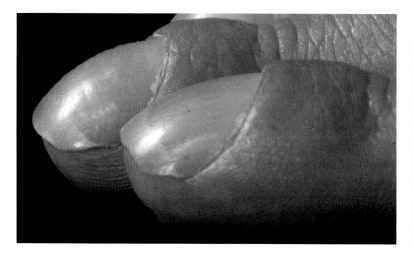

Fig. 14.33 Clubbing

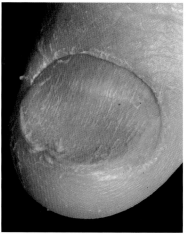

Fig. 14.34 Koilonychia

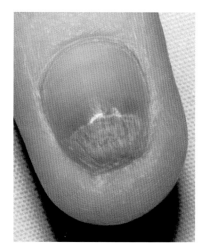

Fig. 14.35 Pachyonychia congenita

INGROWING TOENAILS

Penetration of the lateral nail fold by the nail itself or a spicule of the nail causes redness, tenderness, pus formation and later the development of granulation tissue. The great toenail is most commonly involved. It is due to wearing shoes that are too tight and cutting the nails in a half-circle instead of straight across. Similar changes can occur as a side effect of the retinoid drugs.

TREATMENT: NAIL LICHEN PLANUS

Longitudinal ridging (*see* p. 438) needs no treatment. If pterygium occurs, which will cause permanent scarring of the nails, prednisolone 30 mg/day started as soon as possible will often switch it off. Give this dose for 2 weeks and then gradually tail it off over the next month.

LOSS OF NAILS

WITHOUT SCARRING (TEMPORARY)

- Trauma especially to the great toenails. It can occur to fingernails too after a large subungual haematoma.
- Beau's lines after a severe illness. The nail may break off at the line (*see* p. 437).

WITH SCARRING (PERMANENT)

- **Lichen planus**: the cuticle grows down over and through the nail plate, resulting in permanent scarring. This is called **pterygium**.
- **Genetic** abnormalities: all rare.

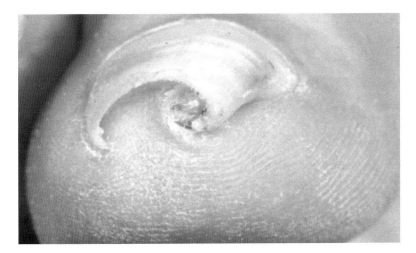

Fig. 14.36 Ingrowing toenail

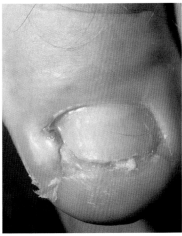

Fig. 14.37 Ingrowing toenail with infection of nail fold

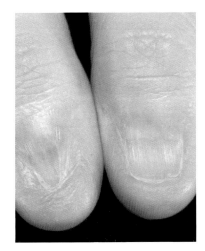

Fig. 14.38 Pterygium of thumbnails due to lichen planus

LUMPS AND BUMPS AROUND THE NAIL

1. **Viral warts**: small skin-coloured, grey or brown papules with a rough, warty surface may occur on the skin around the nail. At this site these are difficult to remove and may grow under the nail. The best way to remove them is by curettage and cautery, but sometimes some of the nail plate may need to be removed.

2. **Myxoid (mucous) cyst**: a round, skin-coloured papule on the dorsal surface of the distal phalanx. If pricked it discharges a sticky clear fluid. These are due to the joint capsule herniating into the surrounding skin. It is best that a hand surgeon carries out the removal, since recurrence is likely unless the capsular defect is sealed. If a fibroma or myxoid cyst occurs over the nail matrix, the pressure on the matrix can cause a longitudinal groove in the nail plate (*see* Fig. 14.42).

3. **Swelling of the distal interphalangeal joint** can occur in gout or osteoarthritis (Heberden's nodes).

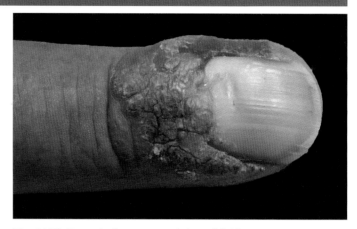

Fig. 14.39 Bowen's disease around the nail fold

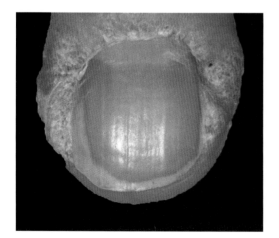

Fig. 14.40 Viral warts around nail fold

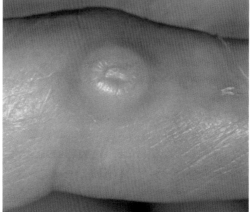

Fig. 14.41 Myxoid cyst lying over distal interphalangeal joint

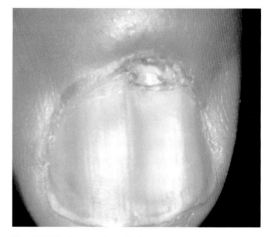

Fig. 14.42 Groove in nail due to pressure on matrix by a myxoid cyst

4. **Subungual and periungual fibroma**: small firm pink or skin-coloured papules protruding from the posterior nail fold or from under the nail occur in patients with tuberous sclerosis (*see* p. 267). They appear after puberty.

5. **Subungual exostosis**: this is a localised outgrowth of bone that presents as a subungual skin-coloured papule. If in doubt, X-ray the digit.

6. **Tumours**: rarely squamous cell carcinoma and malignant melanoma can occur around the nail. Any inflammatory condition around a single nail that does not improve with treatment is an indication for biopsy.

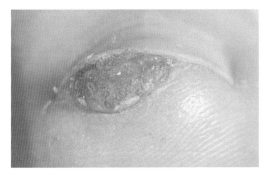

Fig. 14.43 Subungual fibroma

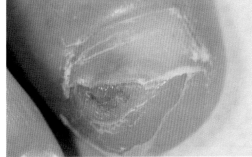

Fig. 14.45 Subungual exostosis

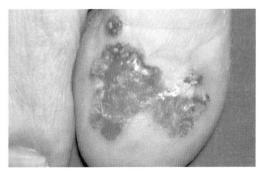

Fig. 14.47 Malignant melanoma in nail bed

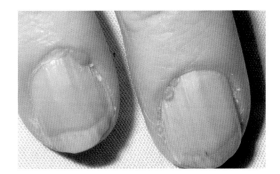

Fig. 14.44 Periungual fibromas in patient with tuberous sclerosis (*see* also p. 267)

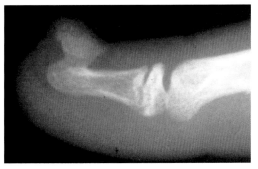

Fig. 14.46 X-ray of subungual exostosis

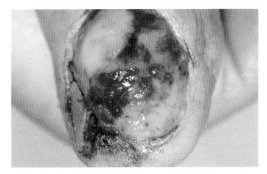

Fig. 14.48 Tumour under nail: a biopsy will be needed to make a diagnosis

General index

List of drugs and associated drug reactions

ACE inhibitors	Erythrodermic	**β-blockers**	Lichenoid
	Exanthematous		Psoriasis
	Lichenoid	**β-carotene**	Orange discolouration
	Lupus erythematosus	**bleomycin**	Flagellate erythema
	Pemphigus		Pigmentation
ACTH	Acne	**bromides**	Acne
allopurinol	DRESS	**busulphan**	Hyperpigmentation
	Erythrodermic	**calcium-channel blockers**	Lower leg oedema
	Purpura	**(amlodipine etc.)**	(eczema)
	Toxic epidermal necrolysis		Lupus erythematosus
	Vasculitis		Pruritis (elderly)
aminophylline	Eczematous	**carbamazepine**	Erythrodermic
amiodarone	Hyperpigmentation		Exanthematous
	Phototoxic	**carbimazole**	Hair loss
ampicillin	Erythrodermic		Purpura
	Exanthematous		Toxic epidermal necrolysis
	Vasculitis	**chloroquine**	Bleaching of hair
androgens	Acne		Blue nails
anticonvulsants	DRESS		Erythrodermic
antifungals	Lupus erythematosus		Hyperpigmentation of skin
aspirin	Histamine release		Lichenoid
	(urticaria)		Phototoxicity
barbiturates	Erythrodermic	**chlorpromazine**	Erythrodermic
	Fixed drug reaction		Lupus erythematosus
	Purpura		Photoallergic
	Toxic epidermal necrolysis		Purpura (thrombocytopenia)
benzodiazepines	Exanthematous	**chlorpropamide**	Eczematous
	Fixed drug eruption		Lichenoid

ciclosporin	Hypertrichosis	**isotretinoin**	Dry lips, nose and eyes
	Non-melanoma skin cancers		Hair loss
	Sebaceous gland hyperplasia		Photosensitivity
cimetidine	Erythrodermic	**lithium**	Acne
clofazimine	Pigmentation – red/pink		Psoriasis
codeine	Histamine release (urticaria)	**mepacrine**	Lichenoid
contraceptives	Erythema nodosum		Yellow discolouration
	Pigmentation of face (chloasma)		of skin
coumarins	Skin necrosis	**methyldopa**	Lichenoid
cytotoxics	Hair loss		Lupus erythematosus
	Purpura (thrombocytopenia)	**minocycline**	DRESS
dapsone	DRESS		Pigmentation – blue/grey
	Pigmentation – blue-grey		Lupus erythematosus
diazoxide	Hypertrichosis	**minoxidil**	Hypertrichosis
diclofenac	Pemphigoid	**nalidixic acid**	Erythrodermic
doxycycline	Photosensitivity		Phototoxic reaction
furosemide	Exanthematous	**nitrofurantoin**	Serum sickness (urticaria)
	Phototoxic	**NSAIDs**	Erythema multiforme
gold	DRESS		Exanthematous
	Erythrodermic		Fixed drug reaction
	Lichenoid		Phototoxicity
	Pigmentation of face – blue-grey		Pseudoporphyria
	Purpura (thrombocytopenia)		Toxic epidermal necrolysis
	Vasculitis		Vasculitis
heparin	Hair loss	**opiates**	Histamine release
	Vasculitis		(urticaria)
hydralazine	Lupus erythematosus	**penicillamine**	Hypertrichosis
	Vasculitis		Lichenoid
imatinib	Lichenoid		Pemphigus
iodides	Acne	**penicillins**	Anaphylaxis (urticaria)
isoniazid	Acne		Exanthematous
	Erythrodermic		Serum sickness (urticaria)
	Pellagra	**phenolphthalein**	Fixed drug eruption

phenothiazines	Exanthematous		Fixed drug eruption
	Phototoxic		Lichenoid
	Serum sickness (urticaria)		Purpura
phenytoin	Acne		Serum sickness (urticaria)
	Erythrodermic		Toxic epidermal necrolysis
	Hyperpigmentation		Vasculitis
	Toxic epidermal necrolysis	**sulphasalazine**	Lupus erythematosus
procainamide	Lupus erythematosus	**tetracyclines**	Photo-onycholysis
promethazine	Photoallergic		Phototoxic
protease inhibitors	DRESS	**thiazides**	Eczematous
	Stevens–Johnson syndrome		Exanthematous
	Toxic epidermal necrolysis		Lichenoid
psoralens	Hypertrichosis		Purpura
	Phototoxic		Serum sickness (urticaria)
retinoids	Dry lips, nose and eyes		Vasculitis
(acitretin)	Hair loss	**thioureas**	Hair loss
(alitretinoin)	Photosensitivity		Vasculitis
rifampicin	Pemphigus	**tyrosine kinase antagonists**	Acne
	Purpura (thrombocytopenia)		Palmar hyperkeratosis
steroids, anabolic	Acne		Rosacea
cortico-	Acne	**vancomycin**	Anaphylaxis (urticaria)
	Easy bruising		Red man syndrome
	Perioral dermatitis		Stevens–Johnson syndrome
	Skin atrophy and striae		Toxic epidermal necrolysis Ashton
	Telangiectasia	**vemurafenib**	Keratoacanthomas and squamous
sulphonamides	DRESS		cell carcinomas
	Eczematous		Photosensitivity
	Erythrodermic	**warfarin**	Hair loss
	Exanthematous		Skin necrosis

Emollient products: how and when to use

Type	Class	Oil (%)	Examples (this list is not exhaustive)	Definition	Usage	Patient groups
Leave-on emollients Use as routine moisturiser anywhere	Ointment (no water) Aerosol spray	100	White soft paraffin (Vaseline), 50/50 white soft/liquid paraffin, Diprobase ointment, Epaderm/Hydromol/Emulsifying oints, Dermamist, Emollin spray	100% paraffin base (no preservative required)	Very dry skin Use twice a day Useful at night-time Greasy – may put off some patients	Severe atopic eczema Ichthyosis Sprays useful in the elderly and in hard-to-reach areas
	Occlusive cream	30–70	Oily cream/hydrous ointment (lanolin), QV intensive, Unguentum M, Lipobase (used as a diluent in Lipocream).	Water-in-oil emulsion (oily/cold creams) and 100% lipid ointments	Dry skin Trunk and limbs 2–3 times a day	Moderate atopic eczema or psoriasis
	Emollient gel containing *glycerol*	30	Doublebase gel, Doublebase Dayleve gel	Water and oil emulsion with humectant Water held in stratum corneum by humectant (glycerol or urea)	Very dry skin Use 3–4× a day, or 2× a day for Dayleve	Very dry skin Psoriasis, Ichthyosis
	Emollient cream containing *urea*	5–10% urea	Aquadrate, Balneum cream, Calmurid, E45 Itch Relief, Eucerin intensive, Hydromol intensive, Nutraplus.		Dry skin Use twice a day	Useful in older patients and in psoriasis
	Emollient cream (others without urea)	11–30	Aquamax, Aquamol, Aveeno cream (colloidal oatmeal), Cetraben, Diprobase cream, Epaderm cream, E45 cream (lanolin), Hydromol cream, Oilatum cream QV cream (contains glycerol), Ultrabase Zerocream, Zerobase cream, Zeroguent	Oil-in-water emulsion (vanishing cream) (*Note: tubs can become contaminated – prescribe pumps*)	Normal to dry skin conditions Face and flexures Good patient compliance 3–4x a day	Mild/moderate atopic eczema Other dry skin conditions such as psoriasis and endogenous eczema
	with antimicrobial		Dermol cream, Eczmol cream	Product contains benzalkonium chloride, and/or chlorhexidine	Useful in preventing flares of atopic eczema Use lotions as a soap substitute	Infected/colonised atopic eczema Healthcare workers Folliculitis
	Emollient lotion *with antimicrobial*	5–14	Dermol lotion			
	without antimicrobial		Aveeno lotion (colloidal oatmeal), E45 lotion (lanolin), QV lotion	Oil-in-water emulsion with low oil content Lighter than creams	Easy to apply 4x day Hairy areas (e.g. trunk, scalp) Summertime use	Poor compliers (teenagers, men)
	Antipruritic emollient		Balneum Plus cream, E45 Itch Relief cream	Product contains antipruritic agents (lauromacrogols)	Pruritus, especially if due to dry skin	First-line therapy for itching (especially in the elderly)

Adapted from Moncrieff G, Cork M, Lawton S, *et al.* Use of emollients in dry-skin conditions: consensus statement. *Clin Exp Dermatol.* 2013; **38**: 231–8.

Wash and bath emollient products: how and when to use

Type	Class	Oil (%)	Examples	Definition	When to use	Patient groups
Wash products Use only for washing, do not leave on the skin	Emollient wash products	15–30	Aquamax cream wash, Doublebase shower gel, E45 wash cream, Hydromol bath and shower emollient, QV gentle wash, Oilatum shower emollient.	Products contain emulsifiers Should NOT contain harsh detergents such as sodium lauryl sulphate (e.g. aqueous cream)	Instead of soap, which is an irritant and therefore should be avoided in any dry skin conditions	Atopic eczema Hand dermatitis and psoriasis
	Antimicrobial wash products	2–50	Dermol shower/wash/lotion, Eczmol cream.	Emollient wash product containing topically active antimicrobial agents (such as benzalkonium chloride and/ or chlorhexidine)	Useful in managing and preventing flares of atopic eczema	Recurrent infections or relapses in atopic eczema and hand dermatitis
Bath emollients Add to bath water, can be used to wash with	Bath oil: Semi-dispersible oil or dispersible emulsion	50–91	Aveeno (colloidal oatmeal), Balneum, Cetraben, Dermalo, Diprobath, Doublebase bath additive. E45 bath oil, LPL 63.4, Oilatum, QV bath oil, Zerolatum, Zeroneum	Deposits a layer of oil on the surface of the water that leaves a slick around the bath; non-foaming and fragrance free Oil disperses evenly through the bath water	All patient with moderate-very dry skin (atopic eczema, ichthyosis) Bathing in water alone is drying; bath oils should not be rinsed off	Use as part of complete emollient therapy in all dry skin conditions (*see* p. xx)
	Antimicrobiol bath oil	50–55	Dermol bath, Emulsiderm, Oilatum Plus, Zerolatum Plus	Bath oil containing topical antiseptic agent	Prevention of infection.	Atopic eczema with recurrent infections
	Antipruritic bath oil	85	Balneum Plus bath oil (soya oil)	Bath oil containing topical antipruritic agent	Protection of the skin barrier during bathing if pruritus is a problem	Should be used in conjunction with an antipruritic emollient

Classification of topical steroids by potency

Group	UK brands	USA brands	Clinical indication
Weak[UK] Group 6–7[USA] Potency = 1% hydrocortisone	Hydrocortisone 0.5%, 1.0%, 2.5% (*Dioderm, Mildison*) Fluocinolone 0.0025% (*Synalar 1:10*) cream	Hydrocortisone 0.5%, 1.0%, 2.5% (numerous products) Alclometasone 0.05% (*Aclovate*) Desonide 0.05% (*Desowen/Tridesilon*)	Eczema on the face Eczema at any site in infants
Medium potent[UK] Group 4–5[USA] Potency = 2.5 (×1% hydrocortisone)	Betamethasone valerate 0.025% (*Betnovate RD*) Clobetasone butyrate 0.05% (*Eumovate*) Fluocinolone .00625% (*Synalar 1:4*) Fluocortolone 0.25% (*Ultralanum plain*) Fludroxycortide 0.0125% (*Haelan*) Hydrocortisone 17-butyrate 0.1% (*Locoid*)	Clocortolone pivalate 0.1% Desoximetasone 0.05% (*Topicort LP*) Fluocinolone 0.025%* Fluticasone 0.005% (*Cutivate*) Flurandrenolide 0.05% Hydrocortisone butyrate 0.1% (*Locoid*) Hydrocortisone valerate 0.2%* Hydrocortisone probutate 0.1% Prednicarbate 0.1% Triamcinolone 0.025%* (*Kenalog*)	Eczema (atopic) on the trunk and limbs, or flexures (both adult or children) Seborrhoeic eczema on trunk Flexural psoriasis
Potent[UK] Group 2–3[USA] Potency = 10 (×1% hydrocortisone)	Betamethasone dipropionate 0.05% (*Diprosone*) Betamethasone valerate 0.1% (*Betnovate*) Diflucortolone valerate 0.1% (*Nerisone*) Fluocinolone acetonide 0.025% (*Synalar*) Fluocinonide 0.05% (*Metosyn*) Fluticasone propionate 0.05% (*Cutivate*) Mometasone furoate 0.1% (*Elocon*)	Amcinonide 0.1% (*Cyclocort*) Betamethasone dipropionate 0.05% (*Diprolene*) Betamethasone valerate 0.1% (*Beta-Val*) Desoximetasone 0.05% (*Topicort*) Diflorasone diacetate 0.05% (*Apexicon*) Fluocinonide 0.05% (*Lidex*) Halcinonide 0.1% (*Halog*) Mometasone furoate 0.1%* (*Elocon*) Triamcinolone 0.5%, 0.1%*	Lichenified atopic eczema Discoid eczema Varicose eczema Scalp eczema Hand and foot eczema or psoriasis Lichen planus
Very potent[UK] Group 1[USA] Potency = 50 (×1% hydrocortisone)	Clobetasol propionate 0.05% (*Dermovate*) Diflucortolone valerate 0.3 (*Nerisone forte*)	Clobetasol propionate 0.05% (*Temovate*) Fluocinonide 0.1% (*Vanos*) Halbetasol propionate 0.05% (*Ultravate*)	Lichen simplex Resistant discoid eczema Discoid lupus erythematosus Lichen sclerosus et atrophicus

Note: *cream in a lower potency group; the ointment and cream base may result in differing groups for same molecule.

Index of algorithms

ERYTHEMATOUS LESIONS

Surface changes	Type of lesion		Number of lesions	Face/bald scalp	Truck/arms, thighs	Axilla/groin	Lower legs	Dorsum hand	Dorsum foot
Acute erythematous lesions/rash									
Normal/smooth	Macules/patches/ papules/ plaques		Progressive rash	166	166	166	166/372	166	166
			Multiple lesions/rash	98	170	170	372	404	170/372
			Transient lesions	171	171	171	171	171/404	171
	Papules/nodules		Single/few (2–5)	177	177	177	177	177/404	177
	Generalised rash			190	190	190	190	190	190
Crust/exudate	Vesicles/bullae			104	179	179	179/372	404	179
	Pustules			183	183	183	183	183	183
	Erosions/ulcers			104	186	186	186/385	186/404	186
Chronic erythematous lesions/rash									
Normal/smooth	Macules			112	202	202	202	202	202
	Papules,	small (<0.5 cm)	Single/few (2-5)	262	262	344	262	262	262
			Multiple lesions/rash	114	196	336	196	196	419
		large (>0.5 cm)	Single/few (2–5)	262	213	344	213	213	213
			Multiple lesions/rash	114	202	336	202	202	419
	Pustules			114	201	201	201	201	201
	Patches & plaques		All lesions <2 cm	126/130	202	336	336	404	419
			Some lesions >2 cm	126/130	208	336	375	404	419
	Nodules			126	213	344	375	410	213
Scaly/ hyperkeratotic	Papules			133	222	336	222	407	222
	Patches & plaques		Single/few (2–5)	133	218	336	218	218	218
			Multiple lesions	224	224	336	224	224	419
	Nodules			329	325	344	325	325	325
	Generalised rash			244	244	244	244	244	244
Crust/exudate/ excoriated	Papules, plaques & small erosions (no blisters present)			138	245	245	202/245	245	245
	Vesicles/bullae/large erosions			255	255	255	382	407	255
	Nodules			329	329	329	329	329	329
	Ulcers			138	329/387	387	386/7	387	386/7

NON-ERYTHEMATOUS LESIONS

Surface changes	Colour of lesion(s)	Type of lesion(s)	Face/bald scalp	Truck/arms, thighs	Axilla/groin	Lower legs	Dorsum hand	Dorsum foot
Normal/smooth	Skin coloured/light pink/yellow	Papules – isolated lesions	262	262	262	262	262	262
		– multiple similar lesions	263	263	346	346	346	346
		Plaques	270	270	270	270	270	270
		Nodules	272	272	346	272/375	410	272
	White	Macules & small patches (<2 cm)	278	278	278	278	278	278
		Papules	278	278	278	278	278	278
		Large patches & plaques (>2 cm)	281	281	281	281	281	281
	Brown	Macules & small patches (<2 cm)	288	288	346	346/399	288	288/399
		Large patches & plaques (>2 cm)						
		present at birth/before age 10	292	292	292	292	292	292
		appears after age 10	295	295	346	399	295	346
		Papules & nodules	300	300	346	300	300	300/399
	Blue/black/ purple	Macules, papules & nodules	310	310	310	310	310	310
		Patches present before age 10	292	292	292	292	292	292
	Red/orange	Macules & papules	314	314	314	399	314	314
		Nodules	213	213	344	213	213	213
Warty	Brown/skin coloured	Papules & nodules	316	316	316/346	316	316	316
Scale/keratin		Multiple lesions / rash	322	322	336	322	322	322
		Single/few lesions	325	325	325	325	325	336
Crust/ulcerated bleeding surface		Papules, plaques, nodules	329	329	329	329/387	329	329/387